# Rogers' Scientific Art of Nursing Practice

# Rogers' Scientific Art of Nursing Practice

### Mary Madrid
### Elizabeth Ann Manhart Barrett

Editors

National League for Nursing Press • New York
Pub. No. 15-2610

*To the memory of Martha E. Rogers.*

*To the registered nurses*
*who will participate in the creation of changes in health care*
*by using the Science of Unitary Human Beings*
*to revolutionize nursing practice.*

# Contents

CONTENTS

# Contributors

**Martha Raile Alligood,** PhD, RN
Professor, College of Nursing
University of Tennessee
Knoxville, TN

**Marcia D. Andersen,** PhD, RN, CS, FAAN
President and Project Director
Personalized Nursing Corporation, P.C.
Plymouth, MI

**Elizabeth Ann Manhart Barrett,** PhD, RN, FAAN
Professor and Coordinator
Center for Nursing Research
Hunter–Bellevue School of Nursing
Hunter College of the City University of New York
New York, NY
Private Practice in Health Patterning

**Eileen M. Bens,** MSN, RN, PNP
Children's Hospital Medical Center
Cincinnati, OH

**Martha Hains Bramlett,** PhD, RN
Research Scientist, Postdoctoral Fellow
Gerontology Center
University of Georgia
Athens, GA

**Howard Karl Butcher,** MScN, RN
Assistant Professor
School of Nursing
Pacific Lutheran University
Tacoma, WA

**Cynthia Caroselli,** PhD, RN
  Assistant Professor
  New York University
  New York, NY
**Jiafang Chen,** PhD
  Research Scientist, Postdoctoral Fellow
  Gerontology Center
  University of Georgia
  Athens, GA
**Wanda Daniels,** MSN, RN
  Assistant Professor of Nursing
  Georgia Southern University
  Statesboro, GA
**Jacqueline Fawcett,** PhD, FAAN
  Professor, University of Pennsylvania School of Nursing
  Philadelphia, PA
**Nancey E. M. France,** PhD, RN
  Assistant Professor
  Murray State University
  Department of Nursing
  Murray, KY
**Maryanne Garon,** MSN, RNC
  Clinical Services Director
  Outpatient Department
  San Diego Veterans Affairs Medical Center
  San Diego, CA
**Joanne Griffin,** PhD, RN
  Associate Professor, Division of Nursing
  School of Education
  New York University
  New York, NY
**Sarah Hall Gueldner,** DSN, RN, FAAN
  Professor and Director
  Center for Nursing Research
  College of Nursing
  Medical University of South Carolina
  Charleston, SC
**Judith Haber,** PhD, RN, CS, FAAN
  Private Practice
  Stamford, CT

**Judy Heggie,** MS, RN
Associate Chief, Nursing Services/Education
San Diego Veterans Affairs Medical Center
San Diego, CA

**Bela Horvath,** MA, RN
Assistant Nursing Care Coordinator
Smithers Rehabilitation Center
New York, NY

**Margie Johnson,** MSN, RN
Assistant Professor of Nursing
Georgia College
Milledgeville, GA

**Lisa Keegan-Jones,** BSN, RN
Children's Hospital Medical Center
Cincinnati, OH

**Ann Kelly,** MSN, RN, CS
Clinical Nurse Specialist
San Diego Veterans Affairs Medical Center
San Diego, CA

**Mary Kodiath,** MS, RNC, ANP
Adult Nurse Practitioner
San Diego Veterans Affairs Medical Center
San Diego, CA

**Dolores Krieger,** PhD, RN
Professor Emerita
New York University
New York, NY

**Mary Madrid,** PhD, RN, CCRN
Clinical Nurse Associate
New York University, Tisch Hospital
New York, NY

**Violet Malinski,** PhD, RN
Associate Professor and Graduate Specialization Coordinator
Psychiatric-Mental Health Nursing
Hunter-Bellevue School of Nursing
Hunter College of the City University of New York
New York, NY

**Nancy J. Morwessel,** MSN, RN
Clinical Nurse Specialist
Pediatric Cardiology and Cardiac Surgery
Children's Hospital Medical Center
Cincinnati, OH

**Margaret A. Newman,** PhD, RN, FAAN
Professor
University of Minnesota
Minneapolis, MN
**Rosemarie Rizzo Parse,** PhD, RN, FAAN
Professor and Niehoff Chair Nursing
Loyola University
Chicago, IL
**John R. Phillips,** PhD, RN
Associate Professor, Division of Nursing
School of Education
New York University
New York, NY
**Marilyn M. Rawnsley,** DNSc, RN
Professor and Assistant Dean for Graduate Studies
University of South Florida College of Nursing
Tampa, FL
**Martha E. Rogers,** ScD, RN, FAAN
Professor Emerita, Division of Nursing
School of Education
New York University
New York, NY
**Sherron Sargent,** MSN, PhD candidate, RN
Assistant Professor
Kent State University
Kent, OH
**Maranah Sauter,** MSN, RN
Associate Professor of Nursing
La Grange College
La Grange, GA
**Geoffrey A. D. Smereck,** JD
Vice President and Associate Project Director
Personalized Nursing Corporation, P.C.
Plymouth, MI
**Dorothy Woods Smith,** PhD, RN
Assistant Professor
University of Southern Maine School of Nursing
Portland, ME

**Justine A. Taddeo,** MA, RN
  Assistant Professor
  Department of Nursing
  College of Mount Saint Vincent
  Riverdale, NY
**Brenda Talley,** MSN, RN
  Assistant Professor of Nursing
  Armstrong State College
  Savannah, GA
**Cynthia A. Tudor,** MSN, RN, CNS
  Children's Hospital Medical Center
  Cincinnati, OH
**Linda K. Tuyn,** MA, RN, CS
  Lecturer/Clinical Specialist
  Decker School of Nursing
  Binghamton University
  Binghamton, NY
**Patricia Winstead-Fry,** PhD, RN
  Professor of Nursing
  University of Vermont
  Burlington, VT

# Foreword

The current of evolution of human consciousness is flowing at a steady pace. Consciousness and action—being and becoming, spirit and matter—are artificial dichotomies. They are all manifestations of a single unitary energy that generates, supports, and evolves. Basic science and applied science cannot be separated; they develop together. The approaches to nursing practice described in this book provide impressive testimony of this. The creative thinking of Rogerian science is transforming nursing practice into an independent, health-promoting, noninvasive, energy-based therapeutic system.

Rogerian science maintains that reality is nonlinear. Nonlinear implies circular, cyclical, or, as Rogers says, rhythmical. Thirty years ago, "love" became the theme of the "new consciousness." Now, in the principal of integrality basic to Rogerian science, we see this theme returning as we begin a new cycle of cosmic awareness. Integrality means unity, and unity is love. The work of Rogerian nurses is part of the rhythmical world-process, which is moving toward the highest-frequency, most powerful energy in the universe—love. This book describes the beginning transformation of nursing practice into its full potential—the potential inherent in living integrally with all.

At a recent regional meeting of the Society of Rogerian Scholars, participants gathered at the foot of the sacred Mount Cuchama, in East San Diego County. One of the nurses shared with us her fear of the rattlesnakes that abound in the area. Dr. Rogers' response illuminated for us all the deep and radical implications of integrality,

"When you realize integrality, you realize you are not separate, and there is no fear. You can only fear what is separate from you."
May each of us realize integrality in our lives!

Barbara Sarter PhD, FNP
Associate Professor
University of Southern California

# Preface

The most beautiful thing we can experience is the mysterious.
It is the source of all true art and science.

ALBERT EINSTEIN

The most frequent question posed to Rogerian scholars is "How can we use Rogers' system in nursing practice?" The continuous demand for practice applications prompted both this book and the Fourth Rogerian Conference, held in June, 1992 at New York University. Some papers presented there were revised for inclusion here, and others were added.

This book provides a glimpse of the state of the scientific art of Rogers' work as currently practiced. The term *scientific art* was chosen to describe the inseparability of the art of Rogerian nursing practice from the philosophical and theoretical tenets of the Science of Unitary Human Beings. The art is integral with and exists through imaginative use of the science.

The contributors are Rogerian scholars who are designing and implementing innovative practice applications. In addition to use by nurses practicing around the world, this text will find a home in schools of nursing, nursing centers, and other health care agencies that ground their programs in Rogers' science. In undergraduate and graduate courses in nursing science, students will welcome the increasing ability of authors to describe Rogers' work in less abstract, more easily understandable language.

Four units provide the book's organizing framework. Unit I contains an update of the Science of Unitary Human Beings from a theoretical perspective, a debate of issues of science-based practice, and a discussion of the political context of Rogerian science in the changing health care scene. Unit II develops in-depth presentations of a wide range of human health conditions that served as a focus for Rogers' scientific art of nursing practice. Unit III provides examples of the frustrations and the joys of operationalizing nursing care delivery systems based on the Science of Unitary Human Beings. Unit IV expands the pedagogical foundations of the science, answers questions concerning theory development and appropriate research methods, and concludes with the unveiling of a unique Rogerian research methodology. The poetry in the epilogue illustrates one of many diverse creative art forms that serve as vehicles of expression for Rogers' scientific art.

The potential for Rogers' science to contribute to changes in health care is powerful; it is a participatory model whereby consumers and health professionals form knowledge-based alliances to promote health and well-being. People have become aware of the limitations and the benefits of the mainstream patriarchal, profit-driven health care system of noncaring. Complementary holistic modalities, often less costly, are being explored by unprecedented numbers of consumers searching for ways to participate more meaningfully and effectively in their health. Several chapters in this book provide vignettes of some of the health patterning modalities presently being used in advanced practice nursing of unitary human beings.

Health care delivery requires a structure that doesn't exist. The nursing profession must be instrumental in constructing a new foundation that recognizes the unity of the human being in integral process with the environment. Holistic world views and theories are arising in numerous and diverse disciplines. Beyond love of the intellectual enterprise, applications of this rapidly developing knowledge base are essential for designing future human health and illness care systems. Rogers' science provides an avenue for traversing this terrain.

The current turmoil of change presents both opportunity and responsibility for using Rogerian science to maximize nursing's contribution to changing the system of health care. Never before in our country has such attention been focused on health-related matters. Consumers, health professionals, administrators, health insurance representatives, economists, legislators, and other groups are engaged in dialogue and political debate related to issues of access, quality, and cost. Even without congressional actions, many changes have already transpired. Registered nurses have engaged in the dialogue and the changes to an unprecedented extent.

For many years, Rogers has proclaimed that, in the future, most nurses will not work in hospitals; rather, autonomous nursing practice will be community-based. Today, nursing education is gearing up for the shift of predominant focus from sickness in the teritary care setting to a health promotion and wellness focus of primary and secondary care to be delivered in homes, schools, and workplaces. Nurse-managed nursing centers will emerge as the nexus from which these activities arise. Such centers will also provide a caring environment for delivering other health services.

These are exciting times for health care providers involved in the making of health care history. This book is a basic navigation chart for nursing's voyage into uncharted waters. In the unpredictable future, wherever there are people, there will be nurses taking actions to create changes that foster human health and well-being. We, the editors, invite you to seize the moment and become nursing pioneers. Participate in the development and use of the Science of Unitary Human Beings for the betterment of humankind. This challenge to Rogerian artists, scientists, and revolutionaries presents infinite possibilities. Together, we can make a difference!

We thank Allan Graubard, Director of NLN Publications, for his encouragement and guidance. We also thank Martha E. Rogers for her legacy to nursing—The Science of Unitary Human Beings.

Mary Madrid and Elizabeth Ann Manhart Barrett

# Unit I

# *THE SCIENCE AND ART OF NURSING PRACTICE*

# 1

# Nursing Science Evolves

*Martha E. Rogers*

Since evolution is continuous, new ideas about the Science of Unitary Irreducible Human Beings will continue to emerge. It is necessary to clarify important directions and changes that have brought us to the threshold of a new reality, a new world-view. We are just about at the critical mass that will trigger major change.

This new reality, whether called new age science or a similar expression, represents the foundation on which the science of nursing is built. The new reality is one of synthesis and holism and gives a broadened perspective of science in the future. Traditional science has focused on analysis; as the coming century approaches, the emphasis is moving rapidly to synthesis. Nursing knowledge is rooted in the new reality and emerges as a synthesis of this new science and metaphysics.

The field about which I am writing, the study of unitary human beings, is not designed either *to replace* or *not to replace* any other endeavor. That which identifies a particular science is the phenomenon of its concern. The uniqueness of nursing lies in its focus on unitary, irreducible human beings and their environments. This particular science provides a unique view of people and their world. The focus of this science is different from that of any other field's phenomenon of concern. A science of unitary or irreducible human beings is unique to nursing.

Holistic trends are becoming more common and are being incorporated into new ways of thinking, as manifested in new ways of perceiving people and their world. From these beginnings, new ways of organizing knowledge can be expected to emerge.

A paradigm for nursing is rooted in that new reality. I have been updating definitions and materials in the past year or so. One of the most significant updates was the replacement of the term *four-dimensional* with *pandimensional*. The definition that had been changed two or three years earlier continued to be correct, but pandimensional was the more appropriate term. Suddenly, one morning about 3:00 A.M., I *knew* that pandimensional was the right word.

Holism is a concept that continues to plague a great many people. Perhaps the idea is difficult for us to grasp since we have grown up in a segmented world in which we have had to deal with parts when we wanted to add them all up. Wholes are irreducible and do not exist as the sums of the parts. If we add up humans' physical, biological, psychological, and social attributes, we do not identify an irreducible human being. I cannot get a holistic human being by adding up parts any more than I can get a cake by adding up the ingredients of flour, sugar, vanilla, and eggs and proclaiming that I now have a cake.

The science of nursing is characterized by an organized abstract system, a synthesis of facts and ideas, a new product. The organized abstract system generates principles and theories. The principles of homeodynamics have undergone only revisions in writing, so that their meaning would be clearer.

The principles of resonancy, helicy, and integrality are very practical. They postulate the nature of change, which is significant in understanding human evolution and providing guidelines for the development of nursing practice. Nurses throughout the world are deriving theories from this organized abstract system and are engaging in research.

There is a potential for deriving a multiplicity of other theories. This paradigm studies, holistically, human beings as energy fields. The development of any new reality or paradigm for nursing must include outer space and beyond. We are no longer planet-bound and it is likely that eventually we will meet one another on Mars or on another galaxy.

Students of nursing are earning doctoral degrees for studies in which the content and dissertation focus is on the science of unitary human beings. As we begin to accumulate research data, a broader picture emerges. The focus is not limited to *Homo sapiens* and *Homo spacialis.* What is of interest is that this organized abstract system enables us to see and understand beyond the planet Earth.

One needs to differentiate between the body of knowledge that is nursing and the use or study of that knowledge. At times, there is confusion between using knowledge and knowledge itself. If nursing is a science, then nursing has its own unique phenomenon: nursing is an organized abstract system that uses its knowledge in practice. In its creative use of its knowledge, manifested in the art of practice, nursing begins to achieve its recognition as a truly important human service.

Practice is not nursing; rather, it is the way in which we use nursing knowledge. Nursing, as a science, designates the term *nursing* as a noun and signifies that nursing is an organized body of abstract knowledge. Traditionally, the term nursing has been used as a verb. Nursing, the science–noun, indicates that there is a body of knowledge specific to nursing. Many people practice "something." The tasks that a biologist performs in a laboratory are of themselves not biology; rather, they are tools a biologist may use in the study of biological phenomena. It is important to remember that practice is not nursing; practice is the use of nursing knowledge.

Education, research, and practice are ways in which nursing knowledge may be used, but in themselves they are not nursing. As we approach a new world-view, many nurses will say, "I knew that; what is *new?*" It is amazing how, when something happens, we all tend to say, "Oh yes, of course." When we begin to address education, one might raise the question, Education for whom?

Nightingale (1992) established two levels of preparation in nursing, and she differentiated these levels according to knowledge. One was the more educated group that might be referred to as "university nurses." Another group was trained to use the knowledge and skills that were developed by those who were more knowledgeable. Today's nurses have two major entry levels to practice, both of which are important. When I write about education, I will be writing about the more learned, university-educated group, those whose broad foundation of general knowledge includes communication skills, history, literature, the world's religions, and so on.

All students, not only those in nursing, need to have a broad education. Every college and university student should have courses in astronomy, politics, and the creative arts. Some observers may say that if educators are going to put in all of this "fine tuning," something is going to have to give. When we speak about nursing, engineering, or any other field, as· times change, requirements change.

In today's nursing curriculum, there are courses that are not needed for the practice of nursing as a holistic science. Perhaps these courses could be reduced in number. Anatomy and physiology might be combined into a one-semester course. Students need to communicate with other people and to know how people's knowledge has developed. They need courses that will teach them this process. They are not going to be practicing physiology or anatomy; they are going to be working with people. That gives us some food for thought: other fields do not work with the whole person, they work with some segments of the person. There is nothing wrong with that approach, but we have to differentiate it from nursing. If for someone who wants to be an engineer, the major area of study is engineering, not some other field. As we move on into synthesis, there will be major changes in how we organize our thinking and our approach to various phenomena. In the meantime, we must concern ourselves with the phenomenon central to nursing.

Several years ago, I was interested in Bennett's work, which came out of the Office of Education: professional fields began their preparation at the baccalaureate level. We are going to need more than the traditional four academic years. The proposal was five years. I think it can be done extremely well in five years, but we shall have to make the most of our educational resources. Most of our professional education is properly placed at the baccalaureate level, although there are some generic master's and doctoral programs. The nature of the degrees being given all over the country varies. Nursing has to look at what is required as preparation for being a learned professional. One needs to know thoroughly not only the science of nursing but also how to use it and how to take advantage of an opportunity to discuss, with knowledgeable faculty, the relationship between the use of knowledge and the knowledge itself. Education prepares a person to commence; it does not produce a finished product. Real education will continue for the rest of our lives.

When we begin to look at practice, many people say, "All that ivory tower theory is fine, but what are we going to do with it?"

In answer, I sometimes use this analogy. Theoretical physicists, engineers, and plumbers all use principles out of the physical world. The nature and the amount of what they know are different from the way in which they use their knowledge. A plumber is not an engineer, an engineering technician is not an engineer, and some engineers are theoretical engineers. Each uses differently the knowledge gained during preparation. We need appropriately prepared nurses to work in basic research in nursing, but it is important to let go of the idea that everybody has to do research.

In terms of practice within a holistic system, we are talking about noninvasive modalities. It has been noted in the literature for over three decades that the twenty-first century is going to be emphasizing noninvasive modalities—a very interesting prediction in view of growing technology. We sometimes forget that technology is a tool we use; it is not nursing, law, medicine, or any other discipline. More and more, nurses are using noninvasive modalities as tools of practice. Therapeutic Touch is one of these tools. Meditation, imagery, and humor additional tools. In some schools, Therapeutic Touch has become standard instruction for all students. We are beginning to recognize that much is going on that we have not understood, but what is going on lends itself to investigation using the framework of Rogerian science. This makes a tremendous difference when we approach some areas that have not previously lent themselves to scientific investigation. There is a critical need for viable theories to be developed using this framework.

There is a difference between knowledge and the use of knowledge; caring is a good example of how we can confuse the two. Caring is not nursing any more than it is any other field. At a recent conference, one speaker announced that her mother was a lawyer and that she would dare anybody to try to argue that her mother did not care as much as anybody. She was very busy doing a great deal of pro bono work and providing service to her clients. The speaker was quite right. So are those who protest, "Who are nurses to think that they care more than someone else?" We need all people to care, especially all health professionals.

Caring is very important, but everyone cares according to his or her own knowledge base. Lawyers care according to their knowledge of law; doctors, according to what they know about medicine; nutritionists, according to their knowledge of nutrition; and nurses, according to their knowledge of nursing science. Caring is doing, it is practice. Caring is a way of using knowledge, and we should be using knowledge in all that we do and all that we talk about doing. The world is full of opportunities for creative thinking in the use of nursing knowledge.

If we do not think in terms of real knowledge, we have no place in higher education. Our knowledge must be nursing knowledge. Sociology is a fine field of study, but theories derived from sociology, regardless of who derives them, are still sociological theories directed toward sociology. Some nurses have derived theories from other disciplines. There is nothing wrong with that crossover, but the theories contribute nothing to nursing knowledge because they are not studying the same phenomenon.

We extend our knowledge of nursing through research. Our education teaches us different categories and divisions of research, and analytical approaches to problem solving—often, I think, making the research process overly complex. There are really two kinds of research: (1) basic and (2) applied. Basic research is solid, theoretical investigation. If one is going to push back frontiers of knowledge, it helps to get near the frontiers. That means doctoral study *in nursing.* A PhD in methodology is not nursing. Many people take courses in and use methodology, but methodology is not the content of a given field, nor does it earn a doctorate in some other field. There are still nurses who are committed to the idea that there is nothing to know in nursing and, therefore, nurses should study other fields. If that were true, we would not need higher education in nursing since nursing would not require graduate or undergraduate study.

As we get into discussion of research, there are many arguments about qualitative and quantitative methods. Bacon and Descartes had battle lines drawn about deductive versus inductive thinking. Initially, people said, "You can't have both; it has to be either-or." Eventually, they understood that both have their benefits—as do qualitative and quantitative research. The point is that none of these ways of thinking is adequate for moving into a new reality. This does not mean that we throw them all out; rather, we begin to look for additional ways of thinking that will be more congruent with the nature of what we want to study. Nothing says that one way of thinking is going to be right for holistic views and wrong for something else. I emphasize this because I have heard people say that quantitative methods would not work in Rogerian science. That is not true. Basic research, however, is the theoretical research that adds new knowledge. Applied research tests knowledge that is already available.

Students at the master's level—and even some bright undergraduates—will look at the manner in which they use knowledge. There are many different ways of looking at what this means in terms of (1) human services and (2) comparing ways of doing things. When one is curious and reads the literature critically—that does not necessarily mean one reads it with a negative approach. Your liking or not liking the literature is irrelevant. The point is to look at it intelligently and ask, "What does this mean? Do I agree with it or not, in terms of its meaning?" Answers here may require careful discernment as new ideas and new theories are circulated.

As we move into the twenty-first century, new ways of thinking will emerge. Robinson and White (1986) propose that, after two generations of space living, *Homo spacialis* will evolve. We are dealing with a whole new potential, an evolutionary change of people living in space. New frontiers continue to open as nurses move into the future. Their responsibility for knowledgeable nursing and human services also grows. The opportunity is there for nurses to use their infinite potential.

## REFERENCES

Nightingale, F. (1992). *Notes on nursing: What it is and what it is not* (Com. ed.). Philadelphia: Lippincott. (Original work published in 1859.)

Robinson, G.S., & White, H.M., Jr. (1986). *Envoys of mankind: A declaration of first principles for the governance of space societies.* Washington, DC: Smithsonian Institution Press.

# 2

# The Open-Ended Nature of the Science of Unitary Human Beings

*John R. Phillips*

We live in a rapidly changing universe. Rogers (1970) stated, nearly 25 years ago, that "Sweeping changes taking place throughout the world emphasize life's creativity and challenge the most visionary to foretell the days ahead" (p. vii).

Other people's concerns with the nature of change have echoed this statement. An example is the early writings of Toffler (1970, 1980), who brought the significance of change to the attention of the public. More recently, Toffler (1984) noted that diversity is occurring everywhere, giving heterogeneity to all of society. More importantly, he observed, "But diversity in the ordinary sense is only part of the story. There is another important factor as well, and that is the speed of change itself" (Toffler, 1984, p. 166). Rogers addresses this factor in her theory of accelerating change.

Recently, Browne (1992) reported that new galaxies are forming billions of light years away from Earth. Such information brings to the forefront new thinking: the process of change itself is changing. Change is no longer seen as a linear process, but as nonlinear with sudden pattern change (Ferguson, 1980).

This new view of change is captured in current theories that are concerned with the "flows within flows within flows" (Gleick, 1990, p. 11), the changing patterns that are unpredictable. Within this whole change process, there is "the ability to grow from acknowledged uncertainty" (Briggs & Peat, 1989, p. 180). In fact, "The

scientists of change have learned that the evolution of complex systems can't be followed in causal detail because such systems are
holistic: Everything affects everything else" (p. 110).

Change of this nature is revolutionary. Rogers recognized this
when she created her Science of Unitary Human Beings. Recently,
Rogers (1992) presented some of her cogent ideas about science and
change. For Rogers, both science and change are open-ended; they
signify wholeness, and they flow in novel ways to create endless patterns of potentialities. Rogers gave a clear image of the relationship
of science and change when she stated, "Since science is open-ended
and change is continuous . . . the development of a science of unitary human beings is a never-ending process" (p. 28). This process
creates new knowledge and provides new insights (Rogers, 1992)
that help one to "see" and experience the patterns of the pandimensional wholeness of the universe.

From the foregoing, the question is, "What are the basis and insights of an 'open-ended' nature of 'a science of unitary human beings'?" Even though Rogers (1992) used a multiplicity of knowledge
to create the Science of Unitary Human Beings, only current pertinent knowledge that relates to the open-ended nature of the Science
of Unitary Human Beings will be described and presented in this
chapter.

When we seek greater understanding of the open-ended nature
of the Science of Unitary Human Beings, a broad vision of the creative potentials of everything in existence requires us to transcend
the science under exploration. This means we look anew at the universe to identify its defining attributes. In this exploration, we must
consider the infinite potentials of the universe. In fact, the potentials are so numerous that the universe appears to be completely
full, making most of the potentials hidden to the naked eye. This
overabundance of fullness is sometimes perceived or experienced as
full–empty, a paradoxical phenomenon. From this fullness–empti-
ness, the open-ended nature of science and the open-ended nature
of the Science of Unitary Human Beings are manifest. A simple example of full–empty can be shown through the use of a clear overhead transparency on which, at the top, the words UNIVERSE OF
ENERGY are printed. This sheet of plastic is completely filled with a
wave pattern, yet its pattern is not visible to the naked eye and the
sheet appears to be otherwise empty. This prompts the question,
"What are the attributes of the full–empty open-ended nature of the
universe?"

First, the universe is energy, a flowing whole that is indivisible and mostly invisible. (Consider again the UNIVERSE OF ENERGY transparency.) Bohm (1980) referred to this as "a universe of unbroken wholeness" (p. xv), where "everything is changing and all *is* flux" (p. 48). Contemporary scientists and writers see the universe as being multidimensional (Maas, 1990) and without borders (Bohm, 1980). The infinite nature of the pattern of the universe, being nonlinear, gives endless complexity where there is limitless creativity. The pattern is unpredictable where "order and chaos are bound together in a dialectic" (Hayles, 1990), "patterned unpredictable" (p. 216) nonlinearity that keeps the pattern from repeating itself. Such a universe of full–empty potentials gives "a science of process rather than state, of becoming rather than being" (Gleick, 1987, p. 5).

Such attributes are required for an open-ended view of science, and these ideas are quite evident in the current literature. However, Rogers created her Science of Unitary Human Beings beginning in the 1950s and 1960s. During that period of history, these ideas lay primarily hidden in the literature. Rogers used her pattern-seeing pandimensional spectacles to "see" and experience the hidden ideas and concepts of the pattern. She then synthesized them to create her Science of Unitary Human Beings. Fortunately, she continues to give greater clarity to her vision to make more evident the open-ended nature of her science and the universe.

What are some attributes that relate to the open-ended nature of the Science of Unitary Human Beings? Rogers' Science of Unitary Human Beings emerges from the universe; thus, it has attributes of the universe, as discussed above.

Rogers has chosen to deal with two energy fields: (1) the human energy field and (2) the environmental energy field. Both are manifestations of the universe. The open-ended nature of the universe of energy does not flow around the human being (Rogers, 1970, p. 49), nor does the environmental energy field flow around the human field. Both the universe and the environment flow through the human field, and the human field flows through the environmental field and the universe. In other words, the energy of the universe, of the human field, and of the environmental field continuously flows through each. Each is integral with the other; there is no separation of the energy fields. This is essentially the dynamic, indivisible wholeness of the universe, the human field, and the environmental field. This dynamic, ever-changing process is captured in Rogers'

(1992) principle of integrality—the "continuous mutual human field and environmental field process" (p. 31).

It needs to be emphasized that *integral* means something cannot be separated into parts; the human field cannot be separated from the environmental field. This integral nature can be represented by a red overhead transparency with the words ENVIRONMENTAL ENERGY FIELD printed on the right side, and a yellow overhead transparency with the words HUMAN ENERGY FIELD printed on the left side. Each of the two fields has its own unique pattern. The red ENVIRONMENTAL ENERGY FIELD transparency and the yellow HUMAN ENERGY FIELD transparency can be overlaid simultaneously on the clear UNIVERSE OF ENERGY transparency. A new pattern emerges as manifested in a new shade of color. The uniqueness of the pattern of the human field and the pattern of the environmental field is still present. Yet they are inseparable and they are integral with each other and the universe of energy, as evident when all three transparencies are seen as a whole.

From this perspective, the word *integral* uniquely conveys this inseparability. *Interconnect* and *interconnection* signify the joining of two things (an example would be the closing of a zipper), the connection of two parts where the connection is still visible. *Interpenetrate* does not capture the inseparability or the wholeness conveyed by the word *integral;* instead, *interpenetrate* conjures up an image of the separation of two things. When an arrow penetrates a piece of wood, the arrow is embedded in the wood but it is not integral with it from a traditional point of view. The same can be said for Rogers' deletion of the words *complementarity* and *interaction.* Because they connote two separate parts, Rogers replaced them with *integral* and *mutual process,* respectively.

The idea of integral—the principle of integrality—is critically important in comprehending the open-ended nature of science. However, the idea of the human field and the environmental field being integral is confusing to some people. In their attempt at clarification, people frequently say, "If the human field and the environmental field are integral, then they are one." This misconception can be related to literature that frequently describes humans as being one with the universe. Rogers has cogently shown that they are *not* one. She states that a pattern distinguishes each of these two fields; yet, even though each field has a pattern, there is no separation of one field from the other. Instead, the energy fields, with their patterns, are integral with each other, as was illustrated previously with the overhead transparencies.

Changes in pattern signify the open-ended nature of the Science of Unitary Human Beings. As a pattern changes, there is a continuous, innovative, unpredictable, increasing diversity in the pattern of the universe, the human field, and the environmental field. This is Rogers' (1992) principle of helicy, which underwrites the open-ended nature of the Science of Unitary Human Beings. The changing patterns of this growing diversity involve lower and higher wave frequencies, with the general acceptance that higher wave frequency patterns are more diverse than lower wave frequency patterns. This idea of lower to higher frequency still retains some elements of linearity. As greater clarity is given to the open-ended nature of the Science of Unitary Human Beings, we may find that growing diversity of pattern is related to a dialectic of low frequency–high frequency, similar to that of order–disorder in chaos theory. When the rhythmicities of lower–higher frequencies work together, they yield innovative, diverse patterns.

Thus, the open-ended nature involves (1) continuously changing patterns that are becoming more diverse, and (2) Rogers' (1992) principles of homeodynamics, where helicy is the nature of change, integrality is the process by which change takes place, and resonancy is how change takes place.

These changes signify the revolutionary, evolutionary, open-ended nature of the Science of Unitary Human Beings; one cannot portray it except through helping a person to create images. Earlier, it was noted that the universe, human field, and environmental field are infinite; a flowing whole; creative, endless patterns without limitations; unpredictable and nonlinear. When one synthesizes all of these and other concepts, a dimension is created that encompasses everything. This is the meaning of *pandimensional:* everything in the universe is nonlinear and infinite, and time as a linear concept is no longer relevant. To be more specific, Rogers (1992) says pandimensional is "a nonlinear domain without spatial or temporal attributes" (p. 29). Gleick (1990), in describing chaos, speaks of processes that "flow toward infinity in a way that the mind has trouble conceiving" (p. 23). Rogers captures pandimensionality through such images as "an infinite now" and a "relative present." Imagine a clear transparency with PANDIMENSIONAL printed down the middle. When the PANDIMENSIONAL transparency is placed on top of the UNIVERSE OF ENERGY, the HUMAN ENERGY FIELD, and the ENVIRONMENTAL ENERGY FIELD transparencies, the unit conveys the integral nature of a universe that is pandimensional; both the human field and the environmental field are integral and pandimensional.

This brief, incomplete picture of the open-ended nature of the Science of Unitary Human Beings is intended to further understanding of the elegance of Rogers' Science of Unitary Human Beings. One of my basic purposes is to help create images and new insights that contribute to the knowledge base of nursing science.

Among the new insights that emerged as the open-ended nature of the Science of Unitary Human Beings was explored was one related to the process by which knowledge is created. Frequently, the literature states that knowledge is generated through objective and subjective approaches to science. This process is often represented as dichotomous or involving polarity:

Objective - - - - - - - - - - - - - - Subjective

The definition of *objective* includes "experience independent of individual thought . . . : having reality independent of the mind," "perceived without distortion by personal feelings" (Webster's 1986). Burns and Grove (1987) stated that quantitative researchers see objectivity as detachment from a study so as not to bias it with their perceptions and values. Essentially, there is an attempt to isolate the observed from the observer. Such a perspective cannot occur with Rogers' principle of integrality.

It is currently recognized in some of the literature that the observer does influence the observed. Capra and Steindl-Rast (1991), in their new paradigm of thinking, stated that "the 'objective viewpoint' is illusory" because, in a total reality, "no one can be a 'detached observer'" (p. 161). We are active participants in the world. It is interesting to note that Rogers, in 1970, stated that "the real world encompasses observer and observed, with both contributing to any ascribed situation" (p. 87). One of the characters in Crichton's *Jurassic Park* (1990) says, "Linearity is an artificial way of viewing the world. Real life isn't a series of interconnected events occurring one after another like beads strung on a necklace" (p. 171). However, some scientists still hold the view of Galileo (cited in Capra, 1989) that "whatever cannot be measured and quantified is not scientific" (p. 133), which now means, "what cannot be quantified is not real" (p. 133).

The dictionary defines *subjective* as "relating to or determined by the mind as the subject of experience" and "arising out of . . . one's perception of one's own states and processes." Burns and Grove (1987) stated that qualitative research involves a researcher who is actively involved. "The findings . . . are influenced by the researcher's values and perceptions" (p. 36) in order to understand human experiences. The question may be, "Can there be subjectivity with integrality, and if so, how is it different?" Subjectivity may exist only in the sense of the physical body being seen as separate from the human field, particularly if the focus is primarily on the mind and not on the integral process. It might be interesting to speculate whether integral subjectivity and integral objectivity are possible, and if so, what are their characteristics?

Harman and Rheingold (1984) noted that only recently have some of the beliefs "approved" by science been challenged. As an example, "There is a clear distinction between the objective world, which is perceivable by anyone, and subjective experience, which is perceived by the individual alone in the privacy of his or her own mind" (p. 61).

My challenge is that neither subjectivity nor objectivity alone gives a unitary view of people and their environment. We need to transcend the subjective/objective limitations and adopt a view that looks at the mutual human field and environmental field from which all manifestations emerge—the open-ended nature of the universe. The concept of *unitive* is characterized by union, which means the uniting of two or more things into something that is then made one. We can refer to objective and subjective as objective-subjective to represent that they are integral with each other. This can be illustrated by putting the two words together in alternating-letter sequence, with objective beginning first:

OSBUJBEJCETCITVIEVE

or subjective beginning first:

SOUBBJJEECCTTIIVVEE

This combination appears at first glance to be chaotic, but subjective-objective lies hidden in a new pattern. The following diagram depicts the relationships among science, knowledge, objective–subjective, and unitive:

Science
|
Knowledge
|
Objective–Subjective
|
Unitive

When objective–subjective is replaced by unitive, the diagram becomes:

Science
|
Knowledge
|
Unitive

where the sequence no longer deals with the dichotomous nature of objective and subjective.

The concept of unitive is significant to the open-ended nature of the Science of Unitary Human Beings, especially when one reads Moody's (1990) quote of Bronowski, "Science is nothing else than the search to discover unity in the wild variety of nature or . . . in the variety of our experiences . . ." (p. 18). The unity of concern in the Science of Unitary Human Beings is the "mutual human field and environmental field process" (Rogers, 1992, p. 31). The idea of unitive was supported elegantly by Bohm and Peat (1987), who stated, "Knowledge of reality does not therefore lie in the subject, nor in the object, but in the dynamic flow between them" (p. 67). They went on to say that this flow is not the ordinary visual or tactile flow but an awareness that is "everywhere and nowhere" (p. 224), which can be called Rogers' pandimensionality, or, more specifically, pandimensional awareness.

The idea of unitive has support also from Dilthey (cited in Ermarth, 1987), who created the idea of human science and who said the world is in us, and "in inner experience there is no separation of appearance and reality, subject and object" (p. 78). The words *mutual process* can be substituted for *inner experience,* to convey the meaning of unitive as presented here. Ermarth (1987) also said that relativity is not incompatible with objectivity and that "there is only relative or 'correlative' objectivity in the human sciences . . ." (p. 86). Such views of unitive were echoed by Capra (1989): ". . . the science of the future will no longer need any firm foundation, . . . the metaphor of the building will be replaced by that of the web, or network, in which no part is more fundamental than any other part" (p. 66). Capra bluntly stated that scientists "deal with limited and approximate descriptions of reality" (p. 67) and that "all natural phenomena are seen as being ultimately inter-connected, and in order to explain any one of them we need to understand all the others . . ." (p. 67). This certainly is getting at Rogers' integrality and the open-ended nature of the Science of Unitary Human Beings. Rogers helps us to transcend the subject–object division (Guenther, 1989) and to deal with the unitary nature of the universe through mutual process and pandimensionality—the unitive approach to science. More importantly, determinism becomes obsolete when there is union of the subjective and objective. However, subjective–objective gives only surface knowledge of the universe of energy, whereas unitive is concerned with the wholeness of the universe of energy.

Mitchell and Cody (1992), in their examination of the meaning of human science to nursing, stated, "There is no subject–object dichotomy; reality is viewed as cocreated with the universe and others while experienced uniquely by the person" (p. 60). The open-ended nature of the Science of Unitary Human Beings calls for the unitive approach to develop nursing science. The unitive approach, open-endedness, and pandimensional awareness give us communion with information and patterns that transcend mind–body and subjective–objective (Peat, 1991). Since unitive is pandimensional, it transcends subjective–objective to experience the whole, which gives rise to more meaningful patterns than either subjective or objective.

One of the beauties of the open-ended nature of the Science of Unitary Human Beings is its ability to free us from the domination and control that are characteristic of the mechanistic and reductionistic views of the universe and human beings. It shows us "the ultimate futility of trying to control and manipulate the world in a machine-like manner" (Peat, 1991, p. 162). Peat goes on to say that, in a mechanistic universe where everything is fixed, a person cannot be described as being free. In an objective world, there is little room for subjective human values such as freedom and creativity.

The assumption is that "all events *must* be the result of some preceding events and that there is no possibility of genuinely creative, self-initiated acts" (Westcott, 1988, p. 15). In essence, then, free will is not congruent with predictability. In fact, in a mechanistic, reductionistic universe, freedom is an illusion. When humans are viewed as machines, there can be no free will, and the future is rigidly determined (Davies, 1990). When God is seen as omniscient and omnipotent, the controller of the universe, then all acts by people are by God and free will in people is "a false presumption" (Westcott, 1988, p. 11).

The open-ended nature of the Science of Unitary Human Beings provides for the experiencing of the fullness of one's free will. With the attributes of an open-ended nature of science, particularly the Science of Unitary Human Beings, free will/freedom emerges from the mutual process of people with the environment. Free will is possible where one transcends the person–environment separation and experiences integrality with the environment. Capra (1982) noted, "If I *am* the universe, there can be no 'outside' influences and all my actions will be spontaneous and free" (p. 270). Free will/freedom can be present in an integral universe where there is unitive rather than subjective or objective knowledge.

Pandimensionality is of great significance in one's sense of free will and freedom, especially since it offers a "nonlinear domain without spatial and temporal attributes" (Rogers, 1992, p. 29). Since human beings and the environment are integral and pandimensional, unpredictability is present, negating determinism with its cause-and-effect relationship. As such, Rogers' principle of integrality allows for free will and freedom. Pandimensionality gives freedom to one's awareness of integrality and the union of subjective–objective—a unitive picture of one's wholeness.

Rogers' principles of homeodynamics make freedom possible in the open-ended nature of the Science of Unitary Human Beings. As noted, these principles address the increasing diversity of patterns that change through mutual process to evolve higher-frequency wave patterns, whereby there is greater expression of the creative potentials of people. The literature supports this view of free will by emphasizing that more complex systems are farther away from cause and effect (Briggs & Peat, 1989), which gives an awareness of unpredictability in a pandimensional world. From a Rogerian perspective, free will and freedom become more manifest with growing diversity. Capra (1982) also discussed Teilhard's "Law of Complexity–Consciousness" which states that "evolution proceeds in the direction of increasing complexity, and that this increase in complexity is accompanied by a corresponding rise of consciousness, culminating in human spirituality" (p. 304). In this quote, pandimensional awareness can be substituted easily for the word *consciousness*.

Thus, freedom increases with each upward shift of attention; in this instance, pandimensional awareness gives the experience of free choice (Koestler, 1978). Pandimensionality gives the possibility of more choices since there is awareness of the integral nature of the universe. The nonlinearity of pandimensionality opens the possibility for freedom of the will and helps one to "escape the determinative constraints of the physical laws governing the physical body" (Dossey, 1989, p. 7). Other writers use the openness of the universe to argue for the reality of free will (Davies, 1990), and the Science of Unitary Human Beings certainly is open. Once we understand, to a greater degree, the open-ended nature of the Science of Unitary Human Beings, then we can express our creative potentials to experience fully our free will in a pandimensional universe. As such, pandimensional awareness enables us to peer into unseen patterns to discover relationships and ideas in mutual process, which give new ideas and insights. This helps to shed the shackles of a mechanistic-reductionistic universe.

Exploration of the open-ended nature of the Science of Unitary Human Beings can provide for sudden, astonishing insights. One of these relates to a question that is frequently asked of Rogers, "How is the Science of Unitary Human Beings related to the concept of God?" For some unknown reason, many people believe that the assumptions of her science do not allow for the existence of God. It seems that, in some instances, this question is based on the belief that Rogers' science evolved from physics. This belief is a fallacy.

The open-ended nature of the Science of Unitary Human Beings supports the existence of God, by whatever name a person uses to identify God. Capra and Steindl-Rast (1991) used a new paradigm in thinking to make interesting relationships between science and theology. A mention of some of these should provoke us to rethink our concept of God.

Earlier, it was stated that the universe is energy. God is also energy, along with human and environmental fields. All are integral with one another, as seen in the open-ended nature of the Science of Unitary Human Beings. In the new paradigm of thinking in theology, "the cosmos, God, and humans are interrelated" (Capra & Steindl-Rast, 1991, p. 101). With the open-ended nature of the Science of Unitary Human Beings, it is easy to accept that "[i]f we belong to God, God belongs to us; we are in a relationship" (p. 107).

This integrality is seen sometimes by scientists as an indivisible web (Bohm, 1980), a concept that supports the new paradigm thinking that the "structure" of God is a dynamic web of relationships and the spirit of God fills the whole universe and holds it together (Capra & Steindl-Rast, 1991). In essence, then, "the universe is God" (Capra & Steindl-Rast, 1991, p. 99).

The attributes of mutual process and pandimensionality of the open-ended nature of the Science of Unitary Human Beings give the freedom to participate in and also to create all the changes that occur in human beings, the environment, and the universe. Then, according to Capra and Steindl-Rast (1991), we create God in our image, and God creates us in God's image. This idea is present in other writings where "God would be at every moment involved in a mutually creative dialogue with His world" (Zohar, 1990, p. 226). It would then be acceptable to say that, in the open-ended nature of the Science of Unitary Human Beings, "God evolves as the universe evolves" (Rayl & McKinney, 1991, p. 48). This makes God holistic—or, as Rogers would say, unitary—and not a mechanistic or reductionistic God who changes in the mutual process of the universe, human beings, and the environment. The human being and the environment are manifestations of the universe. Acceptance of this fact enables one to say that human beings are manifestations of God, and God is a manifestation of human beings. God is pandimensional, and once we are aware of pandimensionality, we can experience our integral nature with God in new ways.

These new ideas of God are integral to the other concepts discussed. For example, Arnold (1989) stated that free exercise of will enables one to have a keener awareness of a higher power. This process certainly involves pandimensional awareness of one's integral nature with the universe. Harman and Rheingold's (1984) quote of Alan Watts connects many of these ideas. "True freedom . . . lies in the clear knowledge that the will of the Self is principally one with the will of the ultimate Reality, and thus with its infinite freedom" (p. 203).

Rogers stated in 1970 that "the capacity of life to transcend itself . . . predict[s] a future that cannot be foretold" (p. 57). More recently, she stated that "human beings are on the threshold of a fantastic and unimagined future" (Rogers, 1992, p. 34). Could Rogers be saying that life will evolve where there is infinite knowledge (Rayl & McKinney, 1991)? If so, then, as human beings of the universe of energy, we must be knowing participants in the creation of this knowledge. The open-ended nature of the Science of Unitary Human Beings helps us to think in new ways and to create the nonlinear knowledge of the full–empty universe. The unitive approach will help us to generate this knowledge and use the full potentials of our free will/freedom in our mutual process with the universe of energy. As Koestler (1978) said, "[A] true science of life," as the Science of Unitary Human Beings is, "must let infinity in and never lose sight of it" (p. 239). We cannot let people's fear of infinity destroy the open-ended nature of the Science of Unitary Human Beings, since it is through pandimensional awareness that we participate in the integral nature of the universe and human beings and their environment (Rucker, 1984).

We are all manifestations of Rogers' Science of Unitary Human Beings. Using the relation of God and the universe and the relationship of people with the universe in the open-ended nature of the Science of Unitary Human Beings, we can say that God and Rogers are in each of us and each of us is in God and Rogers and with each other. We must continue to explore the full potentials of the open-ended nature of the Science of Unitary Human Beings to participate in creating optimum life for all, including transhumans wherever they may be, or as Rogers (1992) would say, *Homo spacialis*. Through the open-ended nature of the Science of Unitary Human Beings and the unitive knowledge it gives us, we have the freedom to transhumanize the universe as we dance infinitely with God through the universe. Transhumanity will be infinitely grateful for Rogers' contributions to science. As William Blake, the poet, said, "If the doors of perception were cleansed, everything would appear to man as it is, infinite" (cited in De Selincourt, 1971, pp. 109–110).

## REFERENCES

Arnold, E. (1989). Burnout as a spiritual issue: Rediscovering meaning in nursing practice. In V. B. Carson (Ed.), *Spiritual dimensions of nursing practice* (pp. 320–354). Philadelphia: Saunders.

Bohm, D. (1980). *Wholeness and the implicate order.* Boston: Routledge & Kegan Paul.

Bohm, D., & Peat, F.D. (1987). *Science, order, and creativity.* New York: Bantam.

Briggs, J., & Peat, F.D. (1989). *Turbulent mirror.* New York: Harper & Row.

Browne, M.W. (1992, June 12). Clues point to young planet systems nearby. *New York Times,* pp. A1, D17.

Burns, N., & Grove, S.K. (1987). *The practice of nursing research: Conduct, critique and utilization.* Philadelphia: Saunders.

Capra, F. (1982). *The turning point: Science, society, and the rising culture.* New York: Simon & Schuster.

Capra, F. (1989). *Uncommon wisdom: Conversations with remarkable people.* New York: Bantam.

Capra, F., & Steindl-Rast, D. (1991). *Belonging to the universe.* New York: HarperCollins.

Crichton, M. (1990). *Jurassic Park.* New York: Ballantine.

Davies, P. (1990). Chaos frees the universe. *New Scientist, 128*(1737), 48-51.

De Selincourt, B. (1971). *William Blake.* New York: Cooper Square Publications, Inc.

Dossey, L. (1989). *Recovering the soul: A scientific and spiritual search.* New York: Bantam.

Ermarth, M. (1987). Objectivity and relativity in Dilthey's theory of understanding. In R.A. Makkreel & J. Scanlon (Eds.), *Dilthey and phenomenology* (pp. 73-94). Washington, DC: Center for Advanced Research in Phenomenology & University Press of America.

Ferguson, M. (1980). *The aquarian conspiracy: Personal and social transformation in the 1980s.* Los Angeles: Tarcher.

Gleick, J. (1987). *Chaos: Making a new science.* New York: Penguin.

Gleick, J. (1990). *Nature's chaos.* New York: Viking.

Guenther, H.V. (1989). *From reductionism to creativity.* Boston: Shambhala.

Harman, W., & Rheingold, H. (1984). *Higher creativity: Liberating the unconscious for breakthrough insights.* Los Angeles: Tarcher.

Hayles, N.K. (1990). *Chaos bound: Orderly disorder in contemporary literature and science.* Ithaca, NY: Cornell University Press.

Koestler, A. (1978). *Janus: A summing up.* New York: Random House.

Maas, T. (1990). David Bohm. In C. Tisdall (Ed.), *Art meets science and spirituality in a changing economy* (pp. 54-56). s'Gravenhage, Amsterdam: SDU Publishers.

Mitchell, G.J., & Cody, W.K. (1992). Nursing knowledge and human science: Ontological and epistemological considerations. *Nursing Science Quarterly, 5,* 54-61.

Moody, L.E. (1990). *Advancing nursing science through research, volume 1.* Newbury Park, CA: Sage.

Peat, F.D. (1991). *The philosopher's stone: Chaos, synchronicity, and the hidden order of the world.* New York: Bantam.

Rayl, A.J.S., & McKinney, K.T. (1991, August). The mind of God. *Omni,* pp. 43–48.

Rogers, M.E. (1970). *An introduction to the theoretical basis of nursing.* Philadelphia: Davis.

Rogers, M.E. (1992). Nursing science and the space age. *Nursing Science Quarterly, 5,* 27–34.

Rucker R. (1984). *The fourth dimension: Toward a geometry of higher reality.* Boston: Houghton Mifflin.

Toffler, A. (1970). *Future shock.* New York: Bantam Books.

Toffler, A. (1980). *The third wave.* New York: Morrow.

Toffler, A. (1984, October). Artificial intelligence. *Omni,* pp. 42, 106.

*Webster's ninth new collegiate dictionary.* (1986). Springfield, MA: Merriam-Webster.

Westcott, M.R. (1988). *The psychology of freedom: A human science perspective and critique.* New York: Springer-Verlag.

Zohar, D. (1990). *The quantum self.* New York: Quill/Morrow.

# Reflections on "The Open-Ended Nature of the Science of Unitary Human Beings"

*Patricia Winstead-Fry*

It is a pleasure to respond to Professor Phillips' exciting paper. My comments will be grouped into three areas. The first is disagreements, the second is ethical issues, and the third is future development.

## DISAGREEMENTS

Toward the end of his paper, Professor Phillips dips into theology, announcing "God is also energy." Professor Phillips goes on to present some ideas, derived from Capra and Steindl-Rast (1991) about freedom and free will, which Phillips seems to equate. I am against mixing theology and nursing science, for scholarly and political reasons. From a scholarly perspective, nurses are generally not educated in theology. The laws of proof and argument in theology are not those generally used in scientific nursing circles.

### Free Will

Professor Phillips' treatment of free will is a good example of what goes wrong when we go beyond our scholarly preparation. He cites Wescott (1988), a psychologist, who states free will is "a false presumption" if God is omnipotent and omniscient (p. 11). Wescott's conclusion is simplistic. The idea of free will was discussed and debated in early Christianity. The Church Fathers addressed the argument that people's fate, with regard to heaven or hell, is predestined because God is omniscient, and they decided that free will did exist (St. Augustine, 1960).

That humans have a free will was upheld throughout medieval times (Goodwin, 1965; Tillich, 1967). The early Christian Church did away with divine determinism a thousand years before scientific determinism was advanced. Belief in free will has been a consistent component of Eastern and Western Catholicism.

With the Protestant Reformation, the issue of free will was again raised, and some of the reformers decided that human free will was a fallacy (Tillich, 1967). Phillips cites Davies (1990), who offered that, if humans are machines, there can be no free will. We must remember that only in the past several hundred years have persons come to be viewed as machines, and that belief was not universally held.

Schlan (1991), who traced the development of art and science, concluded that science did not replace religion as the dominant social force until the eighteenth century. By that time, the issue was being debated in the form of mind versus matter by Locke, Berkeley, and other philosophers of the day. While these philosophers debated, William Blake wrote poetry depicting all of us as divine beings, called science the "Antichrist," and rejected Euclidean space and Newtonian sequential time. In *Auguries of Innocence,* Blake composed:

> To see a World in a Grain of Sand
> And a Heaven in a Wild Flower,
> Hold Infinity in the palm of your hand
> And Eternity in an hour.
>
> [Erdman, 1976]

### Theology and Science

From a different perspective, Wilber (1984), in *Quantum Questions,* presented a strong argument against using physics for theological purposes. He argued that the failure of physics to answer the basic questions about reality had compelled physicists such as Eddington, Schroedinger, and Einstein toward mysticism. *Quantum Questions* presents the mystical insights of some of this century's greatest physicists.

Wilbur's central argument can be summarized in the following paragraphs from *Quantum Questions:*

> The central mystical experience may be fairly (if somewhat poetically) described as follows:
>
> in the mystical consciousness, Reality is apprehended directly and immediately, meaning without any mediation, any symbolic elaboration, any conceptualization, or any abstractions, subject and object become one in a timeless and spaceless act that is beyond any and all forms of mediation . . . beyond words, symbols, names, thoughts, images (p. 7).
>
> . . . when the physicist "looks at" quantum reality or relativistic reality, he is not looking at the "things" in themselves, at noumenon, at direct and nonmediated reality. Rather, the physicist is looking at nothing but a set of highly abstract differential equations—not at reality itself, but at mathematical symbols of reality (p. 8).

Capra (1975), LeShan (1966), and Zukav (1979) presented similarities between physics and mystical experiences. It is interesting in these writings that comparisons are made, for the most part, between physics and Eastern mystical thought. Whether these authors avoid Western religion (mainly, Christianity) for personal or political reasons or because Eastern yogis and Zen monks have been amenable to scientific study is a matter for conjecture. The fact is, Eastern traditions do not have at their core a personal God to Whom humans relate—a central aspect of the major Western religions: Judaism, Islam, and Christianity. Whether the insight of physicists or Rogers applies to the Christian tradition needs more debate and more development than Phillips has offered.

Capra and Steindl-Rast (1991) discussed spiritual implications of contemporary science. Steindl-Rast is a Roman Catholic brother. The conversation in the book touches many topics, but is careful to avoid criticizing central theological tenets of Christianity. For example, the authors discuss the Trinity from a historical perspective, citing insights from the fourth century that the doctrine had to do with the divinization of humans. They do not suggest that the doctrine will change with new paradigm thinking. Their use of historical arguments is always from linear time, not pandimensionality.

My arguments against nurses doing theology, presented above, prompt me to wonder why Phillips cited Teilhard de Chardin (1961), who relates evolution to human spiritual development but in a linear manner. According to Teilhard de Chardin, evolution is advancing to the Omega point, a teleological end. How does a belief in one teleological end point (Christ) mesh with a pandimensional, continually creative perspective? To use Teilhard with Rogers, Phillips needs to discuss teleology in the light of pandimensionality.

I have nothing against including Rogers' ideas in personal spirituality. However, to advance the Science of Unitary Human Beings as a spiritual discipline is a broad jump. It is also an intellectual disservice since nurses are not educated in theology. If Phillips wants to pursue this line of inquiry, he needs to reconceptualize free will or freedom and define each to be in line with Rogers' conceptual model.

### Political Consideration

My second objection to Phillips' approach is political. If nurses can do theology, where does scholarly identity lie? No group has worked harder than nurses to overcome our own anti-intellectualism and to convince other disciplines that we are a real science. If we can do theology, can theologians do nursing?

Are there any boundaries? I think the answer to this last question is, "Yes." Rogers (1970, 1990), from the "purple bible" to current writing, always describes nursing as a science concerned with persons and their environments and health. Rogers never suggests that other sciences or religions are not valuable. They are not nursing, which is her concern.

The old world-view set rigid boundaries that created specialized sciences. These sciences can no longer answer the questions they are raising. Old-view adherents are recognizing that their scientific categories are not functional anymore. Such strange terms as "psychoneuroimmunology" demonstrate their need to merge bodies of knowledge that were artificially defined at the beginning. Whether the paradigm is old or new, we should respect disciplinary traditions of knowledge and methods for developing knowledge.

### ETHICAL ISSUES

I am not too sure how one does genealogy in a pandimensional universe. However, Rogers began to promulgate her ideas in the 1950s and 1960s. Can those of us who learned from her in the 1970s be considered second-generation Rogerians? Whatever we are, I think there are enough of us who have been using Rogers' open-ended nursing model as a basis of our practice and research to identify issues that we need to discuss and debate. I call these ethical issues for want of a better phrase.

Ethical understandings we deal with today come from the horrors revealed at the Nuremberg trials after the Second World War. At these trials, as the facts of the slaughter of millions of people unfolded, it became clear that physicians, and others, behaved with little regard for the persons who were the subjects of their experiments (Bandman & Bandman, 1990). A set of behavioral guidelines for the ethical conduct of human research was developed. Debates and refinements of these guidelines continue. Whatever our individual understanding of ethics, there is general agreement in our society that concern must be given to the consequences of researchers' actions on others.

One of my favorite recollections of the early days of Therapeutic Touch research at New York University is the Institutional Review Board's response to the research. Related to the influence of Nuremberg on the development of ethical standards in research, one of the major concerns is what is *done* to the research participant. *Done* generally connotes either handing the participant a pencil-and-paper test, a relatively minor action, or doing something relatively major, such as a surgical procedure.

Therapeutic Touch does not require actual touching. Many nurse researchers, during this early phase (mid-1970s), made it a point to highlight the fact that Therapeutic Touch would be done at a distance of six inches from the body. This distance stretched the imagination of my fellow reviewers, most of whom were fine old-view persons. In a Newtonian universe, one cannot do anything at a distance. To overcome inertia, one hits a billiard ball with a cue stick; one ignites an engine to start a car.

The Institutional Review Board faced a quandary. One option was to say that Therapeutic Touch research did not have to come before the committee because it did not "fit" the requirements for human research. The committee could not make that determination because humans were the research subjects, and federal rules required a review. I did not make any converts to the new world-view during these discussions. However, members of the committee were offered the experience of Therapeutic Touch and could report to our colleagues that it was not harmful or dangerous.

## The Questions

I learned two things from the Therapeutic Touch–Institutional Review Board experience. One is how difficult energy-based thinking is for materialists, and the other is a growing sensitivity to the complexities of using oneself as the tool of change. Over the 20 years since these questions began to occupy me, I have clarified some of the questions I think we Rogers-based practitioners need to address. I call them ethical primarily because they involve our conduct toward our fellow human beings.

As one practices and grows in using Rogers' concepts, much of the growth is experiential. I have learned to consciously transcend my relative present and to become aware of my pandimensional nature when I wish. As one gains such proficiency, issues arise. For example, what was my responsibility to a stranger who was my seatmate on an airplane, when I knew from observing the person as a nurse, that death was only a couple of days away? *Knowing,* as I use it here, is the quality that Gnostics talk about: in the core of one's being, one knows that something is true. The first couple of times I experienced this knowing, I thought I was being overly dramatic. However, when the obituary columns contained my fellow passenger's name, I had to question my responsibility, if any, in these circumstances.

A corollary of Rogers' open-ended model is that persons who practice from it can have knowledge of environmental field phenomena through the mutual process. In the example above, my stranger–companion was a component of my environmental field, so the fact that I apprehended this knowledge is not surprising. What to do with the knowledge is another question.

I have talked with nurses who work in critical care areas and who apprehend the same type of knowledge about their patients. For example, nurses often know a patient will live through the night. These nurses can use that knowledge to reassure an exhausted family that their loved one will have a good night. The nurses can suggest that the family members take a night off and go home for a good night's sleep. Such behaviors make sense in a critical care situation where the nurse knows the family. Do we have a responsibility to persons for "precognitions" that involve them when we have no relationship with them?

The same type of knowledge can come when a particular student decides to pursue a research topic such as incest or rape. I know that the student was a victim of rape or incest, but the experience is not in the awareness of the student's relative present. What is faculty members' responsibility in this situation? On the one hand, we know that adult learners do best when allowed to follow their own ideas, with the faculty providing tools for learning. On the other hand, we know that students can get mired in topics that are very personal to them and may not be able to accomplish their learning objectives.

I have my own answers to the questions I raise here: I believe we have a responsibility to deal with these issues. We have accepted a model that posits so-called "psi phenomena" are not only possible but are expected, depending on the state of the person–environment mutual process. Conventional ethics does not deal with these phenomena. We need to address these questions because our science raises them.

## FUTURE DEVELOPMENT

### Unitive Knowledge

Phillips' delineation of "unitive" knowledge is an important topic to develop within the Science of Unitary Human Beings. Whatever definition of science one uses, science has to do with knowledge of something. In order to pursue the development of these embryonic ideas, I recommend that Phillips stop dealing with what it is not. By beginning with the subject–object duality, Phillips overlooks the role of the tacit dimension in all knowing (Polanyi, 1962).

Phillips may have selected the word "unitive" prematurely. As Korzybski (1950) pointed out, whatever we say a thing is, is not what it is. When we use words to describe something, we have stepped away from the essence of the thing. Phrased differently, the map is not the territory. Words give a partial expression of what we are trying to get across, but they do not convey the essence of the thing itself. Rogers posits a Science of Unitary Human Beings. If we use "unitive knowledge," such a phrase could be misunderstood as a part of a unitary human being.

The choice of "unitive" to express this kind of knowledge needs further specification. When Phillips cites Mitchell and Cody (1992), who stated that ". . . a reality is viewed as cocreated with the universe and others while experienced uniquely by the person" (p. 60), he does not clarify his ideas because "experienced uniquely by the person" reads as subjective knowledge. If unitary is simply another way of saying subjective, then there is no point to be made.

If unitive is meant to express a way of knowing that flows from the nature of unitary human beings, then it seems logical to begin with questions such as: What constitutes knowledge in a scientific sense in a pandimensional universe? Is pandimensional awareness the same as scientific knowing? Are they different? What are the guidelines for determining facts in a universe of increasing complexity and accelerated evolution? Are scientific laws possible in the Science of Unitary Human Beings, or should all research findings be held as temporary guideposts? Is knowledge synonymous with pattern seeing?

## Patterning Process

Understanding the patterning process seems to be an important next step in explicating Rogers' ideas. Cowling (1990) offered a template of constituents to develop pattern-based nursing practice. The essence of Cowling's presentation is that the nurse and client, in mutual process, develop a field wherein mutual respect of the uniqueness of both is acknowledged, and the promotion of harmony in health-related events is pursued as defined by the client. Madrid and I (1986) also offered some ideas on appraisal parameters consistent with the Science of Unitary Human Beings.

In my experience, the most direct understanding of the patterning process in healing is through Therapeutic Touch and other nonmedical modalities. A recent workshop teaching Therapeutic Touch illustrated some of the patterning process issues and highlighted the importance of the nurse–client mutual process. In this particular workshop, a woman was learning Therapeutic Touch for the first time. She was appraising me. When she reached the area of my right ankle, she jumped away from me and shouted, "Don't step on me!" This outburst brought the workshop to a halt while we sorted out what she had experienced in her appraisal.

The woman stated that she knew I was about to crash my right foot down. As we explored the insight more, she realized that she wasn't sure that I was going to step on her, but the sense of the foot crashing down was so strong that she reacted to it.

Needless to say, my teaching techniques do not include stepping on students. The incident illustrated the pandimensional nature of the Therapeutic Touch appraisal. Several months before the workshop, I had broken my right ankle by stepping down hard in an attempt to prevent myself from falling head-first into a ravine. The woman rightly appraised an event in my life, but, being new to the timelessness of experience, she misinterpreted it as something that was about to happen to her. Along with illustrating pandimensionality, the incident showed the need for the creation of a therapeutic field wherein the client's wishes, goals, and experiences are integrated into a mutual planning for health concerns. The woman could have concluded that I was hostile or dangerous if we had not been able to explore the mutual meaning of her experience.

In *The Future of the Body* (1992), Murphy explored all of the many experiences recorded for centuries about the human body, including stigmata, healing, and extraordinary attributes. The book makes clear that the "stuff" we learned in anatomy and physiology is only the tip of the iceberg when it comes to the capabilities of this remarkable aspect of ourselves. The place of embodiment in the science of energy fields certainly needs more development. To start the dialogue, I propose that the aspect of the human energy field we experience as our body is a receiver/transmitter that facilitates experience of the self-environment mutual process.

## CONCLUSION

If a piece of scholarship can be judged by the issues it raises and the questions developed from it, Professor Phillips' article is a masterpiece. The questions and problems it allowed me to explore in these reflections are issues we need to debate as we develop the science and as we practice within the Science of Unitary Human Beings.

## REFERENCES

Bandman, E.L., & Bandman, B. (1990). *Nursing ethics though the life span.* Norwalk, CT: Appleton & Lange.

Capra, F. (1975). *The tao of physics.* Boulder, CO: Shambala.

Capra, F., & Steindl-Rast, D. (1991). *Belonging to the universe.* New York: HarperCollins.

Cowling, W.R. (1990). A template for unitary pattern-based nursing practice. In E.A.M. Barrett (Ed.), *Visions of Rogers' science-based nursing* (pp. 45–66). New York: National League for Nursing.

Davies, P. (1990). Chaos frees the universe. *New Scientist, 128*(1737), 48–51.

Erdman, D.V. (Ed). (1976). *The selected poetry of Blake.* New York: Meridian.

Goodwin, R.P. (1965). *Selected writings of Thomas Aquinas.* New York: Macmillan/Library of Liberal Arts.

Korzybski, A. (1950). *Science and sanity.* Lakeville, CT: International Neo-Aristotelian Press.

LeShan, L. (1966). *The medium, the mystic & the physicist.* New York: Viking.

Madrid, M., & Winstead-Fry, P. (1986). Rogers' conceptual model. In P. Winstead-Fry (Ed.), *Case studies in nursing theory* (pp. 73–102). New York: National League for Nursing.

Mitchell, G.J., & Cody, W.K. (1992). Nursing knowledge & human science: Ontological & epistemological considerations. *Nursing Science Quarterly, 5,* 54–61.

Murphy, M. (1992). *The future of the body.* Los Angeles: Tarcher.

Polanyi, M. (1962). *Personal knowledge.* Chicago: University of Chicago Press.

Rogers, M.E. (1970). *An introduction to the theoretical basis of nursing.* Philadelphia: Davis.

Rogers, M.E. (1990). Nursing: Science of unitary, irreducible, human beings: Update 1990. In E. A. Barrett (Ed.), *Visions of Rogers' science-based nursing* (pp. 5–12). New York: National League for Nursing.

St. Augustine. (1960). *The Confessions of Saint Augustine.* J.K. Ryan (Trans.). New York: Image.

Schlan, L. (1991). *Art & physics.* New York: Morrow.

Teilhard de Chardin, P. (1961). *The phenomenon of man.* New York: Harper Torchbooks.

Tillich, P. (1967). *Systematic theology, vol. 2.* Chicago: University of Chicago Press.

Wescott, M.R. (1988). *The psychology of freedom: A human science perspective and critique.* New York: Springer-Verlag.

Wilber, K. (1984). *Quantum questions.* Boulder, CO: Shambala.

Zukav, G. (1979). *The dancing Wu Li masters.* New York: Morrow.

# 3

# Current Issues of Science-Based Practice

*Dolores Krieger*
*Margaret A. Newman*
*Rosemarie Rizzo Parse*
*John R. Phillips*

In this chapter, the following issues concerning science-based practice are considered:

- What is science-based practice and is it different from theory-based practice?
- What is seen as the primary issue of a science-based practice?
- What are the issues/problems in implementing a science-based practice?
- What are some of the unique characteristics of Rogerian science-based practice?
- How will practice differ when based on the Science of Unitary Human Beings, especially when the center of health services moves to the community?
- From the perspective of the Science of Unitary Human Beings, what is the relevance of nursing diagnosis—general or specific—to practice?
- It has been predicted that noninvasive modalities will predominate in the twenty-first century. In relation to the practice of nurses, how do these modalities emerge out of the Science of Unitary Human Beings?

- Considering these modalities, how can nurses help clients participate knowingly in the promotion of well-being?
- How is this kind of practice important to nursing?
- Pasteur stated, "Chance favors the informed mind." It has also been said, "'A nurse is a nurse is a nurse.'" Relate this to differentiated practice. In other words, what is the nature of the differences in Rogerian science-based practice according to educational level?
- There is a range in diversity of practice using the Science of Unitary Human Beings. What are the differences in caring for individuals, age groups, or specific groups of persons?
- How will the Science of Unitary Human Beings contribute to punctuational change in science-based practice?

The three nurse scholars who participated in the panel discussion on Issues of Science-Based Practice were chosen because of their scholarliness and their unique contributions to nursing. Each is unique in her own right and each holds a different opinion about what nursing is. Phillips developed the discussion questions and gave the following descriptions of the background of the responders.

Dr. Dolores Krieger, Professor Emerita, New York University, is world-renowned for her work as the originator (with Dora Kunz) of Therapeutic Touch. Her first book, *Therapeutic Touch: How to Use Your Hands to Help or Heal* is in its twenty-third printing. She has published other books, including *Accepting Your Power to Heal: The Personal Practice of Therapeutic Touch* (1993).

Dr. Margaret A. Newman has created a theory of health—the theory of expanding consciousness. She sowed the seeds in 1978 for this theory, subsequently published in her book *Theory Development in Nursing* (1979). She is currently known for her published work, *Health and Expanding Consciousness* (1986). Her research began with a qualitative study of nurse–client interaction, moved to experimental and quasi-experimental tests of the movement–time–consciousness relationships posed in her theory, and, more recently, has focused on a heuristic, dialectic approach to pattern recognition. She considers her current research as praxis.

Dr. Rosemarie Rizzo Parse created the Theory of Human Becoming, originally published in 1981 as *Man–Living–Health: A Theory of Nursing.* She has since published other books, specifically two on paradigms in nursing science and qualitative methods in nursing research. She has developed research and practice methodologies congruent with new theory.

*Dr. Phillips.* When I spoke with some of the panel members, a question was asked of me: "What is an issue?" The definition that I think would be appropriate is "a matter that is in dispute between two or more parties; a point of debate or controversy." For the past several decades, nursing has been concerned with building a body of knowledge, a nursing science. We have come to the point where we are more concerned with the practice of nursing. The issues to be addressed relate to aspects of practice.

There is a theme emerging in the literature that relates to practice. It is one of those themes that requires clarification as to what it means. Are we talking about a science-based practice or a theory-based practice? Are these terms the same, or are they different? What is theory-based practice? What is science-based practice? We ask the members of the panel to present their views.

*Dr. Krieger.* There should be a clear distinction between science-based practice and theory-based nursing practice.

Essentially, the term *science* derives from the Latin word *scientia,* which means knowledge that is based on a systematized study to determine principles based on fact, as opposed to intuition. Valid relationships are logically derived by a process that analyzes assumptions, or universally agreed-upon beliefs for underlying laws or principles and for theorems that express hypothetical relationships. It is these hypotheses that can be tested, and it is the findings of these studies that become the core knowledge base upon which scientific practices proceed. It should be noted that, in the theory building per se, hypotheses, which lie at the heart of the process, may be heuristically derived from an intuitive insight.

*Dr. Newman.* I don't know what science is, and I don't know what theory is. I would imagine that we would have as many definitions of science and theory as we have people in this room. I disagree with my colleagues all the time about what is the meaning of science and what is the meaning of theory. I would say that, for me, science is *knowing,* the process of knowing. There are many ways of knowing. Theory, for me, is a powerful unifying idea. So when you ask the question about science-based or theory-based practice, I almost have a picture in my mind of some kind of platform that we base our practice on. I don't think that is the way it is. My recent experiences convince me that whatever it is that we are talking about in terms of science-based or theory-based has to do with where the person, who is the practitioner, is in his or her thinking. I heard someone talking about teaching and saying that it had to do with "being the theory," so to speak, and interacting with others so that they can experience the theory with you. I think that is what it is in practice also.

I had an experience with some nurse case managers at St. Mary's in Tucson and was interested in their practice because I thought it was consistent with my theoretical ideas. I spent some time interviewing them to find out what was most meaningful to them about their practice. The themes that emerged were themes of process, the importance of the relationship. That was number one. Sensing into the pattern of the person and following the agenda that that pattern dictates were also important. The nurse managers talked about how they, in their own maturation as practitioners, were able to see things that they had not been able to see before. They were able to embrace the whole, so to speak. I had a student say to me, "I think you just live your theory." I think that is true. I think theory-based practice or science-based practice is the transformation of the practitioner in terms of a particular world-view that gets communicated and played out in practice. That may seem too simple, but it is not. It is very complicated.

*Dr. Parse.*     So what you are saying, Margaret, is that it is the belief system of the nurse that is lived in practice. I would agree with that, but that belief system comes from nursing science or nursing theories. I also think that the terms *science-based* and *theory-based* are too broad. As a matter of fact, nursing has been science-based; it has been *medically* science-based and not *nursing* science-based. So I think that when we leave the term nursing out of science-based or theory-based, we are talking too generally about nursing. When we talk about nursing, people say, "We have always based our nursing practice on principles." They can give you principles, but the principles come from another science. It would be wonderful if, when we say *nursing practice,* we would all mean that we are living the frames of reference that are from our own knowledge base.

It does not mean that at this time. Nursing practice means something different to each of us. What the nurse believes about the human being, health, and the human–universe process is what is lived in practice. Should that be called nursing science-based practice or nursing theory-based practice? The term *nursing science* really grew out of Rogers' work and did not really mean nursing practice of various theories. Are all nursing frameworks referred to in the phrase *science-based practice?* Should it be *theory-based practice,* or should it be *Rogerian science-based practice,* in order to identify exactly what the belief system of the nurse is in that particular area? I think we first have to be specific about nursing.

Is it nursing science-based or nursing theory-based practice? What do we mean by nursing science? There are many situations now where nurses are evaluating theories in practice from both the totality and simultaneity paradigms. In those settings, they are called Roy-based practice or Rogerian-based practice.

*Dr. Krieger.*   I think that practice is derived, not based, whether it is science or theory. There is a big difference between science and theory. Theory is a logical derivation. There is something interesting in that, essentially, science is considered to be a systematic study of fact-derived principles as opposed to intuition. Theory really comes from hypotheses that are logically derived. One of the interesting things is that hypotheses can very often be theoristically derived from theories. I think that is a mistake. We think that if something is science-based, anything that touches the concept of intuition is a "No-No." It is about time we have that clarified.

*Dr. Parse.*   Science is a rational–intuitive process. It is not *either* rational *or* intuitive; it is an all-at-once rhythmical process, different sides of the same rhythm.

*Dr. Krieger.*   But when you talk about it, you are not necessarily talking about intuition of vice versa. When you talk about intuition, then you are talking about something that is pulled through the higher order of self. It is something that is impersonal, and the easiest way to say it is that it is an insight. A belief system may or may not be an insight.

*Dr. Parse.*   How can you support the unitary phenomenon if you separate belief system and intuition? I can never separate those.

*Dr. Krieger.*   The thing that holds them together is the individual, the unitary self.

*Dr. Parse.*   How they are lived out in the person is through the intuitive–rational process, which is an all-at-once process. I do not separate the belief system from the intuition; I see those as simultaneously co-creating each other. The insights I get also come from some rational process that I have going on within me, all-at-once, in the various realms of the universe that are "me."

*Dr. Krieger.*   There are always these kinds of "tussles" with one's rational self. If you look at the literature on intuition, the one thing that holds up through time is that, invariably, the following thing happens in a very classic way. The person has exhausted all the rational avenues and literally gives up. Then, lo and behold, the "Aha!"

*Dr. Parse.*   All of the rational–intuitive is intertwined.

*Dr. Krieger.* I think what we have to be careful of, in getting into this discussion, is that "everything is everything." I think that there is enough fiber in what we are about that we can discuss this without resorting to generalized terms.

*Dr. Phillips.* What is the ground for the practice? You mentioned the sensing patterns of the person. You are talking about living, about what is going on, about being involved in the process. Is that enough, or do you need a knowledge base of some kind from which you can interpret or view your living this process and sensing? Is what you are trying to get at science-based or is it theory-based?

*Dr. Newman.* I want to agree that we don't have to separate those things out, but we do come to the point of practice with knowledge that we have been learning all our lives. We do use knowledge from the medical model and from other disciplines. But it is not one of those things where we kind of "lay this theory" on the client, so to speak. Sometimes we may be conscious of the fact that "I'm using this theory right now," but most of the time we are not. All that knowledge comes together through the lens of this particular viewpoint. It will look different from practitioner to practitioner because each has a particular perspective. We use a lot of the same knowledge that, for instance, the physician uses, but we see it differently through our eyes, and the client sees it differently through his or her eyes.

*Dr. Parse.* Should it be knowledge-based practice then or nursing knowledge-based practice, rather than science or theory?

*Dr. Newman.* I think it is probably a function of where we are in our development as a discipline that we have to worry about these words.

*Dr. Parse.* That's why I wish it could just be nursing practice.

*Dr. Newman.* Yes, since as a discipline, it is assumed that we have a knowledge base.

*Dr. Parse.* It is just that we may not agree on what that knowledge base is.

*Dr. Newman.* Another thing about this is that we can see the whole from any one of these perspectives. There is a quotation about seeing the universe "in a grain of sand," and if you are looking for the whole, you can see the whole from any knowledge base. That might be controversial.

*Dr. Parse.* Do you mean there are other disciplines that have as one of their paradigmatic perspectives the idea of wholeness? I would agree with that, but I think that there is a distinct difference between a unitary perspective and a nonunitary perspective or totality perspective.

*Dr. Newman.* That is what I am saying. There is a perspective that organizes the knowledge and provides the meaning in the knowledge.

*Dr. Parse.* If the view is unitary and there are certain principles in Rogerian science that make up the nursing substance or content, how would one approach clients in practice? It would be different from how one would approach them if there was another knowledge base. If you teach undergraduate students the medical model system, when they approach persons for nursing care, the practice is medical-model based. In a sense, it is antagonistic to a unitary perspective.

*Dr. Newman.* I think that we have some responsibility to understand the knowledge that comes from other disciplines in practice. I'm speaking of all the knowledge—the prior knowledge that comes from the resources in the community, and knowing which ones you can use, and so forth. I am thinking of an example of a nurse working with a person whose respiratory system was depressed. There were a number of restrictions. She could not go home or to a rehabilitation facility because she did not have enough lung capacity. They were trying to keep her in the hospital, and all she wanted to do was to go home and die, if that was the next stage in her development. The nurse was looking at it from a holistic perspective and from the perspective of the client. She was able to facilitate the client's agenda rather than the medical agenda. Some of the knowledge in that situation was the same for all practitioners involved, but each one saw it differently.

*Dr. Parse.* But the major nursing perspective was unitary, and the strength of the knowledge base in nursing was the unitary perspective, not the medical model perspective.

*Dr. Newman.* But there is a lot of knowledge involved.

*Dr. Parse.* I would agree, but I think that nurses need not only knowledge from the medical sciences but from the humanities and from the social sciences. That is where the broad base resides. Nurses need a strong base in liberal arts and sciences just like lawyers, theologians, and physicians. Our unitary perspective is our unique view.

*Dr. Krieger.* The primary issue of science-based nursing practice is that most programs have really been composed of overlays of knowledge gained in other fields which have been slanted and shaped into a rationale amenable to, but not necessarily valid for, professional nursing practice. This occurs because of the misinformation that nurses are not supposed to be able to think for themselves.

Many years ago, before there was a nursing science, I wrote a book that was based on an integration of concepts about the human life process. Publishers loved it, but their salesmen rejected it because they said, "Nurses can't think in abstract terms and wouldn't understand it." A few years later, at the urging of Professor Rogers, I parlayed its contents into the first Matrices of Nursing Science course, which was based in the Rogerian conceptual model. I taught that course for almost two decades, and, consistently, students found it personally challenging and transforming and were greedy for more. It became a continuing "Aha!" experience.

*Dr. Phillips.*   The issue here may be that if you are drawing knowledge from a particular discipline to look at what you are doing as far as your practice is concerned, some of the knowledge you are drawing from may be really inconsistent with the basic ideas of the Science of Unitary Human Beings. So, can you bring this knowledge into the Science of Unitary Human Beings, or should the knowledge that you are using be generated from the system itself? I can hear Dr. Rogers saying over and over again, "You cannot just add up sociological, biological and physical, and so forth, and say that you are dealing with a unitary human being." What kind of knowledge are you talking about?

*Dr. Newman.*   I don't think either of us is saying "add up." The knowledge, the perspective—it is hard for me to use words since it seems that when we say "knowledge" and "theory" and "science," there is something out there that we can get our hands on. What helps me in practice comes from Rogers' basic assumptions. It is the concept of pattern. The pattern is very hard to get your hands on, but that is a guiding theme in terms of practice. We are looking for a pattern of the whole so that all of that knowledge is organized or synthesized, or whatever you want to say, through pattern recognition—pattern recognition on the part of the practitioner and pattern recognition on the part of the client. When this process occurs—when there is insight, intuition, whatever you want to call it, into the pattern—then the light goes on. I guess that is knowledge.

*Dr. Parse.*   Your basic belief system, Margaret, has to do with integrality, resonancy, and helicy. That is the belief you have about the human-universe process. It comes out through you, Margaret, as the human being who is with the other in practice, and you are in the pattern, the mutual pattern. Pattern appraisal and a deliberative mutual patterning process are derived from that belief system. That is how you give life to the Rogerian framework.

*Dr. Newman.* It is not that clear to me. You repeat it as though you somehow logically go through those steps.

*Dr. Parse.* I think that it is the intuitive–rational process that you live out through the "who that you are," which would be very different from someone else living the process because of all the experiences that he or she brings to it.

*Dr. Newman.* It does become different with each person who is in this evolutionary scheme of things. As the theory becomes part of each person and of his or her life and life experiences, it is different. That is something that I had to learn in terms of working with students. As the students would take the theory and apply it in their research and in their practice, it would look different to me, and I would say something like, "That is not quite it," but I have learned that it *does* become different with each person. I think that we, as teachers and as theorists, have to be open to that. We have to be open to how the theory enlarges and expands with each person who picks it up.

*Dr. Krieger.* I would like to suggest that it is the concept of mutual process that is even more fundamental; it is the dynamite word in this whole thing. Without a doubt, the greatest gift the Rogerian conceptual framework gave to nursing was to clearly define the essence of concern in professional nursing practice—unitary human beings in mutual process with their environment. The second unique feature is the clear declaration of the proposition that nursing is a learned profession that is based on a body of knowledge used imaginatively and creatively for human betterment. A proposition, of course, is an assignment, but such heritage of learning had never been assumed before. It made perfect sense, and Professor Rogers parlayed it into a revolution in nurse education. This promoted change for the profession itself.

Another singular perspective is that of unitary human beings and environment as dynamic energy fields in mutual process. The individual is perceived as an energy field with a personal totality or integrity, and the energy field of the environment is seen as encompassing all events that are "other."

My most recent "Aha!" helped me appreciate how astute this insight is. The instance that I was considering was that of the nurses' first meeting with a client. Reaching back into my own experiences, my mind pictures the following vignette: As the RN (Rogerian Nurse, of course) is about to approach the client, Energetica Patternosa, she brings to the moment everything relevant to her totality as a unitary being. She is about to tap her energy field potentials so that she can appropriately help Energetica fulfill her own latent possibilities for health or healing. In this vignette, we can see the RN stands posed as a unitary human field in mutual process with her environment—which is to say, Energetica Patternosa—and simultaneously integral with all events around her. She, herself, is manifest as a physical person with emotions, thoughts, memories, aspirations, and so forth, as well as all else that she is related to—significant people, places, and situations. Thus, actual events and perceived relationships all configure into sets of energy patterns within the environmental field at this moment. It is the totality of this energy field that is in pandimensional mutual process with the therapeutic energy field dynamics which is that unitary being, here known as RN. For a nanosecond, what a stunning tableau! The knowledgeable Rogerian Nurse is the Possible Nurse, for she can call upon the whole spectrum of her unitary nature as she engages in mutual process, and, vital energy field to vital energy field, she can call out an infinitude of potentials from the environment that harbors Energetica and all her concerns.

What happens is that simultaneous mutual process occurs. Everything is in complete flow, and out of that flow, the multitudinous patterns arise. It is not so much that they arise as that they are continuously patterned. There is always pattern: wherever you have energy, you have flux; and wherever you have flux, you have pattern, chaotic or not, ever-changing, always in transference. It takes a major effort to interfere with this mutual process. Such interference invokes stress, the major harbinger of illness.

*Dr. Phillips.*    An issue may be that there are differences in the diversity of the pattern. The diversity of the pattern could be related to differences in the knowledge base of the person—the *Rogerian* knowledge base of the person. When you start dealing with the knowledge base and differences in the knowledge base of the person, it is getting at what Dr. Newman was talking about; that is, differences between what she saw and what students saw, because they were coming with a different base of knowledge, a different diversity of pattern. Am I reading into things?

*Dr. Newman.*    The students are at a different maturity level in terms of their own development or system of knowledge.

*Dr. Parse.* I don't see those as two opposites. I think it is just explanations in a different way.

*Dr. Phillips.* Dr. Rogers is talking about nursing as a science and an art. The science is the knowledge you are talking about, and the art is the creative use of that knowledge. She said this back in 1970, so we were touching on the possibility of how, with the use of the Science of Unitary Human Beings, it gives you differences in the practice of nursing.

*Dr. Krieger.* I think this is one of the areas of our weakness as faculty. We have talked a great deal about history, about the principles of the Science of Unitary Human Beings in Rogerian nursing science. We have talked about some research findings, some of which are very consistent. I mean, they are taking stage A, then B, then C. When you are a doctoral student (which was where a great deal of the testing of the Rogerian conceptual model has come from), you select what is going to work for your dissertation. The important thing is what you do after the dissertation, not before. So there are discrepancies as a faculty. I don't think we have gone through that next step, taking students into clinical situations that may be diametrically opposite from the sheltered atmosphere of the university. Some of this material must be put in the practicality of the clinical area.

The issues and problems in implementing science-based practice, in specific regard to the Rogerian conceptual frame, find their core, I believe, in that we, as faculty, have not thoroughly explored the full spectrum of responsibilities to our students. Too frequently, it is the case that we do not fully extend ourselves beyond the mere presentation of principles, ideas, and world-view. We have not been adequately clear to students about the next stage, the appropriate in-depth application of this mindset into the artistry of nursing science practice. Since this is so, too frequently they flounder about, once cut off from the "academic apron strings," until each makes his or her own peace with the system. We have been weak in demonstrating specifically, rather than only talking about, how Rogerian nursing science provides organizing principles for compassionate, considerate, and creative nursing practices.

*Dr. Parse.* There probably should be a Rogerian center for nursing where students could practice. As Dr. Barrett has suggested, a practice methodology specific to the Rogerian framework includes pattern manifestation appraisal and deliberative mutual patterning. I think that those two major aspects of the methodology ought to be taught to the students who are learning Rogerian science. They should then go to practicum settings where they can see the methodology in operation. It is very difficult when students are taught one thing in the classroom and then placed in situations where they cannot practice what they have learned. We are moving to situations in practice settings now where various theoretical frameworks are being tested. There are places where persons can go to see pattern manifestation appraisal in practice.

Dr. Cowling has elaborated on Dr. Barrett's pattern manifestation appraisal. He talks about three areas: (1) experience, (2) perception, and (3) expression. I think those are areas that would help with a pattern appraisal and lead to mutual patterning that the nurse engages in with clients. I think the Rogerian practice methodology is evolving and will continue to do so as Rogerian scholars and nursing practitioners begin to implement it in practice. I know that there are settings where it has been tested.

*Dr. Newman.*    One of the questions on our list is: What are the issues/problems in implementing science-based practice? My answer to that question is that we need an arena for practice. That is the major issue here, and I think that is happening. My experience with those case managers in Tucson demonstrates this. They work primarily in the community although they include the acute episode of care in the hospital as well. They are free to follow the client wherever the client is. That is a growing trend. I lead a parallel life in terms of my interests and pursuits. One of them has to do with models of practice. I am convinced that we have to develop this case manager role. I realize that it is a terrible title, and I faulted the title for a long time because nurses don't think of people as cases and we don't manage them. But that is the title that is in the legislation and that is the title that nurses will get paid for through federal funding and so forth. So I have learned to live with it and those people in Tucson have learned to live with it. There are a lot of other areas across the country where case management models of practice are being developed. The case manager is free to use the theoretical perspective of his or her education and is free to design his or her practice and make judgments based on that knowledge.

*Dr. Krieger.*    When the center of health services moves to the community, nursing practice based on the Science of Unitary Beings will differ little because the Rogerian Nurse will be able to shift easily between concepts of the environment as a place to live, or to the environment as a lifeway or as an arena for social interaction. Regardless of the context, the field dynamics of the ongoing mutual process within the perspective of the situation under consideration will continue to be the center of concern.

Nevertheless, unless we learn wisely from history, the practice of the Rogerian Nurse, like all else in the community, will, over time, be subject to modification by new economic, political, and philosophical factors to which the community is sensitive. In spite of that possibility, however, the compassionate Rogerian Nurse should encourage the movement of centers of health services to the community, for it is still largely true that, although approximately 80 percent of health problems are in the community, about 80 percent of nurses work in hospitals. A shift in field perspective is long overdue.

*Dr. Phillips.*   I am glad you brought that issue up, because you are integrating what has already happened in our discussion: the living the process and the seeing of things. From this, you are synthesizing, and then you are placing the result within the practice methodology that Dr. Barrett has developed. However, there is an issue still with us that is known as nursing diagnosis. Is this idea of nursing diagnosis, in relation to what we have discussed, appropriate, or should we be advocating the methodology as delineated by Dr. Barrett and Dr. Cowling? Or are they inconsistent?

*Dr. Newman.*   I think nursing diagnosis is a bad word because it is like a label. If we are talking about mutual process, and I think we agree on that, it is hard to put a label on it. The work of the nurse theorist task force with the NANDA group, around the time period from 1978 to 1982, was aimed at explicating the Rogerian point of view in terms of the mutuality of the person and environment process moving toward greater complexity. The idea was that if we are going to have anything called nursing diagnosis, it would be at the level of pattern of the whole, not at the level of the particulate kinds of things. But I can remember very vividly: as we presented this, the bulk of the people at that meeting were into those specific kinds of labels. They had spent a lot of time working on them. Their question to the theory panelists was, "Do we have to give up everything we have done?" Someone said "Yes," and you can imagine how well that framework went over. I thought about it and thought, "No," but I did not think fast enough. I then put together how one could incorporate some of that particulate knowledge into knowledge of the whole. Unfortunately, the bulk of that work has continued to be at those particulate label levels, which I think are not helpful. What we have not taught people is how to look at the pattern of the whole—this process of pattern recognition. Then, the work that went into the nursing diagnosis project could be meaningful, but I think the label detracts.

*Dr. Parse.* We were at the same place but I think that we interpreted it slightly differently, as you would expect with our diverse unitary views. I think that what we were trying to do was to put a simultaneity perspective on top of a totality view. We were looking at the sum of the parts and trying to put a unitary cap on it, and that is not logical. They are two absolutely separate perspectives. It did evolve to a point where the theorists made a comment that we thought we could not put a unitary perspective on top of diagnostic labels. The diagnostic system comes out of an old world-view. It has roots in a medical model and has a particularistic, causal perspective. It just does not fit with the unitary perspective. I think that Rogerian practice cannot be encumbered by the term *diagnosis* because it is a totally different perspective. So I would see that Rogerian nurses would not be able to utilize a diagnostic system. I think that the patterns that the theorists talked about there—valuing, choosing, exchanging, and so forth—were good. We did some very good thinking at that time. Diagnoses are labels, causal in nature, and they put us in a whole different direction. They are the sum of the parts; they are particularistic, and that violates the underpinning values of the unitary perspective.

*Dr. Krieger.* I agree with you because they are antithetical. A conceptual frame is essentially a world-view if you look at it in its basic essence. It occurred to me that the only way a world-view can obviously influence something of a particulate nature (which these labels were) is in terms of the values that are implied in them.

It should be noted that conceptual models, such as the Rogerian frame of reference, refer to global or universal ideas or concepts involving individuals, groups, situations, and events that are of interest to a discipline. These models are made up of ideas and statements that express relationships between these concepts and are highly abstract and, therefore, not directly observable. Therefore, they do not lend themselves to traditional empirical testing. Rather, because conceptual models determine how the world is viewed, they provide a specific context for theory formation. It is the theory per se that can be tested.

According to the NLN definition, a nursing diagnosis is a succinct phrase or word that summarizes sets or clusters of empirical indicators representing patterns of unitary human beings. We

see, therefore, that the nursing diagnosis is an evaluative statement of a situation relevant to nursing practice, and, once formulated, it specifies direction for that practice. The context of the assessment, therefore can be set within the perspective of the
Science of Unitary Human Beings. Since the conceptual frame
around which the Science of Unitary Human Beings has been built
projects a particular world-view, such values will be inherent in the
nursing diagnosis.

*Dr. Newman.*    I think you can transform knowledge. You say
you can't go from that particulate base to a unitary base. I think a
paradigm shift can occur. Our prime example is the Copernican revolution, when Copernicus looked at the planets and the sun and realized that the sun was not revolving around the earth; the earth was
revolving around the sun. The same elements were there, but what a
difference it makes when you see it differently. I think that the same
elements that have gone into the old system can be transformed to
the new system. The question is: How do you bring about that
paradigm shift? This is a question that I deal with constantly in
classes because most of the members come to the class from the old
paradigm. How do I help them make the paradigm shift? I have some
ideas, but I still don't know how that shift occurs. I do think it is possible. I think we have some responsibility to help the nursing community make that shift. Rather than saying, "No, everything you have
done does not work any more," say, "How can this shift to another
perspective?"

*Dr. Krieger.*    Dr. Newman, don't you think that one of the problems is—if I can use the term—that shift is going to have to be pandimensional. Consequently, it is not really transformation. What really
has to occur is transcendence, literally looking at it from a completely different perspective.

*Dr. Parse.*    It *is* looking at the familiar in a new way. I would
agree that it is a transcendence; you cannot find substitute words. It
is not a substitution for what was; it is a whole new system. It is similar to looking through the zoom lens of the camera: you see one
thing. If you put on a wide-angle lens and look at the same scene,
you don't see the same things; you see different things. You can't
have the wide-angle lens and the zoom lens on at the same time.
They are very different. I do think that we have a responsibility to
help nurses to see the unitary view, but it is a different view. It creates different kinds of options. In Rogerian practice, you would be
in a practicum setting with people talking about and doing pattern

appraisal and deliberative mutual patterning. That is very different from assessing them from a perspective of a diagnostic system.

*Dr. Phillips.* Are you saying, then, that coming from the Science of Unitary Human Beings, the process we are talking about is very similar for anyone, whether you are talking about clients, students, or you own "personal relationships"? You are dealing with a mutual process and, in this process, you are helping people to participate. Through this participation, they are recognizing their pattern. That is the whole purpose here—to allow them to see their own pattern. This is where we need to start bringing together what we already have in the Science of Unitary Human Beings. For example, with Dr. Barrett's theory of power, the whole process is involved in helping people to participate and to make choices. Then these choices have intentionality, which is getting at whatever we are trying to do to help people participate in change.

There is another issue that we need to be more aware of and ask major questions about. This is the idea of the differentiation of practice. "A nurse is a nurse is a nurse."

*Dr. Newman.* I have introduced what I call a tri-level model of professional practice, differentiating according to associate, baccalaureate, and graduate degree education. I have designated the graduate level practice as the professional practice level and designed it in such a way that the nurse is free of the institution, in terms of moving with the client across settings, and is free to exercise judgment according to the nurse's theory base.

The model says that the associate degree corresponds to what we usually think of as the staff nurse, one whose work is time- and space-limited and is derived from both the medical and the nursing paradigms. It is a delegated kind of practice. I am not even sure that should be in our professional model, but it is a reality. The advanced degree I saw as the graduate level, the real professional level.

I really did not know what to do with the baccalaureate for a while, until one of my friends had an experience of hospitalization. We saw how fragmented the care was, with the various technical practitioners coming in and out and nobody really knowing what was going on. It seemed to me that there was a need for a liaison nurse between the professional nurse who moves in and out of the hospital and the staff person who is on today and off tomorrow. So I incorporated a practitioner who, in the spirit of the old team leader concept introduced in the early 1960s, is someone whose responsibility is that of an in-house clinical leader: to bring together the practice of all the technical people over the 24-hour span of shifts. The practitioner's role is to coordinate the care that is being given within the acute care setting and translate it into a nursing framework, a nursing perspective. That is a very difficult task.

Here is the professional practitioner, who is free to move about and make decisions according to her or his theoretical framework and does not really have to answer so much to the institution. Here is the technical practitioner, whose work is cut out for her or him in terms of the medical regimen and that little "icing of nursing" that sometimes gets played out. And there is the person in the middle, who has to make sense out of events from a nursing perspective and from a coordinating perspective and be able to communicate to all the parties involved. These are three distinct roles. I would like to not see them as hierarchical; yet, to some extent, there is a hierarchy of education and a hierarchy of judgment involved. That is as far as I have gone with it. That kind of model is in practice in a number of places.

*Dr. Parse.*    I would agree with that as a transition phase, as I said in an article in *Nursing Science Quarterly* when I talked about twenty-first-century nursing. I think that if you are bound to an institution that is run by medicine, then you have difficulty practicing Rogerian science. As along as there are medical "somethingnesses" for the nurse to carry out and there are orders from someone from another discipline, then we are not an autonomous profession. I think that we need to move to situations where we have well-educated persons coming into master's programs and where we can teach them the unitary perspective.

The baccalaureate degree would be a general baccalaureate degree earned with other students from business or prelaw or premedicine. The curriculum would include history, biology, chemistry, space science, and so forth. We would get very educated persons coming into nursing. Then our nursing substantive content would include no technologies; it would not include a medical model perspective. What students would learn would be the specifics of nursing science. If Rogerian nursing science, they would learn about helicy and integrality and resonancy and their meaning in the whole human–universe–health process. The phenomenon of concern would be related to nursing science; it would not be mixed, scattered, or picked up. What students would know from sociology, anatomy, chemistry, and physiology would be similar to what other professional people and other scientists know. We would then be living our science. I think that what I see Dr. Newman talking about is a transitional move. I would see us, in the twenty-first century, moving to a completely and totally autonomous discipline.

*Dr. Krieger.*    I have always thought that if people are going to deal with other persons' lives, then it demands nothing less than expert knowledge. I don't care what level it comes at. I think there are a few things that began to be put into place in our time that give us some sense of *how,* here and now; we can start to use Rogerian nursing science in much more explicit ways. I was just thinking of that field of informatics, and a wonderful idea coming out of Sigma Theta Tau at the Virginia Henderson library. They are going to put on-line a whole system of archives of knowledge whereby the nurse clinician needing such knowledge can immediately tap into it. That gives us some idea of what people have to do. We have to start to think of becoming integrators of these high-tech methods, as well as high touchers of the individual whom we have as the focus of our care.

*Dr. Phillips.*    All of you are talking about nursing science and what Sigma Theta Tau is doing to pull this nursing science together. How much of this nursing science they are pulling together is nursing science? The other component of that would be: How many of our nursing models are nursing models or just pulled from other disciplines with nursing attached?

Dr. Parse, you mentioned the twenty-first century. Dr. Rogers has made the statement that, in the twenty-first century, noninvasive modalities will predominate. Could you address these noninvasive modalities in relation to the nursing science you are talking about and how they emerge from the Science of Unitary Human Beings?

*Dr. Parse.*    Noninvasive modalities would be part of the curriculum. If students would learn Rogerian science, they would learn the noninvasive modalities in terms of the practice of nursing science.

*Dr. Krieger.*    I am not sure about your question. If you are talking about noninvasive modalities emerging from nursing, how will they, or how did they? With all honor to Dr. Rogers, they really predated the 1970s. Some of these noninvasive modalities as you are calling them, are centuries, if not thousands of years old.

The Science of Unitary Human Beings is concerned with the dynamics of human energy field to environmental energy field mutual process. From this point of view, the compact, material "stuff" of the physical body is not the primary site of illness. The problems are in the relationships between the relevant energy fields. Within this context, determinations are made in reference to energy flow: Is it blocked, depleted, diffused, or attenuated? Is the human energy field in overload? Or are there dissynchronies to the rhythms of its flow? Based on these findings, action is taken in diverse ways to return the healee's energy field to harmonic balance. Some of the modalities that lend themselves readily to this field therapeutics are imagery, Therapeutic Touch, and *ch'i gong*. However, energy flow is always in flux and requires a moment-to-moment therapeutic dance between the energy fields of healer and healee. This would mandate that the nursing practitioner, as healer, be in a constant state of mindfulness about the dynamics of the ongoing mutual process. In Therapeutic Touch, we start from a state of consciousness by an act we call centering, and we learn to maintain this centered state of consciousness throughout the entirety of the Therapeutic Touch process.

*Dr. Phillips.* What we are getting at is that many things were originally pulled from other disciplines, even the strategy you used with your own work of Therapeutic Touch. Humor has been used since the beginning of time, but how humor is viewed is quite different when you look at it from the Science of Unitary Human Beings. Humor can be viewed, from a psychoanalytic perspective, as a catharsis, which would be inconsistent with the Science of Unitary Human Beings.

*Dr. Krieger.* You don't mean how *did* it emerge; you mean how *will* it emerge? The philosophical background is there. The one thing that is so exciting and challenging about Rogerian nursing science is that it is where the frontier of knowledge has been happening over the past few decades. That is why Dr. Newman can step alongside Dr. Bohm and, I am quite sure, hold her ground very well. I don't see anything inimicable to it. I do see the recognition that Dr. Rogers brought to our attention: that what we are talking about is in nursing unitary people. We are not talking about any spin-offs that become more techniques.

If you are talking about unitary humans and about noninvasive modalities, that is the way it goes. You don't need a label to use any of these modalities. A great many of them really derive out of a human potential to actualize abilities that are not recognized in our society at this time. Once you learn how to accept them, you find that these come readily to the fore in the mutual process you have with your client. I think you are asking me: How does it happen?

*Dr. Phillips.* Or how do they emerge from the Science of Unitary Human Beings?

*Dr. Krieger.* They emerge naturally because of the fact that they themselves are a natural process. Clients can participate knowingly in the promotion of their own well-being by learning to understand their unitary nature in mutual process with the environment. Their persistent urge toward self-knowledge and their unitary natures will dynamically configure as allies in time of protracted stress or vulnerability.

*Dr. Parse.*     If you believe in the idea of pandimensionality, then there are connections that are at many realms of the universe, ways that we don't even know. We can't even name all of the modalities. In our mutual process, much happens. We don't explicitly know all that is happening when we are with another person. It is happening at a tacit level. Therapeutic Touch, guided imagery, or use of meditation, yoga, visualization, music, or lights as nursing modalities may seem put on, in a sense, almost in a causal way. We must be careful how we talk about these.

I would like to talk a little about what appears to be causal when you do Therapeutic Touch, or when you add lights, or when you guide someone through imagery. What about that in terms of causality, if you have an intention in relation to it? How does that fit with the unitary perspective?

*Dr. Krieger.*     Let me understand you: Are you saying that, because there is intentionality at the core of Therapeutic Touch practice, causality is implied? Noninvasive practices such as Therapeutic Touch allow the RN to call upon the full potency of her own unitary nature and use it therapeutically and compassionately while in mutual process with the unified being, the healee, in service of the healee's needs. The point of entrée is to center one's consciousness in the depths of one's own unitary self, and, from that source of inner strength, reach out to help the person in need to replenish his or her own energetic dynamic, in a mutual process that is initiated by compassionate concern.

*Dr. Parse.*     There is always intentionality, but it is with a particular intention that I come to you at a particular time.

*Dr. Krieger.*     Are you talking about cause and effect?

*Dr. Parse.*     That is a question that is often asked. It arises from the research that has been done, for instance, with Therapeutic Touch—the quasi-experimental studies. Dr. Rogers agrees that quantitative research can be done with her work, but the studies appear causal in nature. People often raise questions about this, and I think that it is something we will not solve here but should talk about.

*Dr. Krieger.*     If you think about intentionality, as I understand the concept and use it, intentionality is not that you expect an end cause—in other words, that you are only pushing with your will, but you see a goal; it is having the knowledge to see the goal that is the important part of that concept. I think that anyone who has gotten into the healing modalities in any way recognizes that it is not the so-called "healer"—call her or him Rogerian nurse or whatever—who is actually doing the healing. What you really try to do is to encourage the immunological response of the patients themselves. Within that kind of framework, I really don't see how you could have a cause-and-effect perspective, for, in the end, it is self-healing that takes place. The nurse–healer is only a human support system.

An instance that comes to mind concerns a television program that I was on. Just before the telecast, one of the people who had been attending a workshop that I had been giving that weekend came to me and told me that she had a problem and asked if I could help her. I thought she was one of the people who had volunteered to be on the television program. I said I would work with her while we were on TV. She gave me a startled glance. I did not know until later that she was not one of the people connected with the program. We got to the point of "action, lights, and camera," and I tried to help her with Therapeutic Touch. The next day, I got a telephone call from her and learned that one of her problems was that she had not had a menstrual period in several years, and she was about to be operated on. Overnight, her menstrual period began. She called again, on the second day, to tell me that she had gone back to the gynecologist and found that the tumor that had been identified by x-ray was no longer there. All of that goes by way of a "miracle," albeit a very minor one. The point of the story is that you can look at this two ways. Either it was just coincidental, a synchronous happening, or the power of intentionality can be seen as a multidimensional, valued thing that one can learn to use consciously; that is intentionality. It is hard to talk about these things, but they happen with a certain frequency in nursing and warrant objective, thoughtful exploration.

*Dr. Parse.* She came to you with her intent of having something from you that would help her in a particular way. The mutual process arose from that intent. It was not that you said, "Let's get rid of the tumor." It was like her offering herself for something that she thought you could facilitate by participating in a mutual process. I could see it that way.

*Dr. Phillips.* A strategy I use to get rid of the cause and effect you are addressing, Dr. Parse, comes back to what we are all talking about. That is knowledge. What is the knowledge base of the person, and how does she or he use this knowledge base to participate in the patterning of the environmental field? It is through the mutual process of the person with the pattern of the environmental field that gives her or him the choices and from which all manifestations emerge. This gets rid of cause and effect completely. The participant is involved in this whole process. You are not causing anything. Participants are choosing themselves. This is what we should be doing in nursing and what Dr. Barrett addresses in her theory of power.

*Question from Audience.* I have great difficulty limiting the Science of Unitary Human Beings to the science of nursing practice because I feel like it has been so transforming in my life—not just my nursing life, but my whole life—and with patients and with staff who have made that paradigm shift. If I learn to look at my patient as a unitary human being, I can't look any differently at my next-door neighbor, my husband, or my child. So when I look at it just in terms of my nursing science practice, it is almost contradictory.

*Dr. Parse.* You live the science that you know. You live your life according to your values. It is not something that we can teach, this deliberate patterning. We can't say, "Here's how you do it." It is "Here is how you know it" and then what you know comes out of you as your values are lived day to day.

*Question from Audience.* I have been thinking, as you have been commenting about nursing knowledge and nursing practice and the relationship between the two, that if nursing practice is mutual process—pattern appraisal—an essential element of nursing practice, therefore, is a therapeutic use of one's self. Dr. Krieger began to address this earlier—the difference between the personal self of the nurse and what Dr. Krieger refers to as the "higher-order self" of the nurse. There are some elements there in relation to this, the difference that Dr. Krieger may have addressed between belief and intuition. I am thinking about this in terms of nursing knowledge, the science and the art.

I began to wonder about nursing knowledge. We think about nursing as scientific knowledge or theory where there seems to be some need in this about the nurse's knowledge of self and what implications this may have for nursing education. How well does the nurse as a pattern in this mutual process become aware of all aspects of his or her self? In this mutual process, in the patterning that arises from this mutual process, how does the nurse differentiate between herself and client? How does the nurse learn to do that? This seems to me an essential element of nursing knowledge and nursing practice that would really need to be addressed. Otherwise, how would the nurse really know about what he or she is doing?

*Dr. Krieger.*    I think there should be a course on "how do you know yourself?", and I mean that quite literally. I don't think that we now do. If you are asking that as a question, there are no touchstones except personal ones. I think that the touchstone that I have always used is, when these occur, am I willing to have someone else do the healing? If I find that indeed I am, then I find that I am working from something deeper than myself, deeper than this simple ongoing interaction. I think that we do lack some way of understanding what it is that operates dynamically within us. Most nurses have called upon those higher orders of self in their initial desire to become a nurse.

*Dr. Newman.*    I think that it has tremendous implications for education. The whole educational process has to be changed from a facts approach to this process approach, the experiential approach.

*Dr. Parse.*    Coming to know yourself as you are with others is important. It is also important to recognize that when you are in practice with persons, much is occurring at all realms of the universe that are lived in this pandimensional relationship, and you will not know all at an explicit level.

*Dr. Phillips.*    A John Phillips synthesis. We were talking about the whole process of science—science-based practice or theory-based practice—and we were trying to couch this within the Science of Unitary Human Beings. We have what is known as science, nursing science, and I think we were beginning to get from our discussion that there is something called nursing science which is more than linear knowledge. What was beginning to come out is that knowledge, real nursing knowledge, is going to come from pandimensionality, pandimensional knowledge. All of this knowledge can be put to use through creative modalities. This is going to involve all of the processes that occur with people in general—not only with clients but with all people. We discussed some of the issues that were involved in this whole process.

Other issues are going to come forward as we start shifting or giving direction for nursing knowledge rather than linear knowledge. Another definition of issue is appropriate at this pint. This definition is: "An issue is the point at which an unsettled matter is ready for decision." John Phillips' decision is that we must participate in changing what nursing science is and what nursing knowledge is so that we can participate in furthering—creating—the Science of Unitary Human Beings.

# 4

# Rogerian Scientists, Artists, Revolutionaries

*Elizabeth Ann Manhart Barrett*

Martha E. Rogers, visionary of these nursing times and trailblazer of a new way of thinking in nursing, has created the Science of Unitary Human Beings as the basis for science-based practice (Rogers, 1970, 1990). Rogers' vision of nursing—her ideas, convictions, and science—have undoubtedly led the profession and discipline in a different direction from what might have been achieved without her. Inspired by her long history as active revolutionary as well as scientist and artist, many have elected to follow her on the road less traveled. These nurses must now provide leadership in health care reform and put the science and art of Rogerian nursing practice into a new mainstream of nursing and health care practice. Indeed, we *can* change nursing by our own acts. At a time when old institutions are breaking down and rigid dogmas provide outmoded guides for dysfunctional systems, the Science of Unitary Human Beings can play a vital role in the restructuring of science and provide vision for long overdue changes in health care.

By developing caring partnerships with consumers, we can participate together in revolutionizing health care. "Never doubt," as Margaret Mead first said, "that a small group of thoughtful, committed citizens can change the world; indeed it's the only thing that ever has" (cited in Barrett et al., 1990, p. xxi).

Throughout her career, Rogers has provided a strong nursing voice and, despite considerable opposition, implemented a radically new view of nursing. "Her aim was to advance nursing as a basic science and a learned profession" (Barrett et al., 1990, p. xxi). Several decades ago, with courage and conviction, she set out on a mission to establish nursing science as the springboard for nursing art. Today, some of the fruits of her labor are evident (Barrett, 1990; Malinski, 1986).

## TODAY'S REVOLUTIONARIES

For some time, a quiet, peaceful, emergent revolution has been picking up momentum. Now, there is a call for participation in a radical change of health care, a call for a new unitary science of wholeness as the basis for health care, and a call for artistry whereby the science becomes translated into practice. We are among many renegades migrating from the medical model of parts to a health model of wholeness. The fire for this revolution is being fueled by the American public; angry, disillusioned, financially frustrated consumers are driving these changes. We must become their partners, now!

No longer can nursing be the sleeping giant of health care. No longer can we wait to actualize our potential power. Nursing *is* becoming more united. Nursing *has* proposed an agenda for health care reform. It calls for the following:

- Universal access to health care;
- Empowerment of consumers;
- Wellness and health as priorities;
- Integration of public and private resources;
- Managed care and primary health care as delivery models of choice;
- Objection to increased health care spending;
- Direct consumer access to a variety of professional health care providers, including nurses (Joel, 1992, p. 5).

Nursing is not alone in these efforts unless we fail to reach out and contact others concerned with wholeness, health, and well-being as the bases for health care reform. Others are there, and they have similar new world-views.

Edgar Mitchell (1992), former Apollo 14 astronaut and founder of the Institute of Noetic Sciences, provided some insight into why and how these changes are occurring. He said that human behavior and conscious action are related to deeply held beliefs and commitments to knowledge. Although all new things begin as ideas that may evolve into visions, only when visions are supported by knowledge and charged with passion do they become translated into action. When people begin to experience, to understand, to believe—and believe deeply—their true meaning and purpose, action will take place automatically (p. 30). Change accelerates as soon as the perception of reality changes; we humans have an almost unlimited capacity for this knowing participation in transformation and transcendence (Mitchell, 1992).

We are a part of this broader movement. We must wake up, stand up, speak out, and participate as leaders in changes that will come before 2000—changes whereby quality, cost, and access issues are addressed in a manner that allows Rogerian nursing science to contribute solutions to health care problems within the broader rubric of Nursing's Agenda for Health Care Reform. To create, to innovate, is to let go of old strategies and solutions so that something more authentic can emerge in the continuous process of becoming.

The idea of "change your mind, change your world" (Mitchell, 1992, p. 30) is manifesting in health care. The old notion of "if you get sick, the doctor will fix it" is giving way to each person's capacity for knowing participation in well-being and being well. Nurses can be key facilitators in this shift from the passivity of consumer powerlessness to the activity of consumer power.

From the reconstruction of science along the lines of new paradigm thinking, a new orientation toward health care emerges. Rogers' science is unique among these new world-views and theoretically foremost in applying this thinking to health. Perhaps it is beyond the cutting edge.

This call to revolution is a call to commitment, to caring, to health promotion, and to the public's well-being. This revolution is directly related to nursing's disciplinary imperative, to our societal mandate to promote and improve the health of the public. Why is Rogerian practice revolutionary? It is revolutionary since it is *not more of the same.* It is not an evolutionary building on the old. Like Rogerian science, Rogerian practice is a new product, an innovative creation.

Rogerians are tomorrow-makers. They are seekers, activists, undogmatic exponents of ever-growing Rogerian wisdom and new paradigm thinking. Rogerians are moving toward a renaissance for the new millennium, a paradigm shift in nursing and the larger society.

Do not confuse Rogerian enthusiasm and commitment—"to live it, to love it, to teach it, and to do it" (J. Haber, personal communication, May 21, 1992)—with dogmatism. Rogers (1990) has defined nursing as the study of "unitary, irreducible, indivisible human and environmental energy fields: people and their world" (p. 6). Rogerian science, as science, is a search for truth that is always emerging, open-ended, never proven, never final. Neither Rogerian science nor revolutionary fervor is to be confused with dogma. There is no room for dogma in this system, nor is the system a secular religion. It does not propose to be the only way to search for truth. What may be interpreted as dogma is an effort to remain true to the science and to interpret it in a manner consistent with the assumptions, postulates, and principles of the science. Critique of the science, however, is essential and invited.

## THE SCIENTIFIC ART OF NURSING PRACTICE

A major focus of Nursing's Agenda for Health Care Reform (Joel, 1992) is on having the public actively participate in its own care and take responsibility for its own health and wellness. The agenda includes consumer freedom of choice concerning providers and settings, in order to promote equitable and cost-effective services. As the primary focus for the delivery of care shifts from the hospital as the tertiary acute care center to homes, workplaces, schools, and other community settings, primary and secondary prevention will receive increasing emphasis, and health promotion will finally become the first consideration rather than the last.

Costs will decrease as the focus of care shifts from acute care to health promotion. The Pew Health Professions Commission attributes the "seven million health workers in 700 different job categories and the projected increase to 10 million workers by the end of the decade to growth of technology, increased specialization, and . . . the hospital as a central focus of health care" (Shugars, O'Neil, & Bader, 1991, p. 74). This is changing and will continue to change since *it simply is not working*. Rogers (1972) foresaw this change when she prophesied 20 years ago that hospitals will become one of a wide range of satellite services (p. 10).

Maraldo (1992a) recently noted the trend toward self-reliance in all aspects of American life and observed that the public is taking health care issues into its own hands. She suggested that modalities that embrace the unitary nature of the person, such as acupuncture, imagery, meditation, yoga, and Therapeutic Touch, will become mainstream and a way of life (Maraldo, 1992a, p. 1).

Maraldo (1992a) also proposed that, related to the new meaning and definitions of health: (1) nurse entrepreneurs will multiply; (2) "home care will become the center of health care" (p. 2); (3) "nurses will need to be educated as knowledge specialists of health delivery" (p. 3); and (4) (perhaps the most important trend) "community nursing centers and community health programs to assist in preventing disease and promoting wellness will spring up all over" (p. 3). She advised that, as nursing's autonomy grows and new forms of independent practice emerge, nursing practices will be examined as never before—especially since physicians will be quick to charge that independent nursing practice is giving the public second-best (p. 4).

Moccia (1992) foretold that the coming years will be characterized by how people are connected rather than, as previously, by how people are divided. The dominance at the foundation of the biomedical paradigm is increasingly dysfunctional. Flawed from its inception and at its core, the biomedical paradigm is increasingly a relic and an artifact from another time (p. 17). Professionals can no longer dominate health care, or any profession, through guarding access to information. Consequently, power of the people is being enhanced, and the client–provider relationship is being transformed.

Currently, there are 100 nurse-managed centers providing nursing care in the United States. As a case in point, Stanhope (1992) reported that, in a nursing center in Lexington, Kentucky, serving 97 percent homeless clients, approximately 80 percent of all client problems could be handled by nurses alone. For the first three years, all care was given by clinical nurse specialists. In 1988, when nurse practitioners were added to the staff, only 5 percent more client problems were handled. She concluded that the contribution of clinical nurse specialists to primary care has been largely overlooked. In this nursing center, only 5 percent were referred to emergency rooms and only 4 percent were hospitalized. Care was approximately $300 per year per client; each individual visit was about half the cost ($44) of an emergency room visit ($79). Master's-prepared nurses, while more efficient, increased the cost of care; the increased cost was related to the greater complexity of their nursing actions (Stanhope, 1992).

## TOMORROW'S REVOLUTIONARIES

In this age of science-based practice, Rogers' science and art cannot claim exclusivity but rather specificity within a broader context. Other nurse theorists, particularly those whose work is reflected in the simultaneity paradigm proposed by Parse, Coyne, and Smith (1985) or the unitary-transformative paradigm proposed by Newman, Sime, and Corcoran-Perry (1991), also view humans as unitary beings in mutual process with their unitary environments.

Similarly, a small nucleus of revolutionaries in all disciplines and professions is embracing what Phillips (1988) has termed a science of wholeness and what we know as the integrality of people and their environments. Indeed, we are witnessing the beginnings of a global paradigm shift in the sciences, the arts, and the humanities; from the mainstream world-view of fragmented, mechanistic absolutism to world-views reflecting the science and spirit of unitary wholeness (Tisdall, 1990). This transition is reflected in global politics, the environmental movement, and multiple academic disciplines. It is increasingly evident in the media—for example, the motion picture *Mindwalk* starring Liv Ullman—and in countless books and articles. On some days, it almost seems as if everything's coming up Rogers.

Indeed, the call to revolution is ringing throughout the world. There can be little doubt that we are living in a period of great transition, of radical change, of major revisions cutting across all aspects of human life everywhere. Change continues to accelerate. We are quickly moving to one people, to one world, to planetary wholeness.

Moccia (1992) noted that "everyday experiences will be increasingly multinational" (p. 14). Similarly, Naisbitt and Aburdeen (1990), in *Megatrends 2000,* proposed that the world is becoming increasingly cosmopolitan and global life-styles are emerging.

Butcher and Forchuk (1990) have described parallels between Rogers' science and White's (1987) concept of the Overview Effect. Both describe the potential for human transformation when humanity is viewed as integral with an infinite evolutionary universe. The Overview Effect proposes that space travel is a transcendental experience triggered by the impact of viewing the Earth as a whole from space. The Overview Effect can also be triggered in lesser degrees in other ways. White (1987) postulated that when 20 percent of the population experience this transformation, an accelerating shift in global consciousness will result in the awareness that there are no real boundaries between people and countries. Rather, there is a sense of the unity of people and nature and of the mutual process of integrality.

Nursing's future in this human matrix is unpredictable and undecided. The past is over, and it is too late to change the present. We can, however, suggest possibilities that might happen in the future; this foresight will allow people to choose with awareness those potentials they want to actualize. Nevertheless, predictions are impossible; human decisions can change the future, and many uncertainties are inherent in the human–environment mutual process.

Nursing's future will emerge through our actions in the years ahead, and each of us will participate in creating the twenty-first century. We must believe in the value of our services. Can we dare to envision ourselves as reflections of both Nightingale and Rogers— strong, autonomous, tenacious, curious, imaginative, compassionate, humorous, and possessing an ever-growing nursing science knowledge base?

In the future, a societal split may occur that will not be based on disciplines; rather, the split will be based on world-view. In such a future, the health care delivery system may not be organized primarily by disciplines such as nursing, medicine, psychology, social work, and so on, but by newer versus older world-views.

Each discipline would then retain a focus on its unique phenomenon of concern. For example, in nursing, the focus is on people and their world, that is, on unitary, irreducible persons in mutual process with their environments (Rogers, 1970, 1992). However, the philosophy, conceptualization, and substantive knowledge base of nursing science as a foundation for practice would reflect the worldview. It is reflected now in the totality–simultaneity paradigms (Parse et al., 1985) and in the particulate–deterministic, integrative-interactive, and unitary-transformative paradigms (Newman et al., 1991). What would be different? Nurses from the new world-view would affiliate with those from other disciplines that have a similar world-view; the same would be true for those with older world-views. For example, rather than schools of nursing reflecting both world-views in a somewhat unarticulated and conflicting fashion, there might be schools of health sciences where disciplines share a similar philosophy and world-view. Differentiation among disciplines would speak to the knowledge base of the disciplines' phenomena of concern.

Currently, the newer world-views consistent with Rogers reflect a pandimensional, negentropic, acausal universe where persons and their environments are integral, and open systems give rise to homeodynamics, mutual process, and growing diversity (Rogers, 1992). This is contrasted with the older world-views, rooted in a three-dimensional, entropic, causal universe where persons and environments are dichotomous and closed systems give rise to homeostasis, adaptation, and dynamic equilibrium (Rogers, 1992).

We have begun to see interdisciplinary groups representing each of these competing paradigms. What is being proposed here is that competing paradigms representing the unitary (whole) perspective and the particulate (parts) perspective may transcend disciplinary boundaries, not only in health care but in the sciences, the arts, the humanities, business, and politics. The Institute of Noetic Sciences is an interdisciplinary group representing newer world-views. These views may have international reverberations and may precede a global paradigm shift to a unitary world-view for this planet as well as for outer space.

O'Neil (1981), in his book *2081,* defined the major drivers of change for the future: computers, automation, energy, communications, and space colonies. Changes ranging from the first human in an aircraft to the first human in a spacecraft have occurred in the span of a person's lifetime. To grasp the changes that have transpired over the past 300 years, consider that the usual speed for passenger travel has accelerated from six miles per hour (mph) (by stagecoach in 1781) to 60 mph (by steam-powered train in 1881) to 600 mph (by jet aircraft in 1981), and may soon reach 6,000 mph by vacuum (projected for 2081). People will travel by underground vacuum tunnels across the United States and by underwater subway systems under the oceans. Colonization of space will constitute the new frontier (O'Neil, 1981).

## SPACE NURSING

In considering the future, no discussion of the science and art of Rogerian nursing practice would be complete without describing how nursing will participate in space. Rogers (1992) proposed that "humankind is on the threshold of a new cosmology transcending an Earth-bound past and . . . *Homo spatialis* looms on the horizon as moon villages, space towns, and Martian communities foretell a new world" (p. 27). Such a view is embraced by a growing cadre of nurses; in April 1992, a Nursing in Space Society emerged from the Third Nursing in Space Conference (Linda Plush, personal communication, April 15, 1992). At the ANA Convention in 1990, Aerospace

Nursing was designated as nursing's newest specialty (D. Goettelman, personal communication, September 22, 1990). The year 1992 was designated International Space Year, and the purpose of Space Week (in July 1992) was to encourage and promote the human exploration, development, and settlement of the space frontier.

It is important that efforts to revolutionize nursing practice on Earth be linked to simultaneous efforts to articulate ways in which nursing practice will promote human well-being in space. Rogerian science brings to the space effort a new world-view that provides a theoretical explanation for understanding humans in a radically different environment, not only as they are now but as they might someday become. Accompanied by a sense of adventure, curiosity, wonder, and awe, a launch window for the development of new health patterning modalities is on the threshold of tomorrow. For example, conceptualized from a Rogerian point of view, the use of virtual reality may provide a means of direct, online, real-time, computer-augmented interactive communication between people in space and their loved ones on Earth.

To those who say, "Let's solve the problems on Earth first," I would suggest that it is not a matter of first and second; rather, both evolve together. As Rogers noted, the terrestrial and the extraterrestrial cannot be separated. Spin-offs from space can lead to more effective services for *Homo sapiens* on Earth. Indeed, 30,000 products have been developed as spin-offs from the space program, "everything from velcro to voice-operated wheelchairs to eyeglasses for the deaf to see sounds and the blind to feel images" (Maurer, 1989, p. 59).

Rogers' creative vision of the next frontier, of a new world in space, may leave an indelible impact on the universe. Imaginative use of the Science of Unitary Human Beings in space may become Rogers' most profound contribution to the well-being of humankind. Rogers is of our time; yet is she not also of another time, a time yet to arrive?

## A ROGERIAN PLAN FOR PARTICIPATION IN NURSING'S AGENDA FOR HEALTH CARE REFORM

Within the broader context of what Maraldo (1992c) called a crossroads of a new destiny for health care reform, this section presents a beginning sketch of a Rogerian plan for participation in Nursing's Agenda for Health Care Reform. In 1988, Rogers wrote that, although both community agencies and hospitals provide meaningful services, it is the broad community-based health promotion services that provide the umbrella (p. 102).

## Primary Care

Primary care—the first contact with a health provider for a specific health event—is not solely the physician's domain. Just as health care is more than medical care, primary care is more than primary medical care. With roots in private duty nursing and public health nursing, nursing needs to reclaim and theoretically underwrite the autonomous, independent practice of *nursing* primary care. Florence Nightingale said it clearly: "Experience teaches me . . . that nursing and medicine must never be mixed up. It spoils both" (Zachary, 1958, p. 121).

Rogers has pointed out that *tools of practice* must not be confused with substantive knowledge for practice. In some instances, what has been called medical care by physicians may indeed be tools of practice that can be as legitimately used autonomously by nurses and other health professionals as by physicians. At one time, taking a temperature or testing blood pressure was the exclusive domain of medical practice; now both are in the public domain. Today, one thinks of physical examination or acupuncture as functions often reserved to medicine, yet these tools of practice are being increasingly recognized as more appropriately within the larger domain of multiple health professionals.

Much of primary care as it exists today is dominated by the medical care system based on the disease model and a philosophy of "doing to" patients and expecting so-called "compliance" with medical regimes. What is being proposed here is a nursing primary care system based on health promotion and underwritten by substantive nursing knowledge and a philosophy of helping clients to knowingly participate as they wish. Another difference between the medical and the nursing perspectives was pointed out by Newman (1991), who said that, for nurses, disease is information about the pattern of the whole person whereas, for physicians, disease is an entity to be eliminated. In gaining information about the pattern of the whole person, the nurse offers information for clients' consideration. Many health difficulties and diseases may be allies rather than enemies; they may serve to signal a need for life-style changes to enhance health and well-being (Manahan & Manahan, 1992). However, it is the clients who decide what values they place on the various viewpoints.

McGivern, Mezey, and Glynn (1990) proposed that health as defined in primary care includes "health promotion, health maintenance, self-care, and health teaching" (p. 163). Within this broad scope, Rogers noted that health is a value and is self-defined by each individual or group.

What strategies will enable us to participate as sculptors in designing and carrying out nursing's unique nursing science-based services? With respect for all disciplines, nursing must claim and develop its territory for the good of the health of people. Many nurses are already engaged in creating this future, but a peaceful and powerful revolution is necessary to achieve a major paradigm shift in health care.

Perhaps the single most important item on the Rogerian practice agenda is to link nursing knowledge with health of the people. Additionally, we must continuously change ourselves. The changes in us will ultimately create a change in the environment in which we practice, for "although we cannot change anything but ourselves, in changing ourselves we change everything" (Boyle, 1985, p. 1). As we explore new ideas and methods for practice, we will do well to remember that, just as doing can't be separated from knowing since what we do is based on what we know, neither can art be separated from science. In our partnership with the public, perhaps the most important health-related idea for consumers to embrace is that *they* have the power to knowingly participate in healing themselves and, most importantly, to participate in ways that they choose. As health professionals, we must also guard freedom, hope, love and laughter; we must use imagination to see things as they might some day become rather than as they are now. In the words of Rogers, "Dream big" (M. E. Rogers, personal communication, September 23, 1976).

## Power and Health Patterning Centers

For both clients and nurses, power (knowing participation in change) is the password in the Rogerian revolution. This view of power is crucial to the work that we are undertaking. Power interweaves awareness, choices, freedom to act intentionally, and involvement in creating changes. "Power is being aware of what we are choosing to do, feeling free to do it, and doing it intentionally" (Barrett, 1986, p. 175). Health patterning is (1) facilitating well-being by assisting clients with their knowing participation in change and (2) a mutual process whereby power is actualized by clients. Clients are health seekers concerned with the quality of their lives. Health patterning facilitates both their search for meaning and their ways of making changes in their health.

Health Patterning Centers (Barrett, 1991) will provide the creative hub for nursing care delivery systems. Rogers reminds us that nursing's concern is all people, whether sick or well. Many of these delivery systems will focus on primary care; others will emphasize secondary or tertiary care. All Health Patterning Centers will be nurse-managed and nurse-operated. Some will be owned by nurse entrepreneurs. Many will offer managed care as the best package of services for a given population at the lowest price (Maraldo, 1992b, p. 3). Referrals to other health professionals will be made as appropriate. Only those professionals ascribing to a philosophy and science of wholeness will be eligible for preferred provider status. Maraldo thinks that community nursing centers ought to be encouraged as the managed care model of choice in high schools, postsecondary schools, and the community (Maraldo, 1992b, p. 3). Moccia (1992) suggested that "a nurse in every school" could not only be a plank in a platform for national health care but could clarify connections between education and the health of individuals and communities.

Yet, there is a major difference between a nurse in a school practicing from a medical primary care "parts" perspective and a nursing primary care "unitary" perspective. Consider the following example:

> A first-grade child came into the [school] clinic with a severe stomach ache, and wanted to go home. The nurse said to the child, "You look so sad. What are you sad about?" The child immediately began to cry and shared her story. Her grandfather had died recently and she hadn't had a chance to say goodbye. After further sharing, the nurse called the mother to let her in on the unresolved grief the child was experiencing. Next, the nurse suggested to the child that she write her grandfather a letter and carry his picture to look at when she missed him. Twenty minutes after the initial crisis, the child went back to class smiling.
>
> This was an example of a (unitary) focus on the whole person. If the child's care had been based on the medical model, she would have been asked, "What did you eat, when did this start, how often does it hurt?," charted, and then sent home. (Till-Tovey, 1992, p. 3)

This example illustrates a major difference between medical primary care and nursing primary care. The medical approach is to find out whether a disease is present. The nursing approach is to find out what is happening with the person. The unitary nurse considers:

> Why is the problem occurring in this person at this time? What can the patient [sic] do to help eliminate the problem or keep it from happening again? How are the patient's [sic] family and co-workers involved and how are they affected? How does the patient [sic] feel about what is happening to him or her? Does the patient [sic] understand what is happening? (Manahan & Manahan, 1992, p. 1)

From a Rogerian perspective, the focus is not on the physical, psychological, social, cultural, or spiritual parts of a holistic person. Rather, all characteristics of the person are pattern manifestations of the whole. The configuration of pattern manifestations presents a different picture of the unitary person. Care is operationalized by means of the Rogerian practice methodology, which consists of pattern manifestation appraisal and deliberative mutual patterning (Barrett, 1988, 1990).

> What we mean by "understanding" or "comprehension" is seeing how parts fit into a whole and then realizing that they don't compose the whole, as one assembles a jig saw puzzle, but that the whole is a pattern, a complex of wiggleness, which has no separate parts. . . . Parts exist only for purposes of figuring and describing and as we figure the world out we become confused if we do not remember this at the time. (Watts, 1966/ 1972)

Health Patterning Centers could be the matrix for these and other ways to reach out to people in their homes, workplaces, and schools. A nurse for every family, with *family* broadly defined, could be part of the managed care options.

In the immediate future, Health Patterning Centers will attract clients by:

1. Providing services for health care difficulties that reflect society's ills and are not being adequately addressed (women's health, the elderly, homelessness and other poverty-induced

conditions, prevention of infant mortality, teenage pregnancy and HIV infection, hospice care);

2. Providing primary care to healthy at-risk populations who are not covered by other services or funding (the uninsured and those ineligible for Medicaid or Medicare) but who are unable to pay the usual fees-for-service;

3. Providing services to populations for whom allopathic methods have not worked (smoking cessation, eating difficulties, alcohol and other substance use, other life-style risks);

4. Providing services not otherwise available (health patterning modalities such as imagery, Therapeutic Touch, meditation, light, color, sound, motion).

Health Patterning Centers will need to be socially and culturally relevant and to target inner cities and rural areas that have chronic shortages of health care (Shugars et al., 1991). Advocacy and education will be central to all services. The centers will serve as clearinghouses for information on health and illness. They will provide information on resources, education, and teaching groups of many types, including negotiation of the health system, choosing among health patterning modalities to assist with life-style and other health changes, and formation of self-help groups. Difficulties in living will not be pathologized as diseases. Understanding and supporting the role of various community agencies will maximize services (Shugars et al., 1991).

Although funding for community nursing centers has not yet been passed by Congress, the Health Care Financing Administration (HCFA) has some funding for demonstration projects staffed and administered by nurses (Stanhope, 1992). Other funding has been and will continue to be necessary. Reimbursement has expanded for direct care services provided by nurses practicing independently.

In these centers of unitary wholeness, there will be no fragmentation of the services or of the person. Nurses will neither be isolated in ivory towers nor buried in bureaucracies. Research will be an integral aspect of Health Patterning Centers. Consumers will be involved in important ways, and the need to educate communities to care for themselves will be addressed (Shugars et al., 1991).

When 3,500 nurses in practice told their stories in 1987 for the *American Journal of Nursing,* they expressed concern and guilt over their inability to surmount system restraints to deliver the care they had been educated to give, and they were distressed by the lack of support from both hospital and nursing administrators (Huey & Hartley, 1988). In Health Patterning Centers, the system will not stand in their way, nor will the findings of the Pew Foundation, which noted that whole sets of skills were often written out of job descriptions because others were not able to perform them (Shugars et al., 1991). Practice will not be reduced to the lowest level of knowledge and skill within the group. Rather, appropriate roles for associate, baccalaureate, master's, and doctorally prepared nurses will exist when nurses write the job descriptions and hold their peers accountable for performing them. Responsibility, accountability, and authority will be vested in nurses, thereby keeping the system both powerful and viable.

## ROGERIAN HEALTH PROMOTION OBJECTIVES FOR THE YEAR 2000

The Pew Health Professions Commission studied health care trends and, in 1991, defined 17 attitudes and abilities needed by health professionals for the year 2005 (Shugars et al., 1991). My challenge to readers is: Put on violet-tinted glasses and work with others to devise ways in which Rogerian scientists, artists, and revolutionaries can address these attitudes and abilities from the perspective of the Science of Unitary Human Beings. As a grass-roots project, many things can be accomplished by many nurses.

The health professional competencies needed for the year 2005 are:

1. Care for the community's health
2. Expanded access to effective care
3. Provision for contemporary (clinical) care
4. Emphasis on primary care
5. Participation in coordinated care
6. Care that is cost-effective and appropriate
7. Practices focused on prevention
8. Involvement of patients and families in the decision-making process
9. Promotion of healthy life-styles
10. Appropriate access and use of technology

11. Improvement in the health care system
12. Management of information
13. Understanding of the role of the physical environment
14. Provision for counseling on ethical issues
15. Accommodation of expanded accountability
16. Participation in a racially and culturally diverse society
17. Continued learning (Shugars et al., 1991, p. x)

A line from the film *City of Joy* describes a challenge: "In this world there are three kinds of people: the runners, the spectators, and the committers." Can we commit to developing a Rogerian science-based view of these abilities? What would they look like?

The 1990s have been proclaimed as a decade of women leaders (Naisbitt & Aburdeen, 1990). The decade promises likewise to be the most exciting in the history of nursing. As we get past the fear of standing up and speaking out at the right times and in the right places, we will actualize the power required to establish the nurse as the key health care provider of the twenty-first century.

## VISIONS OF ROGERIAN NURSING PRACTICE FOR THE NEW MILLENNIUM

Jonathan Swift said, "Vision is the art of seeing things invisible." Rogers' vision provides glimpses of science-based nursing in the coming millennium.

In 1989, Gioiella wrote of Rogers' scientific and professional contributions to professionalizing nursing. She said, "That Rogers was a prophet for professional nursing is unquestioned. Whether she was a prophet crying in the wilderness is yet to be determined. Clearly, nursing has continued, in large measure, to ignore Martha's messages and is suffering the consequences" (p. 61). A plurality of revolutionary voices answering Rogers' cry with Rogerian scientific art is being manifested in many ways in many places. Rogerian science links education, research, and practice, and thereby guides nursing actions. Science is the knowledge of the discipline and provides the potential for practice. Although usually the Rogerian scientist creates the science, it is the Rogerian artist who uses this knowledge for human betterment. The artist's work is creative and innovative; it gives birth to that which has not existed before; the artist facilitates becoming. The Rogerian scientist may also be a

Rogerian artist, but this is not necessarily so. However, for the Rogerian nurse in practice, creating art without the science base is like walking in the dark without a flashlight or trying to make ice cubes without refrigeration.

Avant-garde exemplars of what the nurse does, how it works, and why it is claimed to flow from Rogerian science are increasingly evident in the nursing literature (Barrett, 1990; Malinski, 1986; Sarter, 1988). Propositions linking the postulates, the principles of homeodynamics, and theories derived from Rogerian science must continuously be articulated to demonstrate operationalization in the practice domain. Applying research findings to see whether they are appropriate for particular clients is another avenue from knowledge about the phenomenon of concern to knowledge in the context of the clients' meaning and expression of their lived experiences. In the future, the interface of academia and practice can be strengthened by academicians serving as translators of the science, and practicing nurses can more effectively convert the science into nursing care.

In this system, both person and environment are irreducible energy fields. There is no mind, no body, no spirit, only the inherent unity of all that we are. Nursing care is caring for the unitary person by patterning the environment to promote well-being. Phillips (1992) called the goal of nursing care to see the "wholeness of the living–dying rhythm" (p. 5). This requires metaphorical, analogical, and dialectical ways of thinking, as well as logical and rational decision making. This work is about transforming and transcending ourselves and about our clients' transforming and transcending themselves as we share the mutual human–environment process. It is a nonlinear, acausal, nondeterministic, and unpredictable process of knowing participation in a pandimensional reality without attachment to outcomes.

## CONCLUSION

Looking wistfully back and longingly ahead, Rogers' vision will sustain nursing for more than the next hundred years, just as Florence Nightingale's vision sustained nursing for more than the past hundred years. More and more nurses will walk this road less traveled; the journey will be difficult yet exciting, and the task will be immense yet filled with unimaginable potentials. We will continue to press onward. We will do it deliberately and knowingly, with intention, with excellence, with freedom and choice, and we will be continuously guided by the Science of Unitary Human Beings.

As Rogerian revolutionaries, we will risk encounters at the edgelessness of pandimensional reality. We will face the unknown and learn to trust the process unfolding through our nursing lives. We will do this powerfully. We *will* make a difference in the health and wellbeing of people wherever they may be. It *can* be done. A few years ago, Newman (1979) shared with the nursing community the story of "the 100th monkey phenomenon." On an island in Japan, in 1952, the winter was severe, and the monkey colonies had been given supplementary feedings of sweet potatoes. However, the potatoes fell out of their faulty containers and became coated with sand, and it was difficult to eat them. One day, a young female monkey learned to wash the potatoes in the stream. She taught other monkeys, and slowly the knowledge spread. A critical mass of monkeys, probably 99, had learned to wash sweet potatoes, and 20 minutes later all the monkeys on the island were doing it. By that evening, monkeys on two neighboring islands, despite having had no physical contact, were washing sweet potatoes. The knowledge had reached a critical threshold above which it became common knowledge. This has come to be known as the 100th monkey phenomenon (Newman, 1979).

What has been presented in this chapter is all about preparing for the 100th Rogerian phenomenon. What are we waiting for? Let's get on with it. NOW!

## REFERENCES

Barrett, E.A.M. (1986). Investigation of the principles of helicy: The relationship of human field motion and power. In V.M. Malinski (Ed.), *Explorations on Martha Rogers' Science of Unitary Human Beings* (pp. 173–184). Norwalk, CT: Appleton-Century-Crofts.

Barrett, E.A.M. (1988). Using Roger's Science of Unitary Human Beings in nursing practice. *Nursing Science Quarterly, 1,* 50–51.

Barrett, E.A.M. (1990). Rogers' science-based nursing practice. In E.A.M. Barrett (Ed.), *Visions of Rogers' science-based nursing* (pp.31–44). New York: National League for Nursing.

Barrett, E.A.M. (1991). Space nursing. *Cutis, 48,* 299–303.

Barrett, E.A.M., Doyle, M.B., Madrid, M., Malinski, V.M., Racolin, A., & Walsh, P.C. (1990). Preface. In E.A.M. Barrett (Ed.), *Visions of Rogers' science-based nursing* (pp. xxi–xxiii). New York: National League for Nursing.

Boyle, B. (1985). Professional practice—myth or reality? Unpublished manuscript.

Butcher, H.K., & Forchuk, C. (1990, April). The overview effect: Space travel and its impact on the evolution of nursing science. Paper presented at the Nursing in Space Conference, Huntsville, AL.

Gioiella, E. (1989). Professionalizing nursing: A Rogers legacy. *Nursing Science Quarterly, 2,* 61-62.

Huey, F.L., & Hartley, S. (1988). What keeps nurses in nursing: 3500 nurses tell their stories. *American Journal of Nursing, 88,* 181-188.

Joel, L. (1992, June). Beyond pride: President's perspective. *American Nurse,* p. 5.

Malinski, V. (Ed.). (1986). *Explorations on Martha Rogers' Science of Unitary Human Beings.* Norwalk, CT: Appleton-Century-Crofts.

Manahan, D.J., & Manahan, W.D. (1992, May). The nurse as the primary health care practitioner. *Beginnings: Official Newsletter of the American Holistic Nurses Association, 1,* 4.

Maraldo, P. (1992a, January/February). Trends to watch for in '92: Health highest on American agenda. *Executive Wire: National League for Nursing,* pp. 1-4.

Maraldo, P. (1992b, May). Now is the time to come to the aid of the public. *Executive Wire: National League for Nursing.* pp. 1-4.

Maraldo, P. (1992c). NLN's first century. *Nursing and Health Care, 13,* 227-228.

Maurer, X.A. (1989, January). They came from outer space. *Modern Maturity,* pp. 57-61.

McGivern, D., Mezey, M., & Glynn, P.M. (1990). Evolution of primary care roles. *Nurse practitioner forum, 1,* 163-167.

Mitchell, E. (1992). Consciousness research and planetary change. *Noetic Sciences Review, 21* (1), 30.

Moccia, P. (1992). In 1992 a nurse in every school. *Nursing and Health Care, 13,* 14-18.

Naisbitt, J., & Aburdeen, P. (1990). *Megatrends 2000.* New York: Avon.

Newman, M. (1979). *Theory development in nursing.* Philadelphia: Davis.

Newman, M. (1991, June). *Differentiated practice.* Paper presented at the conference of the Columbia Presbyterian Hospital Nursing Department, New York.

Newman, M., Sime, A. M., & Corcoran-Perry, S. A. (1991). The focus of the discipline of nursing. *Advances in Nursing Science, 14* (1), 1-5.

O'Neil, G. (1981). *2081: A hopeful view of the human future.* New York: Simon & Schuster.

Parse, R.R., Coyne, A.B., & Smith, M.J. (1985). *Nursing research: Qualitative methods.* Bowie, MD: Brady.

Phillips, J. (1988). The looking glass of nursing research. *Nursing Science Quarterly, 1,* 96.

Phillips, J. (1992). Choosing and participating in the living–dying process: A research emergent. *Nursing Science Quarterly, 5,* 4–5.

Rogers, M.E. (1970). *An introduction to the theoretical basis of nursing.* Philadelphia: Davis.

Rogers, M.E. (1972). *Journal of the New York State Nurses Association, 3* (4), 5–10.

Rogers, M.E. (1988). Nursing science and art: A prospective. *Nursing Science Quarterly, 1,* 99–102.

Rogers, M.E. (1990). Nursing: Science of unitary, irreducible, human beings: Update, 1990. In E.A.M. Barrett (Ed.), *Visions of Rogers' science-based practice* (pp. 5–11). New York: National League for Nursing.

Rogers, M.E. (1992). Nursing science and the space age. *Nursing Science Quarterly, 5,* 27–34.

Sarter, B. (1988). *The stream of becoming: A study of Martha Rogers' theory.* New York: National League for Nursing.

Shugars, D.A., O'Neil, E.H., & Bader, J.D. (1991). *Pew Health Professions Commission. Healthy America: Practitioners for 2005, an agenda for action for U.S. health professional schools.* Durham, N.C.: The Pew Health Professions Commission.

Stanhope, M. (1992, May). *Community Nursing Centers.* Paper presented at the Hunter–Bellevue School of Nursing, Hunter College of CUNY, Community Health Nursing Master's Program meeting, New York.

Till-Tovey, M. (1992, June/July). Numbers versus needs. *Beginnings: The Official Newsletter of the American Holistic Nurses Association, 3.*

Tisdall, C. (Ed.). (1990). *Art meets science and spirituality in a changing economy.* Amsterdam: SDU Publishers.

Watts, A. (1972). *The book: On the taboo against knowing who you are.* New York: Vintage Books. (Original work published in 1966.)

White, F. (1987). *The overview effect: Space exploration and human evolution.* Boston: Houghton Mifflin.

Zachary, C. (1958). *Florence Nightingale and the doctors.* Philadelphia: Lippincott.

# Comments on Rogerian Scientists, Artists, Revolutionaries

*Violet Malinski*

In "Rogerian Scientists, Artists, Revolutionaries," Elizabeth Ann Manhart Barrett offers a bold vision of the ways nurses can use their knowledge to transform the health care system. Three notable convictions emerge as central to this vision:

1. There is a knowledge base unique to nursing.
2. Nurses can use it to provide knowledgeable caring.
3. Nurses are capable of assuming responsibility and are accountable for their knowledge and their actions.

Barrett echoes the beliefs of Martha E. Rogers (1961, 1964), who introduced these ideas into the nursing literature in the early 1960s. They bear repeating during a time of rumblings in some quarters about the need to relegate nursing conceptual models and theories to the historical archives in the belief that nurses can find more "useful" knowledge in, say, the Health Belief Model. Barrett is not suggesting that Rogerian nurses simply carry on by providing more of the same kind of health/medical care we already have, simultaneously doing it better and more inexpensively than physicians, but that we participate in a total transformation of the health care system. Four themes emerge in her chapter, and I will address each of them here:

1. The implications of different world-views;
2. The need to develop caring partnerships with consumers in order to revolutionize health care;

3. The increasing focus on community, highlighted by the development of nursing centers;

4. The potential impact of the merging technology of virtual reality.

### WORLD-VIEWS

Barrett describes Rogerian revolutionaries as being "among many renegades migrating from the medical model of parts to a health model of wholeness." As categories of nursing conceptual models and theories, she cites the world-views of the totality–simultaneity paradigm articulated by Parse (1987) and of the particulate-deterministic, integrative–interactive, and unitary–transformative paradigms described by Newman, Sime, and Corcoran-Perry (1991). Barrett notes that the ideas set forth in these world-views are not unique to nursing. Rather, nurses join with other health professionals, scientists, and interested observers from a variety of walks of life who have proposed what can be called, generically, a new world-view, of which Rogerian science offers one perspective. Capra (1982, 1983; Capra & Steindl-Rast, 1991) provides an example of one scientist who has consistently highlighted the importance of world-views and their impact on culture, society, and the disciplines. He described "new paradigm thinking" as characterized by an awareness of interconnectedness and interdependence (Capra & Steindl-Rast, 1991). Rather than using the properties of the parts to understand the dynamics of the whole, new paradigm thinking teaches that parts can be understood only in the context of the whole. Ultimately, parts do not exist: "What we call a part is merely a pattern in an inseparable web of relationships" (Capra & Steindl-Rast, 1991, p. xii). The emphasis shifts from structure to process. Structure is then understood as a manifestation of the underlying process.

Other scientists, such as Bohm and Prigogine (cited by Malinski, 1986, 1990), offer ideas that resonate with Rogerian nursing science; each reflects ideas from the new world-view, the new paradigm thinking. As Barrett emphasizes, nurses who share this world-view need to join with those in other disciplines who also participate in new paradigm thinking. Only in this way can we hope to reach the critical mass that will portend the major paradigm shift capable of transforming the health care system.

Such a shift, a fundamental change in how we perceive the universe, will allow us to shake loose from old expectations and attain the freedom to be creative and innovative.

Barrett suggests that, in the future, we may see a societal split based on world-views, with both interdisciplinary schools of health sciences and the health care delivery system organized according to world-view rather than by discipline. Such a split already seems evident in nursing. The nursing world's perspective of the individual rooted in the totality paradigm is qualitatively different from the perspective in the simultaneity paradigm. Perhaps two different paths based on world-view will emerge in nursing. One will prepare, for example, a specialist in AIDS and in the health manifestations of AIDS. The other will prepare a specialist who explores the meaning of such an experience to the individual, his or her awareness of choices, and other attributes of power to knowingly participate in change. Whether the medical diagnosis is one of AIDS or schizophrenia, whether the experience is one of stigmatization, isolation, or compromised immune functioning, the "wholeness of the living-dying rhythm" (Phillips, 1992, p. 5) will be explored in the nurse-client caring partnership.

## CARING PARTNERSHIPS

Rogers' (1986) principle of integrality specifies the context of change as the human–environment mutual process. Barrett's concept of the caring partnership is an expression of this mutual process, where nothing and no one is separate. All life exists in an integral flow of field patterning.

Presenting another perspective within new paradigm thinking, Fritjof Capra, physicist, and David Steindl-Rast, psychologist and Benedictine Brother, offered the garden as a metaphor for the human–environment relationship (Capra & Steindl-Rast, 1991). Steindl-Rast introduced the view of the human as steward of the garden, charged with the responsibility to tend and nurture rather than dominate and exploit nature. Upon the biblical fall, human beings separated themselves from the garden and embarked on the latter path of exploitation, dominance, and control. Capra and Steindl-Rast suggested that freedom and responsibility are necessary to restore the connection—the freedom to choose and the responsibility to choose wisely. Barrett encompasses a similar idea in the language of knowing participation and choice with awareness. Through caring partnerships, nurses and clients, nurses and members of society, and nurses and other health professionals can knowingly participate together to revolutionize health care. An integral concept of this revolution is enhancing clients' power to make knowledgeable choices in the context of their own life patterns.

The garden metaphor has been used to explore the caring moment in nursing. Jensen, Back-Pettersson, and Segesten (1993) likened the gifted nurse to the gifted gardener, the one with the "green thumb." They identified the green-thumb nurse as "one who recognizes the caring moment" (p. 102), "characterized by mutual attention, harmony, trust, and the experience that 'time stopped'" (p. 102), and "acts consciously on the spur of the moment with competence, compassion, and courage" (p. 102).

The green-thumb gardener is a potent image for nursing. Centuries ago, Hildegard of Bingen coined the word "viriditas," or "greening power" (Fox, 1985). This greening power is the source of growth and creativity that bonds human and nature in an integral, infinite cosmos. To be healthy is to live harmoniously, justly, and with compassion in this organic web. One is then moist, creative, and fertile. Separating oneself from this cosmic unity means becoming barren and dry, wasting away. The nurse, as gardener, tends and nurtures those who come for services, ever mindful of the person–environment mutual process. As Barrett wrote, "Nursing care is caring for the unitary person by patterning the environment to promote well-being." By expanding awareness of choices and facilitating knowing participation in change, "power of the people is enhanced and the client–provider relationship is being transformed" (Barrett). The importance of this client–provider relationship is evident in the writings of Maraldo and Moccia on nursing's health care agenda, as cited by Barrett.

## NURSING CENTERS IN THE COMMUNITY

Barrett emphasizes Rogers' early assertion that nursing takes place wherever people are, whether at home, in the community, at school, or in space. Hospitals are only one potential setting, among many, for the delivery of health care services. In the community, nurses can provide the broadest base of services to enhance well-being. According to the World Health Organization, provision of primary health care involves participation by both the individual and the community in a way that "promotes the idea of self-care and self-reliance within a shared responsibility" (Collado, 1992, p. 411). Farley (1993) discussed the process of building community participation and creating professional–citizen partnerships. She noted that one of the many potential difficulties is the unwillingness of professionals to acknowledge that citizens can participate in solving problems in their own communities, seeing them instead as "unmotivated, inexpert, and uninformed" (p. 248). This view accords with the older paradigm view of nursing and health care, but not with the newer paradigm view as exemplified in Rogerian nursing science. As Barrett so aptly writes, "For both clients and nurses, power (knowing participation in change) is the password in the Rogerian revolution." Health patterning is the process of assisting with this knowing participation.

Barrett correctly notes that primary care is not the sole domain of the physician. Furthermore, as Schorr (1993) noted, what we are discussing in health care reform is not medical care. Medical care is only one aspect of health care, just as nursing is one aspect of health care. Medical care is limited in scope, arising as it does from the biomedical model of parts with an emphasis on disease. Find the broken part; mend it or replace it with a new one. Within Rogerian nursing science, disease is another pattern manifestation. Clients must become experts in their own patterning process. In Barrett's words, "Clients are health seekers concerned with the quality of their lives. Health patterning facilitates their search for meaning as well as ways to make changes in their health."

The premiere issue of *Prism: The NLN Research & Policy Quarterly,* in 1993, focused on nursing centers, noting the tremendous variety of structures and services that exist under this umbrella phrase. One commonality identified was the emphasis on providing care to neglected populations, such as the poor, the aged, children, and minorities. Another is the focus on primary care. Of the centers responding to the NLN's 1991 survey, 48 percent indicated that primary care is their principal service (Staff, 1993, pp. 4–5). Unfortunately, the report also noted that nursing centers are financially at risk for these very same reasons, and may have to reduce services to poor, high-risk clients in the future. The Rogerian revolution needs to guard against what would then be a return to business-as-usual—providing services primarily to those who can pay.

This concern highlights the need, identified earlier, to join with others who share a similar world-view. Health patterning modalities such as Therapeutic Touch, imagery, meditation, light, color, music, humor, and laughter receive little recognition in the biomedical model. Counseling and teaching are not as valued as giving a shot or a medication. The last two take up less time, freeing the practitioner to see more clients with whom he or she spends minimal time while earning more money. Our view of health, health promotion, and health care must undergo a paradigm shift if we are truly to revolutionize health care, providing Barrett's nursing health patterning centers "of unitary wholeness" to our clients.

## VIRTUAL REALITY

Barrett mentions virtual reality in relation to a "computer-augmented interactive communication between people in space and their loved ones on Earth." Virtual reality will also play a role in health patterning centers, whether they be located in space or on Earth, as I have discussed elsewhere in this volume. Virtual reality allows us to choose and participate in mutual process with any environment, any world, any galaxy. We can experience pandimensionality in a virtual world that transcends time and space while teleporting us out of our physical bodies. McKenna (1991), like Rogers, suggested that space exploration will accelerate the transformation of the human species. He went on to speculate that "A technology that would internalize the body and exteriorize the soul will develop parallel to the move into space" (McKenna, 1991, p. 96). Virtual reality is one such technology. What we can imagine can become a virtual experience of total immersion, one where we can see, touch, hear, feel, smell. Virtual reality may be the key to a real understanding of Rogers' contention that the body is only one manifestation of field patterning.

In conclusion, Barrett challenges us to transform and transcend ourselves with our own knowing participation in change. Only in this way can we become the Rogerian scientists, artists, revolutionaries who can participate in transforming the health care system. The 100th Rogerian monkey is already knocking on the door!

## REFERENCES

Capra, F. (1982). *The turning point: Science, society and the rising culture.* New York: Simon & Schuster.

Capra, F. (1983). *The tao of physics* (2nd ed.). New York: Bantam Books.

Capra, F., & Steindl-Rast, D. (1991). *Belonging to the universe: Explorations on the frontiers of science and spirituality.* New York: Harper-Collins.

Collado, C.B. (1992). Primary health care: A continuing challenge. *Nursing & Health Care, 13,* 408–413.

Farley, S. (1993). The community as partner in primary health care. *Nursing & Health Care, 14,* 244–249.

Fox, M. (1985). *Illuminations of Hildegard of Bingen: Text by Hildegard of Bingen with commentary by Matthew Fox.* Santa Fe: Bear & Company.

Jensen, K.P., Back-Pettersson, S., & Segesten, K.M. (1993). The caring moment and the green-thumb phenomenon among Swedish nurses. *Nursing Science Quarterly, 6,* 98–104.

Malinski, V.M. (1986). Contemporary science and nursing: Parallels with Rogers. In V.M. Malinski (Ed.), *Explorations on Martha Rogers' Science of Unitary Human Beings* (pp. 15–23). Norwalk, CT: Appleton-Century-Crofts.

Malinski, V.M. (1990). The meaning of a progressive world-view in nursing: Rogers' Science of Unitary Human Beings. In N.L. Chaska (Ed.), *The nursing profession: Turning points* (pp. 237–244). St. Louis: Mosby.

McKenna, T. (1991). *The archaic revival.* New York: HarperCollins.

Newman, M., Sime, A.M., & Corcoran-Perry, S.A. (1991). The focus of the discipline of nursing. *Advances in Nursing Science, 14,* (1), 1–5.

Parse, R.R. (1987). *Nursing science: Major paradigms, theories, and critiques.* Philadelphia: Saunders.

Phillips, J.R. (1992). Choosing and participating in the living–dying process: A research emergent. *Nursing Science Quarterly, 5,* 4–5.

Rogers, M.E. (1961). *Educational revolution in nursing.* New York: Macmillan.

Rogers, M.E. (1964). *Reveille in nursing.* Philadelphia: F.A. Davis.

Rogers, M.E. (1986). Science of Unitary Human Beings. In V.M. Malinski (Ed.), *Explorations on Martha Rogers' Science of Unitary Human Beings* (pp. 3–8). Norwalk, CT: Appleton-Century-Crofts.

Schorr, T.M. (1993). The term is "health care." *Nursing & Health Care, 14,* 294–295.

Staff. (1993). *Prism: The NLN Research & Policy Quarterly, 1* (1), pp. 1–12.

# Unit II

# SCIENCE-BASED PRACTICE WITH SELECTED GROUPS

# 5

# Participating in the Process of Dying

*Mary Madrid*

Nancy was 33 years old, and this was her first hospital admission. Four years prior to her hospitalization, she had been given a medical diagnosis of leukemia and had been successfully treated as an outpatient. She suddenly developed a "blast crisis," a transformation from a more stable form of leukemia to an aggressive form whereby the bone marrow produces an overwhelming number of premature cells. This was a life-threatening situation, and she was admitted to the intensive care unit for monitoring and treatment.

I was working as a staff nurse the evening of Nancy's first day of hospitalization. On my initial contact with Nancy, her husband was by her side. I noted that their conversation was filled with expressions of mutual love and caring. They were trying to be bright and cheerful. She and her husband made light of Nancy's hospitalization, nervously joking and laughing about her admission (e.g., how her husband was glad to finally get her out of the house and how he couldn't wait to leave). I intuitively sensed an underlying concern that each of them had about Nancy's hospitalization and that neither one of them wanted to bring it out into the open for discussion.

I viewed Nancy as a human energy field in mutual process with her environmental field and set about to identify the pattern of these fields by pattern manifestation appraisal. This appraisal would allow me the opportunity to identify "manifestations of the human and environmental fields that relate to current health events" and to engage in deliberative mutual patterning (Barrett, 1988, p. 50). The appraisal and patterning process would be continuous and began by my focusing on her human field image. This would give me insight into the pattern of her human field and allow me to capture her experience in the relative present. Her human field pattern would be appraised "through manifestations of the pattern in the form of experience, perception and expressions" (Cowling, 1990, p. 52). Perception of Nancy's human field pattern would involve an intuitive awareness of her wholeness as a unitary human being and a sensitivity to her thoughts and feelings and to her verbal and nonverbal expressions of experiences in the relative past and present. Appraisal of the environmental field pattern would take place simultaneously since the human and environmental fields are integral and in mutual process. Pattern information emerging from this mutual process would be organized and synthesized as a guide in the creative use of therapeutic modalities inherent in the art of nursing practice.

Nancy's human field image evolved from the pandimensional patterning process whereby human potentials emerge. As defined by Phillips (1990), human field image represents "the ever-changing relative present that synthesizes the past, present and future. This synthesis involves all the changes that have occurred in past human field images as well as those projected future human field images" (p. 14). Perception of her relative present human field image would help me to understand her human field pattern.

Nancy told me that she had been married for eight years. During this time, she had struggled to complete her education to become an accountant, rearing her family at the same time. She had been successful in accomplishing her goals. She had two daughters whom she and her husband spoke of with pride.

From the time of diagnosis, Nancy had been able to care for her family and continue full-time employment. She had received treatment as an outpatient in the form of chemotherapy and blood transfusions. Nancy recalled the "hard times" she had experienced in regard to her illness and her family and employment responsibilities, but took courage in her ability to rally through them. Her view of reality was that, even though, in terms of her medical diagnosis, the future was uncertain, she could endure whatever hardships came her way.

Her human field image reflected confidence in herself and determination to draw on her inner strengths to see her through this crisis. Nancy saw herself as a loving wife and mother. She knew that she could count on her family to muster up strength and encouragement. Nancy and her husband reached out to hug one another and emphatically stated that they "could handle anything as long as they had each other." One could identify the harmonious integrality of the rhythms of their energy fields as manifested by a resonating pattern of love.

Nancy viewed illness as an expression of the life process and did not really see herself as a "sick person." The need for intermittent blood transfusions and other modalities of treatment had been integrated into her life pattern and taken with what she called "a grain of salt."

Her pattern manifestation appraisal that day reflected courage and tenacity. She was aware of the crisis she was undergoing but was confident that it would resolve and that she would be discharged in a few days. Nancy had "always hoped for the best." She recalled events and crises from the relative past that had been associated with hope. Nancy spoke about the process of hoping and how it had given her the ability to be creative, establish her goals, and remain optimistic about the future. As she faced the new reality of hospitalization and the evolving pattern changes in her energy field, her goal was to overcome the "tired feeling" she was experiencing and to maintain an optimistic view of her life's potentials. My intent was to assist her in accomplishing these goals through the use of deliberative mutual patterning.

After a lengthy visit, her husband left and Nancy appeared exhausted. She was being given blood products. Her body movements were slower and required concentrated effort; the volume of her voice was low. She declined eating dinner. These behaviors were manifestations of her field pattern and indicated a change in the rhythm and frequency of her energy field. I encouraged her to tune into the rhythm of her field pattern so that she would recognize changes in her pattern relative to feelings of tiredness. This would permit her to balance activity with rest. She could participate in the process of enhancing healing by taking periods of quiet relaxation. These restful periods would promote harmony between her human and environmental fields.

She felt that she "overdid it" that day and looked forward to resting. I demonstrated a relaxation exercise, which she readily agreed to perform, and I turned the radio on to play restful music. Nancy drifted off to sleep, and awoke later to see a heavy snowfall drifting down from the sky.

It continued to snow heavily. By late evening, a "snow emergency" had been declared. Travel was at a standstill. The staff could not leave the hospital, and most of the relief shift could not leave their homes. Our unit organized a schedule so that we could have nursing coverage and alternate between periods of sleep and periods of work.

Nancy had a restless night. She would sleep for short periods of time and awaken perspiring profusely. Her temperature fluctuated and went up to 104. At times, her heart rate was fast and pounding. She had a sense of time dragging and thought the night would never end. These physical and behavioral manifestations were indices that identified the changing pattern of her human field.

Deliberative mutual patterning was directed toward promoting rest, refreshment, and mobilization of the healing powers within herself. She was still receiving blood products and would have blood drawn for testing. At times, she would be awakened for this purpose and would find it difficult to get back to sleep. Since staffing was so short, the technical staff was very willing to go along with my offer to draw the blood at a time when she was awake and send it off to the laboratory. This would allow her to have uninterrupted periods of sleep.

I assumed a centered state of awareness as I gave her a tepid bath and back rub several times throughout the night. This aided me in acquiring an intuitive sense of her human field as a unitary whole. She found physical touch to be soothing and relaxing. The cool hand and gentle motions involved in bathing her body and massaging her back promoted sleep. I used Therapeutic Touch (Krieger, 1979) to appraise the pattern of her energy field and facilitate a balanced flow of energy. Her high temperatures declined, and the quality of sleep improved after each treatment.

There was no letup from the snowstorm. By morning, power lines were down, there was no telephone service, and our facility was running on "auxiliary power." Whoever was working in the hospital was there to stay. Physicians were taxied to the hospital by jeep (compliments of the National Guard) to see patients or to handle emergencies.

It was Nancy's second day in the hospital. She began to express concern about her fever and the fact that, throughout the night, she had had intermittent episodes of blood oozing from her nose and gums. I used humor as a therapeutic modality to ease some of the tension she seemed to be experiencing. We joked about the snowstorm and about "hospital food." I bathed her and left for my rest period. As

I left the room, she was peacefully watching the snowflakes fall upon the window.

I came back hours later and found her with a sad look on her face, engrossed in counting the drops of blood as they dripped from the chamber into the infusion line. The change in her human field pattern was characterized by depression and a decelerated field rhythm.

I learned from the end-of-shift report that she had experienced an episode of severe epistaxis. Shortly thereafter, she became hemodynamically unstable, and invasive monitoring and medicated infusions had been initiated. Her fever was high, and she had been placed on a hypothermia blanket. Several physicians had been by to appraise her medically and to write orders. They did not share much information with her about her clinical status.

Manifestations of patterning were continuously changing. In order to initiate practice strategies, it was necessary to appraise these manifestations in the relative present. I could see that she was disturbed and asked her how she felt about what was going on. She expressed difficulty in organizing her relative experience. Nancy recognized that she would be in the hospital for a longer period of time than she had anticipated, and this was disturbing to her. She was experiencing a sense of powerlessness over what was happening to her. She perceived herself as being cut off from her family and support systems and was beginning to have doubts about her ability to cope. Multiple attempts to reach her family were unsuccessful.

Nancy missed not being able to have her husband and family visit. The weather was still the same; the heavy downfall of snow continued. She envisioned her day as being long and dragged out, with little to do to occupy her mind and break the monotony. Her human field image was changing and her behavioral manifestations reflected this change. There was no reflection of the confidence and determination she had displayed earlier. The rhythm of her energy field was not harmonious with the rhythms of the environmental field.

Deliberative mutual patterning involved meaningful presence, empathy, and listening to her expressions of her lived experience in the relative present. In order to increase her awareness of the power she had within herself to create healing change, I suggested that she focus on affirmations that depicted her strengths and accomplishments. I asked her what her specific goals were and told her that I would collaborate with her in proposing pattern strategies to accomplish them. She wanted to just "get through the day and try to put some of my worries out of my head so I can rest." Because I had some tasks to perform and would be in her room, I suggested that we share experiences with each other in the form of story telling. The experiences could be fact or fiction. Together, we could imaginatively experience whatever we chose and travel anywhere in the infinite, timeless universe.

Story telling allowed her the opportunity to participate in the mutual process of patterning the human and environmental fields toward innovative change. Nancy used her imagination creatively. She became free to venture and explore, to bring experiences of adventure, humor, and intrigue alive and real into the relative present. At times, her imaginative story telling touched her experiences in the real world. These experiences were enriched by her telling them to someone. They seemed to be more real and meaningful in the sharing than in the experiencing of them. She was free to travel between fantasy and reality, between objectivity and subjectivity, and she was able to perceive the universe from a nonconventional perspective.

Nancy was able to transcend the relative present and experience phenomena from the relative past and relative future, synthesizing her thoughts and feelings and expressing them so that she experienced a "wholeness" or "harmony of fields" (Rawnsley, 1985, p. 26). Nancy's pattern manifestations characterized the evolving changes in her human field pattern as it became more diverse. She found time passing more quickly. She experienced the integrality of the mutual process between her energy field and the environmental energy field as she told stories that encompassed her husband and children and their experiences as a family.

There was receptiveness in the environment to her verbal expressions as she shared her stories and events. The integrality of our human and environmental fields was felt as we imagined and journeyed together to various places in our infinite universe to experience events in the relative past and future. It was a pandimensional experience for both of us.

As the day advanced, her pattern manifestations indicated that the "blast crisis" was progressing. She would tire more easily, and her breathing became more labored. She required longer rest periods and found it tiring to engage in lengthy conversation. Her eyes appeared dark and sunken and had deep circles around them. The color of her skin was sallow, and she continued to spike high fevers. The oozing from her mouth and nose became more profuse. Several times, she had large amounts of oral and nasal bleeding. Her heart rate was fast, her blood pressure was labile, and she was in renal failure. The amount of blood products being delivered increased. The physicians shared their perceptions with the nurses, stating that "things did not look good."

Nancy apologized for not sharing any more "stories" with me. She stated that she preferred to just lie in bed, trying to relax and reflecting on pleasant experiences in her life. This reflection promoted feelings of wholeness and integrity. Patterning strategies to promote well-being focused on providing comfort and rest.

I went for my rest period late in the evening and came back on duty in the very early hours of the morning. I was surprised to see the change in Nancy. Her pattern manifestations as described before were even more pronounced. I was told that there were indications that her progressive "blast crisis" was irreversible. Although her physicians were still trying to do everything possible from a medical standpoint, there was not much hope that she would make it through this crisis. I asked if anyone had discussed this with her. No one had. Continued attempts to contact the family remained unsuccessful.

When Nancy awoke, she was quiet and concerned. She had sensed that "something was very wrong." The behavioral patterns of the staff and the physicians who came into her room to tend to her had changed. They spent less time in the room with her. It was not that they did not administer proper care to her, but they did not linger. She knew that, because of the weather, they were tired from working extended shifts and were busy and stressed by having an extra work load. Nancy perceived, however, that their pattern manifestations did not reflect stress or fatigue but rather manifested feelings of discomfort when being in her presence. No one seemed to want to "look me in the eye and tell me" what was going on.

Nancy was also tuned into the behavioral manifestations of her human field. She was aware of the increased bleeding, fevers, hemodynamic changes, fatigue, and periods of decreased levels of consciousness. She knew that they were indices of change in the pattern of her human field, and she thought about the meaning of this change. Nancy was struggling to push aside thoughts of death. Intuitively, I knew that she was having difficulty integrating the concept of death into her human field image. Her struggle was painful.

Nancy had the capacity to participate knowingly in the continuous patterning of her human and environmental fields. She had power, including freedom, to act intentionally in creating change. She chose to deal openly with her thoughts and feelings and confronted me with their meaning. She asked me if what she was experiencing meant that she was dying. I reached for her hand, looked into her eyes, and said, "Yes, it seems so."

There was silence and a long pause before she bolted upright to a sitting position, grasped the side rails of the bed, and began to shake them. It was evident that she was angry and frustrated. Neither one of us spoke. I left the room and came back with a basin containing rubber gloves filled with water. I put a bath blanket on the floor against the wall facing her bed and placed the basin on her bed. I picked up a glove and threw it against the wall. It made a "squishy" sound as it burst and fell to the floor. I said the rest were for her and that she should call me when she was finished or if she wanted more gloves. I walked out of the room and closed the door behind me.

Several minutes later, I looked in on Nancy. The basin was empty and she was lying in bed weeping. I entered the room and began to pick up the blanket and gloves. She began speaking and said that she never dreamed that death would come so soon. There was so much she had wanted to do with her life. She expressed concern about the welfare of her husband and children. I suggested that she rest and told her we would talk more when she was refreshed. I gave her a Therapeutic Touch treatment, and she eventually drifted off to sleep.

Deliberative mutual patterning had been initiated so that Nancy could have the freedom to act intentionally. The environment was patterned so that she had the freedom to express her feelings and vent her frustration and anger. Creative change emerged from the mutual process of her human and environmental energy fields. Nancy faced a new reality—the reality of death. Her human field image had reflected that reality. She had a keen awareness of pain and sorrow as she began to deal with the reality of death.

When she awakened, she began to speak openly about her feelings of death. She said again that she never thought it would happen so fast. She wanted to know "how long she had" and "how it would happen." I could not answer the first question, but I assured her that I would do what I could to make her comfortable. I told her about my experience with death from my personal experience at the bedside and from what I read. I shared that those who have had near-death experiences have described it as a beautiful transition. I expected that she would drift off into a coma and that she would feel no pain. She said that she felt a real peace within herself. Nancy was internalizing the concept of death as a developmental process and recognized that "living/dying is a rhythmic manifestation of the life process" (Phillips, 1990, p. 19). She did not want to die, but she had no fear of death.

The snow emergency still existed, and it was not possible for her husband to visit. At the onset of the storm, they had talked by phone to each other several times when service had been temporarily restored. Now, however, telephone service remained inoperable, and it was not possible for them to communicate. Nancy felt that they had much to talk about. She told me that both of them had expected her to live to see their children grown. She had done so well up to this point that they had had no reason to believe that their hopes for the future would not be fulfilled.

Nancy said that she often wanted to talk to her husband about her eventual death, but he refused to participate in a discussion. He would become so upset that she would drop the subject and not pursue it further. She regretted not having had the opportunity in the relative past to tell him what was on her mind.

She told me that she had wanted him to have a happy life when she was gone. She wanted him to feel free to marry again and especially so if she died when the children were young. She wanted her children to have a mother and her husband to have a wife to love and care for him. I asked her if she would like to write a letter to her husband. She was too weak to do it herself, and I offered to write it for her in her own words and give it to him. She was grateful for this opportunity.

She began to find comfort in facing death and began to prepare for that transition. She spoke of the fear she had had of dying; it was mostly the unknown that had bothered her. Now that she had it "out in the open," she felt relieved since it really had always been "gnawing at her from underneath." Before, she had just pushed her feelings of death aside. She had an awareness of these feelings and, by experiencing and expressing them, she was better able to release them.

This conversation was not an easy one. Nancy's pattern manifestations were rapidly changing. She was becoming more lethargic; her words became slurred and, at times, she would drift off in the middle of a sentence. Her kidneys and liver were functioning poorly, and the physical manifestations of her human field gave evidence to the seriousness of the situation. She slipped into a coma, and I continued to talk to her as I worked at her side or administered to her. I was with her when she died.

It was a memorable experience to have participated with Nancy in the process of dying. It was possible for me to observe the accelerated dynamic changes in the pattern manifestations of her energy field as she apprehended and experienced death.

Different modalities were initiated that allowed her the opportunity to conceptualize the dying process and to have the power to knowingly participate in the experience. She was given the freedom to make choices. These choices were supported, and deliberative mutual patterning was directed toward fulfillment of her goals, her hopes, and her dreams.

## REFERENCES

Barrett, E.A.M. (1988). Using Rogers' Science of Unitary Human Beings in nursing practice. *Nursing Science Quarterly, 1,* 50–51.

Cowling, W.R. (1990). A template for unitary pattern-based nursing practice. In E.A.M. Barrett (Ed.), *Visions of Rogers' science-based nursing* (pp. 45–65). New York: National League of Nursing.

Krieger, D. (1979). *The Therapeutic Touch: How to use your hands to help or heal.* Englewood Cliffs, NJ: Prentice-Hall.

Phillips, J. (1990). Changing human potentials and future visions of nursing: A human field image perspective. In E.A.M. Barrett (Ed.), *Visions of Rogers' science-based nursing* (pp. 13–25). New York: National League of Nursing.

Rawnsley, M. (1985). Health: A Rogerian perspective. *Journal of Holistic Nursing, 3*(1), 25–29.

# Storytelling as a Scientific Art Form

*Joanne Griffin*

In the preceding chapter, Mary Madrid reveals her considerable talents as a storyteller. What the reader cannot appreciate is the storytelling gift she shared with the participants at the Fourth Rogerian Conference. I can close my eyes and capture the bright Sunday morning sunlight in the auditorium. The sunlight was streaming in through the curtains which were moving softly as a cooling breeze blew in from Washington Square Park. We had just listened intently to Cowling's intellectual challenge and Malinski's powerful description of her practice. I was anxious because one of the speakers for the next series of presentations had not appeared yet, and I was "responsible." Others in the audience were beginning to stir restlessly. I remember thinking, "We should have scheduled the coffee break earlier." And then . . . Mary caught us all up in this incredible story. We were transported to that snowy time when Mary met this young woman and her husband, and the blizzard came. We heard Mary's increasing fatigue as the snowbound staff spelled each other, and her sadness as Nancy became weaker; we raged with Nancy as she recognized what was happening, and we wept and mourned with Mary when Nancy died.

The irrelevance of three-dimensional time and space was "proven" in ways that even the most rigorous of the logical positivists would have accepted that morning, accomplished in a very human and very ancient form by Madrid. Ordinary narrators would say that we were transported (as on a magic carpet) to that time and place, and popular entertainment on the level of *Back to the Future* would underline the appeal of the escapist notion. But we were not trans-ported there, nor was that time brought into the auditorium in the heart of New York City; we did transcend with Madrid in a mutual process that would seem to this participant to be the epitome of inte-grality as Rogers writes about that principle.

Recently, Sandelowski (1991) wrote convincingly about the im-portance of telling stories as a means of conveying to readers and learners the nature of human experience. "Scholars now see the story in the study, the tale in the theory, the parable in the principle and the drama in the life" (Sandelowski, 1991, p. 161). Bruner (1986) discussed the reciprocal nature of storytelling by suggesting that the story is not what is written (or told) by the storyteller, but what the listener (or reader) hears (or reads); this is a process that qualitative researchers describe as the search for meaning. Most of us who hear a good story think about it frequently and recount it to family and friends. The story changes with each telling, and new meanings are uncovered every time. Interpretation, by both the storyteller and the story reader, has always been recognized as critical to the process.

Learning to listen and to hear the core truth of what is being said is an important clinical skill for all health care practitioners, and Madrid's telling of Nancy's story demonstrates this need vividly. That kind of active listening has always been a hallmark of compassionate practice, and it is a skill that can be taught and learned, as Kleinman (1988) and Brody (1987) have discussed. This particular noninvasive modality, which uncovers the truths of the human experience, needs more attention from Rogerian scholars. The "talking cure" brings much healing to those who suffer, as Nouwen (1992) has reminded us so powerfully in *Beyond the Mirror.*

Sacks wrote of his own experiences as a patient in *A Leg to Stand On* (1984), and he made a strong case for the application of this skill. As a physician himself, he understands the clinical problem and recognizes that he needs more than the diagnostic "professional" techniques from those he would choose to care for him. Sacks also had the honesty to tell us about the ugly feelings of jealousy, rage, and despair he experienced during his illness and convalescence. He described a "well documented phenomenon—the hateful spite of the sick" (Sacks, 1982, p. 177) and went on to admit how difficult it was to write about such reactions. He reminded us that it is easy to write (and to read) about good things like humor, nobility, and courage; the repulsive and distressing feelings and behaviors are much more difficult to recount. The people most nurses work with almost always experience those feelings of "hateful spite," and it is the rare nurse who can see that behavior, recognize its validity, and, in doing so, acknowledge the humanity of the client. Madrid demonstrates that rare ability in her story. She shows Nancy her own power, and helps her to retain her dignity and find peace.

We have recently expended much intellectual effort in attempting to clarify the nature of what Barrett (1990) has called power, and this is an appropriate thing for Rogerian scholars to do. I suggest that Madrid's story offers additional insight into that concept, which can point the way to future researchers who are interested in examining it. In the old world-perspective, no patient could be more helpless than Nancy was, and no nurse—trapped in a snowbound hospital, exhausted by working double and triple shifts, and surprised and distressed by her patient's unanticipated physical decline—could have been more professionally powerless than Madrid. The story shows another outcome altogether, and turns the sorrowful tears of mourning into those of joy. There is much to learn in this story.

Those of us who teach undergraduate nursing students and are charged with introducing them to the Science of Unitary Human Beings have been grateful to Madrid ever since another story, about a person named Roger, appeared in *Visions of Rogers' science-based nursing* (Barrett, 1990). Students who first read Madrid's chapter in that book can usually go on to the contributions by Rogers, and others, and understand them. When students start with chapter one, it just doesn't make sense to them. Now we have Nancy's story to add to the collection and to provide further insight. Thank you, Mary Madrid, and WRITE ON!!!!!

## REFERENCES

Barrett, E.A.M. (1990). Rogers' science-based nursing practice. In E.A.M. Barrett (Ed.). *Visions of Rogers' science-based nursing* (pp. 31–44). New York: National League for Nursing.

Brody, H. (1987). *Stories of sickness.* New Haven: Yale University Press.

Bruner, J. (1986). *Actual minds, possible worlds.* Cambridge, MA: Harvard University Press.

Kleinman, A. (1988). *The illness narratives: Suffering, healing and the human condition.* New York: Basic Books.

Madrid, M. (1990). The participating process of human field patterning in an acute-care environment. In E.A.M. Barrett (Ed.), *Visions of Rogers' science-based nursing* (pp. 93–104). New York: National League for Nursing.

Nouwen, H. (1992). *Beyond the mirror: Reflections on death and life.* New York: Crossroad.

Sacks, O. (1984). *A leg to stand on.* New York: Harper Perennial.

Sandelowski, M. (1991). Telling stories: Narrative approaches in qualitative research. *Image: The Journal of Nursing Scholarship, 23,* 161–166.

# 6

# Health Patterning for Individuals and Families

*Violet Malinski*

In this chapter, I will discuss work with clients in my private practice, which I advertise as Health Patterning for Individuals and Families. When contemplating what to call what I offer, I decided to follow Elizabeth Barrett's (1990) terminology and description of the health patterning process in Rogerian science-based practice. According to Barrett (1990), "Health patterning enhances clients' capacity to transform themselves in creative mutual process with their environments" (p. 33). Through my private practice, I offer clients opportunities to participate in their own health patterning through the field modalities of Therapeutic Touch, meditation, and imagery.

On my business card, I describe health patterning as providing knowledgeable caring to assist clients in actualizing potentials for well-being through knowing participation in change. Some potential clients can relate to this immediately; others are totally at sea, even after we discuss this phrase and what I mean by it. Some people, therefore, choose not to work with me, and I assist with other referrals when possible, if they request this of me. I see this element of therapist choice as an integral aspect of clients' knowing participation in change, and this process starts with my business card and initial contacts with potential clients. Similarly, not everything I will relate here works with everyone. This is not surprising, particularly in Rogerian science where the emphasis is on diversity and the need for individualizing nursing care.

## THE BASIS FOR A PRACTICE IN HEALTH PATTERNING

The basis for a practice in health patterning comes from key ideas in Rogerian science. According to Rogers (1992), human and environment are irreducible, pandimensional energy fields identified by pattern. Pattern flows in higher and lower frequencies, continuously changing in creative and unpredictable ways. Thus, to live is to flow in changing patterns as though one were a kaleidoscope—not looking into the tube of a kaleidoscope but being the pattern that changes colors and configurations.

Everything we see, everything we do is a manifestation of field patterning. As Rogers has indicated, we see and experience manifestations of patterning rather than the field pattern itself. For me, this translates into work with clients that often focuses on the metaphorical or figurative realm. When we deal with the person as physical manifestation or body, we need to remember that we are not dealing with the whole of that person but with what is manifest, or the "presenting portion of the field, whether it's human or environment" (Rogers, 1988, personal communication). Therefore, working in the imaginal realm—the world of image and imagination—through imagery and meditation is particularly useful, along with the health patterning modality of Therapeutic Touch, taught by Krieger and Kunz.

Knowing participation has long been a basic assumption in Rogerian science. People cannot start or stop change, which is continuous (Rogers, personal communication, 1988), but they can change the nature of their participation in change. Barrett (1986) identified this knowing participation in change as power and developed a tool to measure four manifestations of power: (1) awareness, (2) choices, (3) freedom to act intentionally, and (4) involvement in creating changes.

Another key to the health patterning process within the Rogerian framework comes from the world view represented by the Science of Unitary Human Beings. Rogers distinguishes between older and newer world-views, with older world-views characterized by a three-dimensional perspective focusing on cell theory and concepts such as matter, homeostasis, adaptation, and entropy. An example is the world-view represented in the physics of Isaac Newton, with the dominant metaphor of clock or machine. Both the human being and the universe are seen as machines composed of parts and possessing finite energy, inevitably running down from the moment the on-switch is pushed. In this view, find the defective part, repair or replace it, and the machine will continue to run. Illness is acontextual, an attack by an invading army. Thus, metaphors appropriate to nursing and medicine come from the language of war, reflecting mobilization of a defending army.

Newer world-views, including Rogers' science and the physics of David Bohm, are characterized by a pandimensional perspective focusing on field theory and concepts such as energy, homeodynamics, mutual process, and negentropy. The metaphor is the hologram, where an image of a person or object is enfolded in the frequency domain through an interference pattern recorded on a photographic plate. A beam of light, when shone through the plate, produces an image of the person or object in three-dimensional space of though actually there. Any part of the hologram can be used to access the whole. Therefore, the whole is in the part; the word "part" becomes meaningless. Bohm (1980), like Rogers, describes the world as one of undivided wholeness. Illness is not seen as external, something to be warded off for as long as possible or eradicated from the body, but as contextual, another manifestation of the mutual field patterning process. In this view, nurses help people participate knowingly in the patterning process, actualizing potentials most commensurate with well-being. Choice rests with the client. Metaphors capture the essence of flow, of movement and change.

## HEALTH PATTERNING APPRAISAL

I am still evolving the process of health patterning assessment or appraisal in my practice. I obtained permission to use Barrett's (1990) Power as Knowing Participation in Change Tool, a semantic differential tool that assesses the four manifestations of power mentioned earlier, and Paletta's (1990) Temporal Experience Scales, a metaphor scale that assesses the dimensions of time as dragging, racing, and timelessness. I follow the procedure described by Barrett (1990) in *Visions of Rogers' Science-Based Nursing,* looking at the descriptions obtained from clients of awareness, choices, freedom to act intentionally, and involvement in creating changes, and I assess where they feel comfortable, where they identify a desire for change. To my knowledge, use of Paletta's tool in practice has not been described in the literature. I use it with clients to identify the dominant theme in their current life patterns regarding time as a manifestation of field patterning, identified by Rogers (1990) as time experienced as slower, faster, or timelessness. We discuss the theme identified in terms of the client's life experiences, comfort with time experience, and any perceived desire for change.

Integral to the assessment process is a Therapeutic Touch field appraisal. Before we start, I talk a little about centering, which I believe is a way to help people awaken into awareness of integrality. We do an exercise together to facilitate this centered, pandimensional experience. I use breathing and the image of a tree, grounded in and sharing energy with Mother Earth, reaching up and sharing energy with Father Sky in an unbroken circle, the circle whose center is everywhere and whose circumference is nowhere. Following the field assessment, we talk briefly about the process and the client's experience of it, and I then complete the Therapeutic Touch. We talk more about the client's experience, often disclosing images, colors, or sensations experienced by one or both of us.

A common image for me is often evoked with clients as well: the image or feel of water. Water is my most common metaphor for movement and flow. Water can appear solid and bound, like an ice cube; flowing and bound, like a stream within its banks; flowing and unbound, like a river that has crested over its bank. Water can flow gently and calmly or so vigorously and energetically it breaks through log jams. The *Tao Te Ching* (Mitchell, 1988, p. 78) describes it this way:

> Nothing in the world
> is as soft and yielding as water.
> Yet for dissolving the hard and inflexible,
> nothing can surpass it.
>
> The soft overcomes the hard;
> the gentle overcomes the rigid.
> Everyone knows this is true,
> but few can put it into practice.

Another passage in the *Tao*, beginning "The supreme good is like water" (p. 8), is explained in a comment by Emilie Conrad-Da'oud:

> Water is the source of all life, life's matrix and fecundity; it overflows into everything, it moves everywhere. We are fundamentally water: muscled water. And the idea that we ever leave the amniotic fluid is a misconception. The amniotic fluid is the state of total nourishment and unconditional love. It is always

present for us and contains everything we could possibly want. In fact, we *are* that fluid of love. (Mitchell, 1988, pp. 88–89)

Water also represents clarity, the medium we use to wash away dirt, enabling us to clean and to see clearly. Flowing water carries things away once we choose to let them go. When we center, things can move through us rather than attach to us, making it harder for us to get hooked by things like pain, stress, or hassles of daily living. What is flowing is changing, not static. Again, from the *Tao:*

> If you realize that all things change,
> there is nothing you will try to hold on to.
> If you aren't afraid of dying,
> there is nothing you can't achieve.
>
> Trying to control the future
> is like trying to take the master carpenter's place.
> When you handle the master carpenter's tools,
> chances are that you'll cut your hand.
> (Mitchell, 1988, p. 74)

Finally, there are general questions I ask to prompt clients to discuss what they are experiencing and what they hope we can accomplish together. I've tried various ways to obtain descriptions of Rogers' (1990) manifestations of field patterning. For example, one question I routinely ask concerns sleep–wake patterns, hoping to get at field diversity evolving as longer sleeping, longer waking, beyond waking. Pandimensional awareness does not cease when we fall asleep, and sleep is not a state of relative "unconsciousness"; often, we may be most pandimensionally aware when we are asleep. Dreams are important experiences; they transcend space and time, so I try to be sensitive to the words I use. Following something I learned from Oh Shinnah Fast Wolf, a Native American ceremonialist and teacher, I ask, "What do you see when you're awake?" and "What do you see when you're asleep?" Giving equal attention to waking and to experiences many people regard as nonwaking (and therefore beyond awareness) seems to help clients see their dreams in a different light. Often, they become more aware of the potential meaning of dreams.

If people have difficulty with the questions or with verbal descriptions of what they're experiencing, I use imagery as an alternative. Since movement and flow are such key concepts in Rogerian science, I think they can be used to help interpret patterning. One exercise is:

> Imagine yourself as a seed planted in the earth, beginning to grow, moving up through the earth to the surface, and bursting through to the open air. Move as you would if you were this seed sprouting into a stem, growing leaves, and producing a flower.

Some people can show all of this through movement. Others find it helpful to draw an artistic representation of the experience or to describe it in terms of characteristics like size, color, scent. I think this may be one way to get at the manifestation of human field image, defined by Phillips (1990, p. 14) as "an evolving diverse manifestation of the human field pattern that synthesizes all past and projected future images" into a pandimensional picture of the unitary human.

## HEALTH PATTERNING PROCESS

As I was preparing this chapter, it became difficult to distinguish assessment or pattern manifestation appraisal and deliberative mutual patterning, the two phases of the Rogerian practice methodology of health patterning described by Barrett (1990). Pattern appraisal and deliberative mutual patterning flow together as knowing participation in change. Both are ongoing, and one informs the other. In this way, they are similar to the process of Therapeutic Touch, where assessment is an integral aspect of the entire process, not just something that occurs at a point identified as the beginning of the treatment. Understand that what I wrote about earlier is woven through the process of working with a client.

A client I'll call "Mary" was a 29-year-old data processor who saw herself as chronically overweight. She had enrolled in a variety of weight reduction programs since age 17, but had never been successful in maintaining any weight loss. Mary described herself as "big," "slow-moving," "ponderous," and "dense." On Barrett's tool, her awareness manifested as timid, unpleasant, and uninformed. Mary's attention was caught by the bipolar adjective pair of "expanding–shrinking." Physically, she saw herself as constantly expanding in body. Initially, the idea of an expanding awareness made no sense to her. Meditation came to mind as one way to help Mary experience an expanding awareness.

Mary agreed, a little hesitantly, to try it with me. After talking about the experience we shared, we came up with an exercise for her to try on her own. Mary had talked about friends who were the "life of the party" whenever they socialized, describing them as "light," "airy," and "free"—opposites of the way she had described herself. We talked about this, and Mary chose to meditate with a focus on the word *floating,* a word that really appealed to her. Initially, she had difficulty maintaining her focus, often finding herself thinking about food or feeling hungry. Mary was learning to be gentle with herself. Instead of acting on the intrusive thoughts or feelings or becoming angry with herself, she gently tried to set the thoughts aside and focus, using her breath. After a while, Mary found herself thinking of "yellow" instead of food. Going with "floating yellow," Mary experienced a sunburst of color, accompanied by what she later described as a "sunny, bright feeling" that seemed to flare and dissolve into drifting yellow bubbles. She felt buoyed up by these bubbles; she experienced a new, "dreamy, weightless type of floating." For the first time, Mary experienced an awareness of new choices opening to her, along with a new sense of herself as flowing motion. On her own, Mary enrolled in a yoga course and continued to meditate, finding a new relationship to food in the process. She periodically calls to let me know how she's doing and reports a slow but steady weight loss.

Frank, a 68-year-old retired businessman, requested Therapeutic Touch to help with a variety of somatic complaints, including headaches. Discussion revealed that he was having difficulty with retirement and found himself in frequent arguments with his wife of 45 years. Looking back, Frank expressed the fear that he had wasted a good portion of his life doing things he thought he should do but never really wanted to do. He didn't know how to change that life pattern and now felt unsure of himself, "adrift." In addition to Therapeutic Touch, we tried meditation. Following Frank's use of the word "adrift," I encouraged him to think of a flowing river and experience what it felt like to be carried along with its flow. He reported that "he wasn't getting there fast enough." Not surprisingly, he didn't know where "there" was or why he was in such a hurry. He agreed to try meditation on his own and to involve his wife. Since they lived in a wooded surburban area, the couple chose to sit outdoors in their gazebo and listen to the trees, flowing with the rhythm expressed by the swaying and sighing of the boughs. Gradually, both began to experience a drifting that they now identified as pleasurable, filling them with contentment. They actualized this feeling by taking long walks, then going on fishing trips together, and finally joining a local environmental protection group. Over time, they reported a qualitative shift in their relationship, and Frank let go of the somatic complaints.

Another client, whom I'll call "Joe," is 69 years old. A stroke left him with left-sided hemiplegia and some cognitive impairment. He's currently in a rehabilitation center, which is where I visit him. I didn't think either the power or time tools would be appropriate with him. We tried them, but he couldn't relate to either one. I taught him a simple relaxation exercise, which I then put on tape for him. In talking with him, I learned that he loved to fish, so together we worked on an imagery exercise using one of his favorite fishing holes. During Therapeutic Touch, I asked him to visualize an ice cube, to see that ice cube slowly melting, and to think of his affected left side as slowly unfreezing and becoming more fluid, regaining movement. The melting ice then becomes a gentle stream of water flowing through him, down to his feet, passing through his feet to the earth. Because Joe had difficulty with imagery exercises, saying he really couldn't "see the picture" for very long, I used with him a set of three pictures that I pulled from old Sierra Club calendars I had kept. The first depicted a snowbound scene with a river choked with ice. The second showed a lake at sunset, where the ripples and the play of light on the surface suggested gentle motion. The third showed a waterfall cascading down a mountain into a foamy river winding its way through large rocks. I asked Joe to think of himself as water (how he would move and flow) and then to select the picture that he related to the most. As his physical therapy progressed to the point where he could walk using a leg brace, a cane, and parallel bars, his choice moved from the first scene (snowbound) to the second (ripples of motion on the lake). On days when he felt particularly tired after therapy, he tended to choose the snowbound scene.

Therapeutic Touch has been the most useful health patterning modality for Joe. He relaxes fully during the experience and relates that it's the only time he feels he really can relax. In fact, he gets so relaxed that a nurse who happened to enter the room and saw him fully relaxed let out a yell that made us both jump. She thought he had passed out or worse. We've tried other exercises together, but he doesn't seem to find any of them very useful. He rarely listens to the relaxation tape or uses imagery on his own. He does, however, look forward to Therapeutic Touch. Joe enjoys looking at the pictures

I described, but he uses them differently from the way I had originally envisioned. The scenes help him to reminiscence (another kind of flow) and he likes to talk about events and activities from earlier phases of his life, when he traveled around the country.

While using the pictures with Joe, it occurred to me that it might be useful to begin compiling pictures that could be used like a deck of cards, perhaps using the Q-sort technique, to help clients identify current and evolving field images. One client, when I asked her to sort through a set of pictures I had compiled in an attempt to represent the manifestations of change identified by Rogers (1990), including diversity, motion, rhythm, and time experience, brought some of her own selections with her the next time. Her pictures included a photo of a weed-choked, garbage-strewn, inner-city lot, ringed by tenements, and another of a busy city street with vehicles and pedestrians moving along at what appeared to be a rapid pace. For her, they symbolized different aspects of both motion and time experiences. The few clients with whom I've used the pictures relate to the idea enthusiastically, so I may continue to develop my "flow cards," as I've been calling them.

## HEALING ENVIRONMENTS

What I've been describing is a small private practice that is an adjunct to my full-time faculty position. My own "beautiful dream," as Oh Shinnah calls our hopes and aspirations, is to create a nursing center for health patterning that is also a healing environment. Rogerian science defines the environmental field or the environment and describes it as integral with the human field or human being. Thus, "health and healing for humankind are health and healing for the environment" (Malinski, 1991, p. 60). Tending the flow of patterning of the environmental field is equally as important as tending that of the human field.

The images I've discussed and to which I find myself drawn usually encompass nature. Patterning of the environment is manifested through wave phenomena such as light, color, and sound. Nurses have long recognized their importance. More than a century ago, Nightingale (1860/1969) described nursing as "the proper use of fresh air, light, warmth" (p. 8) and so on, and enumerated the elements necessary for a healthy house: pure air, pure water, drainage, cleanliness, and light (p. 24). She wrote, "A dark house is always an unhealthy home. . . ." (p. 28). She identified the importance of color, noting that color "affects" the body as well as the mind, and that the body "affects" the mind as much as the mind "affects" the body (pp. 59–60). When hospitalized, patients should be placed near windows so they can see the sky and have sunlight. Without sunlight, she believed, mind and body degenerate (p. 87). "The sun is not only a painter but a sculptor," she wrote (p. 85). Light, color, sound, and boundaries constructed to allow a flow between indoor and outdoor spaces would be important in the design of the health patterning center.

The principles of building I would follow come from the Center for Environmental Structure in Berkeley, California, and are described in *A Pattern Language* by Alexander and his colleagues (1977). They define a pattern as a commonly recurring problem with the way we structure our environment. They then describe ways to solve the problem. For example, one pattern is "connection to the earth." The problems identified are typical ways of building, say a house, that result in an abrupt separation of inside and outside (Alexander et al., 1977, p. 786). Suggestions to solve the problem focus on ways to make the boundary ambiguous, such as using spaces that open to the outside yet are clearly inside the house. Why is this an important pattern? These architects believe that "our lives become satisfactory to the extent that we are rooted, 'down to earth,' . . . it may just be true that it is helped or hindered by the extent to which our physical world is itself rooted and connected to the earth" (Alexander et al., 1977, p. 787). Light, color, communal spaces, "trees places," cooperative play areas, and sleeping spaces are a few of the other patterns addressed. Their philosophy of building is congruent with Rogerian science. It is based in the belief that

> . . . no pattern is an isolated entity. Each pattern can exist in the world, only to the extent that it is supported by other patterns. . . . This is a fundamental view of the world. It says that when you build a thing you cannot merely build that thing in isolation, but must also repair the world around it, and within it, so that the larger world at that one place becomes more coherent, and more whole; and the thing which you make takes its place in the web of nature, as you make it (Alexander et al., 1977, p. xiii)

I believe that integrating such ideas as those expressed by the staff at the Center for Environmental Structure can help facilitate a unitive awareness of the integrality of the person–environment process. In this way, health and healing for the person would be health and healing for the environment.

Briefly, the health patterning center would be designed to be as open to the light and as fluid as possible, with movable wall panels and alcoves with window seats. Full-spectrum light sources, approximating the wavelength spectrum of sunlight, would be used to provide artificial light when necessary. One room would open into an outdoor meditation area where people could relax while listening to the sound of flowing water.

Although limited to what I can do with my home office, I was very conscious of the way I structured the space. Predominant colors are blue-green (because this color suggests cool water to me) and white. Clients have verbalized that the room feels comfortable and peaceful. It opens onto the back porch, which I keep filled with plants. They often serve as a nesting place for bird families, so, during warm weather, there's usually the music of bird songs.

## VIRTUALLY REALITY

Looking toward the future, we may soon be using another potential health patterning technique: virtual reality (Rheingold, 1991). "Star Trek: The Next Generation" fans will be familiar with virtual reality through the Holodeck on the *USS Enterprise*, where computer-generated images allow the crew to transcend time and space and immerse themselves in any environment or world they choose. The word "virtual" means something that appears to be; it exists to all intents and purposes but is not actually there. "Virtuality" refers to the essence or potentiality of something. A hologram, therefore, is a virtual image that appears to exist in three-dimensional space but in actuality has no extension in time or space. Because the holographic image does not occupy space, one can pass through it.

Similarly, virtual time is the time of rhythm and frequency, of pattern rather than of the clock. In his book, *Drumming at the Edge of Magic: A Journey into the Spirit of Percussion,* Mickey Hart (1990), drummer for the Grateful Dead, wrote of his belief that music carries us to the world of virtual time, where all is in synchrony. "Rhythm is just time, and time can be carved up any way you want" (p. 143).

Virtual images and virtual time seem to reside in the frequency domain of pandimensionality. Computers will provide us with a way to access virtual reality until such time as our accelerating change propels us to where they are no longer needed. Virtual reality offers ways to see and experience the world differently. The observer effect in quantum physics has shown that reality is a participatory process. Change the way we see reality, and reality changes. Research on imagery has shown that the brain does not distinguish between image and reality; the body performs as though the image were the reality. Consider the potential implications if, instead of the usual imagery exercise, the client and computer worked together to generate a virtual reality hologram of the image. Instead of imagining yourself on the beach, you are immersed in the experience of the beach, complete with the sound and smell of the water, the feel of the sun and the hot, grainy sand. For someone who, for whatever reason, cannot make the trip to the beach, the computer can transport them. Someone who needs to experience nature—a stream in the woods, for example—but cannot leave the city because of job and family pressures, can take a quick, refreshing break. Clients at an urban health patterning center can meditate by a waterfall. Virtual reality flow cards can be carried to clients' homes. At the moment, the cost and cumbersome equipment needed to take a virtual reality journey preclude uses such as I've described, but they are on our horizon. There are endless possibilities for virtual reality to facilitate experiences of pandimensionality and integrality.

## CONCLUSION

The practice of health patterning is integral with the flowing unity that is the human–environmental field process. Rogerian science helps us look at our world in a new way, a way consistent with emerging world-views in other disciplines. The idea that the fundamental unit of life is the field, and everything else, including the physical body, is a manifestation of field, resonates with Bohm's view of the implicate and explicate orders. Rogers has identified motion and pattern as inherent in the field. Bohm (1980) described field motion as a flowing process of enfolding and unfolding, "Undivided Wholeness in Flowing Movement" (p. 11). If all is motion, everything is continuously changing; nothing is static. Therapeutic Touch, imagery, and meditation are health patterning modalities that can help clients achieve this awareness and participate in a sense of themselves as flowing motion.

## REFERENCES

Alexander, C., Ishikawa, S., Silverstein, M., Jacobson, M., Fiksdahl-King, I., & Angel, S. (1977). *A pattern language.* New York: Oxford University Press.

Barrett, E.A.M. (1986). Investigation of the principle of helicy: The relationship of human field motion and power. In V.M. Malinski (Ed.), *Explorations on Martha Rogers' Science of Unitary Human Beings* (pp. 173–184). Norwalk, CT: Appleton-Century-Crofts.

Barrett, E.A.M. (1990). Health patterning with clients in a private practice environment. In E.A.M. Barrett (Ed.), *Visions of Rogers' science-based nursing* (pp. 105–115). New York: National League for Nursing.

Bohm, D. (1980). *Wholeness and the implicate order.* Boston: Routledge & Kegan Paul.

Hart, M. (1990). *Drumming at the edge of magic: A journey into the spirit of percussion.* San Francisco: Harper.

Malinski, V.M. (1991). Spirituality as integrality: A Rogerian perspective on the path of healing. *Journal of Holistic Nursing, 9*(1) 54–64.

Mitchell, S. (Transl.) (1988). *Tao te ching.* New York: Harper & Row.

Nightingale, F. (1969). *Notes on nursing: What it is and what it is not.* New York: Dover Publications, Inc. (Original work published in 1860).

Paletta, J.L. (1990). The relationship of temporal experience to human time. In E.A.M. Barrett (Ed.), *Visions of Rogers' science-based nursing* (pp. 239–253). New York: National League for Nursing.

Phillips, J.R. (1990). Changing human potentials and future visions of nursing: A human field image perspective. In E.A.M. Barrett (Ed.), *Visions of Rogers' science-based nursing* (pp. 13–25). New York: National League for Nursing.

Rheingold, H. (1991). *Virtual reality.* New York: Summit Books.

Rogers, M.E. (1990). Nursing: Science of Unitary, Irreducible Human Beings: Update 1990. In E.A.M. Barrett (Ed.), *Visions of Rogers' science-based nursing* (pp. 5–11). New York: National League for Nursing.

Rogers, M.E. (1992). Nursing science: a Science of Unitary Human Beings. *Rogerian Nursing Science News, IV*(3), 7.

# 7

# Healing Groups:
# Awareness of a Group Field

*Sherron Sargent*

Rogers' Science of Unitary Human Beings is theoretically comprehensive and can be applied in a variety of settings (Barrett, 1990; Malinski, 1986; Rogers, 1970, 1990). Rogers' science provided the theoretical basis for the creation and implementation of healing modalities for four groups of people who were living with an AIDS diagnosis or who were HIV positive. These groups were established within a private nonprofit organization in a large metropolitan city.

## SCIENCE OF UNITARY HUMAN BEINGS

According to Rogers (1990), "groups are defined as two or more individuals" (p. 8). Any type of group can be identified as a group energy field with its own unique environmental field. The basic assumptions that apply to the human field also apply to the group field. Therefore, the group field is viewed as a single irreducible field that is open and without boundaries. The reality for this group field is pandimensional, and the field is identified by the manifestation of its pattern. The principles of homeodynamics known as resonancy, helicy, and integrality postulate the nature of change related to the group field (Rogers, 1970, 1986, 1990).

## THE HEALING GROUPS

Initially, two groups were started at two different sites within an organization that provided a wide range of services for people with

AIDS or those who were HIV positive. After four months, two additional groups were offered at two additional sites. Nurses, acting as consultants, were available at various sites to answer questions regarding individuals' health potential. The individuals using these services were concerned about various issues—symptoms, side effects of medication, relationships with significant others, and options regarding treatment. They were also interested in exploring complementary therapies.

The healing groups were developed to offer support for individuals living with AIDS and were open to anyone who wanted to attend. There were no restrictions on the number attending. The groups met on a weekly basis, and the number of participants in the groups ranged from three to twenty.

When applying Rogers' science to a group of individuals, the field can be identified as one group field rather than several individual human fields, each with its own unique environmental field. At first, the healing groups that will be discussed here were viewed by the nurse facilitator as individual human fields within a group setting. Through the continuous mutual process of the human and environmental fields, the nurse facilitator became aware of the group field with its unique environmental field and shifted her perception from individual human fields to one group field.

When the nurse facilitator began forming these groups, Rogers' science provided the conceptual basis for implementing various nursing modalities. The nurse was aware that the group members were in continuous mutual process with the environment, which included the nurse. Together, activities for the group were jointly planned by the group and the nurse.

For the first few weeks, the majority of meeting time was spent in a discussion of group members' symptoms, side effects of medication, and treatment programs. Each week, a guided imagery experience was used to help promote relaxation. Over the weeks, the group began spending more time participating in experiential exercises and less time in group discussion. The activities of the group became more diverse, more creative, and more complex. Activities included relaxation exercises, guided imagery, Therapeutic Touch, meditation, music, and the sharing of written material.

It was difficult to describe the group experience to someone who had not participated in the group. When group members invited other individuals to join the group, they would say, "Just come and try it; come and see what it is like; you will find it helpful."

## PATTERN MANIFESTATION APPRAISAL

According to Barrett (1988), "the major phases of the Rogerian practice methodology are pattern manifestation appraisal and deliberative mutual patterning" (p. 50). Pattern manifestation appraisal is "the continuous process of identifying manifestations of the human and environmental fields that relate to current health events" (Barrett, 1988, p. 50).

While participating in the experiential exercises, the nurse facilitator became less aware of the pattern manifestations of individuals in the group and increasingly aware of the pattern manifestations of the group field. Many of the manifestations of the group field were experienced intuitively, since the nurse had her eyes closed during the exercises and was not visually observing the group. One of the manifestations of the group field pattern was observed by hearing the rhythm of breathing. The breathing was labored and sometimes noisy; often, coughing or the clearing of a throat could be heard. As the group participated in the guided imagery experience, the pattern of the group breathing changed and the rhythm of breathing became slower and deeper.

As the nurse facilitator guided the group through the process of imagery, she noted that the manifestations of her field pattern paralleled the pattern manifestations of the group field. Her voice became hoarse, she felt a tightness in her chest, and she would feel the need to cough. Similarly, the pattern of the group field was tense and tight, and coughing could be heard. Newman (1986) suggested that pattern recognition involves "getting in touch with our own pattern and through it in touch with the pattern of the person or persons with whom we are interacting" (p. 72). Reeder (1986) noted that "a science of humans in the world requires a theory of knowledge (epistemology) in which the knower and the known are integral . . . " (p. 61). The group and environmental fields are integral and do not exist in isolation. Through the mutual process of integrality, the nurse facilitator had an awareness of her own field and an increased awareness of the pattern manifested by the group field.

As she became aware of manifestations of the group field, the manifestations of the individual fields became insignificant; the group field breathed as one. The breathing pattern of the group field signified the integral nature of this group field, and the group breathing signified the irreducible wholeness of the field.

The group was aware that death was imminent. There was a sense of peace in coming to terms with the issue of mortality. The pandimensional view of reality for the group field may have facilitated this peace. Pandimensionality describes a nonlinear domain without temporal and spatial attributes (Rogers, 1992, p. 29). When one accepts the pandimensional view for the group field, death no longer is viewed as an ending. Death is merely the notion of existing in a different way.

Through various exercises, the group became aware that the group field was infinite and without boundaries. The manifestations of the field patterning moved from verbal communication to less verbal and more nonverbal communication, and then went beyond conventional communication. An example of this was when the nurse facilitator was scheduled to be out of town and the group arranged to meet without her. She explained that she would think about the group and send thoughts to them during the time when they were meeting. The group met and practiced what they had learned as a group. Intuitively, the group was able to sense that even though miles separated them, the nurse facilitator was present with them. The group field was characterized by a nonlinear domain without spatial and temporal attributes. The group field was infinite, coextensive with the universe, and not merely situated in a physical place at a given time. The nurse was able to send rhythms in the form of thoughts and colors and sense rhythmicities from the group while she was in a distant location. Also, anyone who had experienced the group field in the past could become aware of that experience in the relative present whenever he or she chose.

## DELIBERATIVE MUTUAL PATTERNING

Deliberative mutual patterning is defined as the "continuous process whereby the nurse with the client patterns the environmental field to promote harmony related to the health events" (Barrett, 1990, p. 36). Pattern-based practice rests on a foundation of knowing participation (Barrett, 1988, 1990).

The individuals who were members of the healing groups needed information that would enable them to participate knowingly in the process of facilitating their healing potential. Initially, the main focus was on finding various ways to promote relaxation, relieve pain, and conserve energy. The nurse facilitator continuously encouraged individuals who attended the groups to explore ideas for the group format. She set forth no preconceived notions, no expectations, and no specific goals for the groups. Throughout this experience, the group format remained flexible, and activities were not predetermined by the nurse facilitator.

Each week, the group began with a discussion of concerns volunteered by members of the group. During this time, the focus was on the collection of individual human fields within a group setting. As the group continued to meet over the next several weeks, the time used for discussion was shortened, and more time was used for experiential exercises. There was a heightened awareness of group field pattern manifestations.

On a weekly basis, the nurse facilitator used a guided imagery experience to enhance relaxation and promote power enhancement (Barrett, 1990). Through the use of guided imagery, the group was able to participate knowingly in the process of actualizing potentials for well-being (Barrett, 1990). Initially, the guided imagery experience began with an emphasis on relaxation of the field. The group engaged in slow deep-breathing exercises. The guided imagery also included directing the individuals in the group to visualize a place in nature where they had previously felt calm and peaceful. Being able to feel as one with nature or to feel integral with nature helps one to understand that human beings do not end at their skin but are coextensive with their environment, and that both fields extend to infinity. The group members were instructed to imagine that they were in this special place and were encouraged to pay attention to the sights, smells, sounds, and feelings associated with it.

Explaining Rogers' ideas to the group helped them to understand their unique wholeness. For example, the physical body could be seated in a chair, in a room, in a building, in a city, while the human field was also manifested somewhere in nature. The manifestations of the group field pattern became more imaginative and more diverse, changing from an awareness of time speeding up or slowing down to an awareness of time standing still or being nonexistent. These examples demonstrate the way in which guided imagery became more complex, more diverse, and more creative as it was used with the group field.

As the group worked more with the guided imagery experience, the individuals in the group would close their eyes and independently go to the place in nature where they felt peaceful and calm. Some said that they had stopped listening to the guided imagery and had stayed behind or gone off on their own. Others said they didn't even hear the nurse facilitator verbally guiding them. The nurse facilitator became aware that the individuals did not need to be guided and had learned to do their own imagery. They had enhanced their power by participating knowingly in change and had actualized their potential for health and well-being. They were now able to use this modality regardless of whether their physical body was present in the group. The nurse facilitator was also able to be aware of her own changing rhythms and those of the group. She was comfortable with the group's independently flowing in its own unique pattern; she became more silent and did less guiding.

As the nurse participated in the continuous mutual process through the modality of guided imagery, she recognized that the group was one. There was no focus on individuals, their roles in the group, or group dynamics. Verbal communication was either absent or minimal.

In one group session, a candle was used as a meditation experience. Everyone sat in the dark and used the candle flame as a focal point. The rhythm of the group field began to resonate with the flame of the candle as the flame flickered and danced in consonance with the currents of air. There was silence throughout the room, and the rhythm of communication was nonverbal, beyond conventional communication.

During another group experience, at the end of the guided imagery experience, a man sang a song he had composed. He asked that the group remain silent and not look at him while he sang. He asked that they either close their eyes or keep their heads down. The group resonated with the vibration of musical sounds, and there was a general feeling of peace and calm during and after the singing. The group was quiet after his song. No one spoke as people gradually began to leave the room.

One night, during a silent meditation, a woman asked if the individuals in the group could hold each other's hands. The members joined hands, closed their eyes, and sat quietly. During this time, the nurse facilitator became aware that one of her arms was being lifted. She felt like her arm was floating weightlessly in the air. Curious as to what was happening, she opened her eyes and saw the resemblance of a wave as members' arms were slowly being raised around the group. Everyone's arms moved as one and everyone had his or her eyes closed. There was, it seemed, a feeling of oneness, or, in Rogerian terms, an awareness of integrality. The group field moved as one. The focus was not on physical bodies but on a feeling of flow without constraints of time and space. The peace and calm experienced in the room extended outside into the dining room and beyond the location of the group meeting. The group and environmental field were integral and in continuous mutual process. The pattern manifestations of the environmental field, peacefulness and calmness, were similar to the pattern of the group field.

Therapeutic Touch, as defined by Krieger (1979, 1987), was taught in the groups by the nurse facilitator. She demonstrated the modality and explained that Krieger (1979, 1987) believes the potential to do Therapeutic Touch is innate. Anyone can learn to use this modality. Krieger (1979) suggested various exercises that help individuals learn to assess an energy field and differentiate various vibrations felt in the field. According to Krieger (1979), these exercises can provide a base for recognizing that the energy field extends beyond the skin boundaries. Understanding the concepts underlying Therapeutic Touch gave the group an opportunity to learn about energy fields, openness, and pattern. When using Therapeutic Touch as a healing modality, the pattern of communication is nonverbal and beyond conventional communication.

Another example of heightened awareness of the group field occurred when one group participated in healing at a distance. The nurse facilitator had a friend whose child was having surgery. She lived 450 miles away from where the group was meeting. The group, using their hands in sweeping motions, collected energy flowing through and around them and formed an "energy ball." As they made this "energy ball," the group was thinking about peace, love, and healing. When everyone was ready, the energy was directed by thought in the direction of the city where the child was hospitalized. There were no boundaries, no time or space constraints; thoughts of peace, love, and healing were sent as a whole. According to Krieger (1987), energy follows intent, and it was the group's intent to help this child heal. Rogers' concept of pandimensionality provides a view of reality in which healing thoughts can be sent from one location to another. A month later, the nurse facilitator was talking to the child's mother and discovered that the child had developed serious complications following surgery. The doctors were not sure whether the child would live. Two hours after the onset of the complications, the child's condition had a remarkable turn and showed improvement. This improvement occurred at approximately the time when the group had sent their thoughts across the miles to this child. This may have been coincidental, but research is needed to investigate such anecdotal events.

Krieger (1987) has participated in experiments in healing at a distance when the healer and healee are removed from each other geographically. She devised her own research design and used vivid visualizations to validate healing at a distance. Her findings suggest that transfer of nonmaterial objects, such as thought, needs to be explained by a view of the physical world that is different from Newtonian mechanics. This is congruent with Rogers' (1986, 1990, 1992) ideas that unitary human beings are irreducible wholes that cannot be known by studying their parts. Unitary human beings are viewed from a pandimensional perspective rather than being locked into a causal world with spatial and temporal attributes.

Another example of the awareness of group field occurred after the nurse facilitator became ill and returned to her home 450 miles away. The group continued to participate in guided imagery experiences facilitated by other nurses. Although separated by space, one member reported having visited the home of the nurse who was ill. He reported that she was sitting on her couch in the living room, watching television, and that she looked well. The group field knows no boundaries; it has no time and space constraints. When the group and environmental fields are placed within a pandimensional view, the past, present, and future are experienced in the infinite now (Malinski, 1986; Reeder, 1986). Since the energy fields are integral, communication can take place in the form of thoughts, images, memories, and dreams.

## PATTERN PROFILE FOR THE HEALING GROUPS

The human field, whether defined as a single individual or a group of individuals, is "a nonspatial, nontemporal, infinite energy field that you perceive according to patterning" (Rogers, 1986, p. 14). The idea of a group field in continuous mutual process with an environmental field is important, however, and more scientific exploration of this phenomenon is needed.

The pattern profile for the group field does not incorporate the reductionist view of scientific inquiry where the observer and the observed are separate entities. Rather, the pattern profile for the group field requires viewing the group as a whole, without reducing the group to its individual members. It also requires perceiving the group field without the constraints of time and space. An awareness of a group field, coextensive with the universe, is in continuous mutual process with the environmental field. The group field does not exist in a room or in a community. It exists without boundaries and extends to infinity. Nursing modalities that include imagery, meditation, Therapeutic Touch, and wave forms of color and music help to transcend a three-dimensional view of a group made up of a collection of individuals. The group field is unique to itself. A pandimensional view of the group field acknowledges that it has the ability to manifest itself in multiple ways. The continuous mutual process of the group and environmental fields provides the potential for healing to occur.

After using the nursing modalities in the experiential exercises, the individuals in the group were more aware of the integrality of the human and environmental fields. They made comments like "I feel strengthened by the group experience." The word *love* was often used to express a harmonious rhythm. Many of the individuals returned to the "healing group," week after week, and encouraged others to attend.

## A POEM

During the time when the nurse was away from these groups and recuperating from illness, she thought about her experience with the healing groups. She became aware of her own healing and the continuous mutual process of the group and environmental fields. An expression of this experience follows:

### Our Healing Group

We have come together as unique individuals each with
  our own strengths and weaknesses to bear.
Sharing, trusting, feeling, experiencing new ways of
  being, new ways to care.
Feeling, hearing, seeing, believing something new, yet it
  was always there.
A glimpse of something unexplained in a poem, a song,
  a smile, a prayer.
This is wonderful, a quick fix, something to make it
  better,
I must get some whatever the cost.

It doesn't come to you that way, it is easy only for those
who have suffered, alone, and lost.

You taught me so much about myself and made me stop
and look at all that is mine.

I searched for a cause, for medicine, I didn't like feeling
like this, I wanted to be fine.

Wait, I reflected, this is a test; do you believe what you
taught—that healing is free?

The strength comes from a unity with others, the sky,
and sea, the earth, a tree.

When I can no longer see you in this form, smile at you,
or look into your face.

I will hear a tune, feel a breeze, know you are there and
rest awhile in this place.

While knowing in a intuitive way with a sense of peace
and without feeling fear,

that you have transcended time and space, as I know it,
to come for a visit and be near.

The miracles occur flowing on and on whether rich or
poor, young or old, healthy or ill.

Your willingness to share, your love, your faith, all that
we have known remains still.

Thank you for believing in me, in yourselves, and in our
ties to each other in love.

Thoughts of joy, hope, peace, and harmony carried
everywhere on the wings of a dove.

## REFERENCES

Barrett, E.A.M. (1988). Using the Science of Unitary Human Beings in nursing practice. *Nursing Science Quarterly, 1,* 50–51.

Barrett, E.A.M. (Ed.). (1990). *Visions of Rogers' science-based nursing.* New York: National League for Nursing.

Krieger, D. (1979). *The Therapeutic Touch: How to use your hands to help or heal.* Englewood Cliffs, NJ: Prentice-Hall.

Krieger, D. (1987). *Living the Therapeutic Touch: Healing as a life-style.* New York: Dodd, Mead.

Malinski, V.M. (1986). *Explorations on Martha Rogers' Science of Unitary Human Beings.* Norwalk, CT: Appleton-Century-Crofts.

Newman, M.A. (1986). *Health as expanding consciousness.* St. Louis: Mosby.

Reeder, F. (1986). Basic theoretical research in the conceptual system of unitary human beings. In V.M. Malinski (Ed.), *Explorations on Martha Rogers' Science of Unitary Human Beings* (pp. 45–64). Norwalk, CT: Appleton-Century-Crofts.

Rogers, M.E. (1970). *An introduction to the theoretical basis of nursing.* Philadelphia: Davis.

Rogers, M.E. (1986). Science of Unitary Human Beings. In V.M. Malinski (Ed.), *Explorations on Martha Rogers' Science of Unitary Human Beings* (pp. 3–8). Norwalk, CT: Appleton-Century-Crofts.

Rogers, M.E. (1990). Nursing: Science of Unitary, Irreducible, Human Beings: Update 1990. In E.A.M. Barrett (Ed.), *Visions of Rogers' science-based nursing* (pp. 5–11). New York: National League for Nursing.

Rogers, M.E. (1992). Nursing science and the Space Age. *Nursing Science Quarterly, 5,* 27–34.

# 8

# Pattern Diversity and Community Presence in the Human–Environmental Process: Implications for Rogerian-Based Practice with Nursing Home Residents

*Sarah Hall Gueldner*

Based within the Rogerian (1970) perspective, the purpose of this survey was to describe characteristic patterns within the person-environmental process of ambulatory, mentally alert nursing home residents, and to compare their patterns with individuals of similar age and state-of-health who live independently within the community setting. Clinical implications are derived from the findings, and recommendations are offered for increasing the diversity of options within the mutual human–environmental process of elders to live in nursing homes.

## RESEARCH BASIS FOR PRACTICE INNOVATIONS

Isolation from life's mainstream poses a major problem for persons living in nursing homes. Barney (1984, 1987), commenting on the public abandonment of our institutionalized elders, pointed out the need for "community presence" in nursing homes. Research findings

This research was funded by a grant from the Division of Nursing, Department of Health and Human Services (Ref. 1R23NU01147).

have shown that the frequency of visitation by relatives and friends drops off considerably for nursing home residents about six months after admission (Barry & Miller, 1980), and that a significant number of nursing home residents have no visitors from the outside (Barney, 1987). These findings are alarming because studies have indicated that nursing home residents who have more visitors enjoy a more positive nursing home experience and have fewer undesirable effects than those who have fewer or no visitors (Barney, 1984; Gottesman & Bourestom, 1974).

Over recent years, numerous authors have proposed ways to provide increased opportunities for nursing home residents to become more interactive with the outside world (Barney, 1984, 1987; Kosberg, 1973). Regardless of compelling efforts on the part of staff, gerontologists, and community volunteers, little or no involvement with the outside community remains a painful and devastating problem for many nursing home residents. This concern provided the impetus for this investigation.

The Rogerian Science of Unitary Human Beings (Rogers, 1970) views both social dialogue (verbal and nonverbal) and physical activity as integral features of the total human–environment process. It was postulated that the opportunity for diverse environmental experiences with other persons may be reduced for the institutionalized elderly.

The design of the study consisted of a matched-group comparison. The sample (N = 81) for the study consisted of 39 ambulatory, mentally alert nursing home residents and a matched group of 42 ambulatory, noninstitutionalized persons of comparable age and health status from two southeastern states. There were 64 (79 percent) females and 17 (21 percent) males, with a mean age of 77.4 years (age range: 61–94 years).

The nursing home residents were recruited from four nursing homes in nonurban communities, and the noninstitutionalized subjects were recruited from community senior citizen groups and elderly housing facilities within the same locale as the nursing homes. All subjects were ambulatory, and approximately the same number in each group used walkers or canes. Sixty percent of the nursing home residents had relatives living in the same town, as compared to 74 percent of the community dwellers who reported family members living in the same town. Almost all subjects (95 percent in both groups) had family living within 100 miles.

Pfeiffer's (1975) Short Portable Mental Status Questionnaire (SPMSQ) was used to screen for disabling mental impairment that might make it difficult or uncomfortable for an individual to respond. An adjusted score of four (4) or less was selected as the cut-off score for participation in this study. If the individual's adjusted SPMSQ was five or greater, the tester thanked the individual for his or her participation and excused the individual graciously without further interview.

Each subject was asked to respond to a short, simply worded, investigator-developed questionnaire that provided demographic information and data related to activity patterns associated with daily living, including: (1) going outside, (2) walking, (3) visiting, (4) receiving mail, (5) using the telephone, and (6) having contact with others outside the nursing home or in the community. Content validity for the questionnaire was established through expert review, and items were piloted with comparable subjects to ensure clarity and accuracy of inquiry. Each subject responded to the questionnaire in a one-to-one setting, with a member of the research team reading each item aloud in an unhurried manner.

Patterns within the human–environmental field process were assessed by asking the residents to indicate: (1) how often they attended group activities (almost every day, one to two times each week, or not very often); (2) how often they went outside (every day, about once every week, not every week, or almost never; and (3) what they usually did when they went outside (walk, sit on porch, ride in a car, other). They were also asked how often they saw their family and how often they received mail (once a week, more often than once a week, less often than once a week, seldom or never). Chi-square analyses were performed to determine the presence of significant between-group differences for each of the pattern manifestations examined. Alpha of .05 was established as the acceptable level of significance.

## RESEARCH FINDINGS

Subjects in the community dwelling group had considerably more years of formal education than the nursing home residents. All of the subjects in the independently dwelling group had been to school for at least one year, whereas four (11 percent) of the nursing home residents had either no formal education or less than one year of schooling. Likewise, almost two-thirds (62 percent) of the individuals living independently in the community had completed high school, whereas only about one-third (36 percent) of the nursing home residents had completed high school. Twice as many community dwellers had attended college, compared to their counterparts who lived in the nursing homes. These findings suggest that education level may indicate whether an elder will enter a nursing home or continue to live a more independent life-style within the community (Gueldner, Clayton, Schroeder, Butler, & Ray, 1992).

Several highly significant between-group differences were identified in patterns within the human–environmental field process. The most notable differences centered around the extent of everyday contact that each group had with the world outside of the building in which they lived. Almost all (90 percent) of the community dwellers had been outside of their houses on either the day of testing or the day before, while fewer than a third (31 percent) of the nursing home residents had been outside of the building during that same time period. The community dwellers were almost twice as likely as the nursing home residents to ride in a car and do errands when they did go outside (Gueldner et al., 1992).

## VISITING PATTERNS

The nursing home residents in the study saw their families less often and had significantly fewer visitors in general than the community dwelling cohort. Three-fourths (76 percent) of the community dwellers, as compared to a little more than one-half (54 percent) of the nursing home residents, said they saw a member of their family weekly. However, almost half (46 percent) of the nursing home residents, compared to one-fourth (24 percent) of the community dwellers, said they saw family members only monthly or less often (Gueldner et al., 1992).

## INDIRECT CONTACT WITH OUTSIDE WORLD

Major differences were also demonstrated in terms of indirect contact with persons who lived outside of their building or residence. For instance, almost all community dwellers (93 percent) said they had used the telephone "today or yesterday"; among the nursing home residents, (36 percent) had used the telephone recently. Follow-up study revealed that none of the nursing home residents in this sample had telephones in their rooms, whereas all of the community dwellers had telephones in their homes. A similar pattern emerged concerning receipt of mail. Almost all (95 percent) community dwellers had received mail "yesterday or today," while fewer than one-half (41 percent) of the nursing home residents had received mail within the past two days (Gueldner et al., 1992).

## PAST ACTIVITY PATTERNS

Past activity patterns were surprisingly similar for the two groups. More than 80 percent of both groups said they had walked a great deal in the past, and more than half of the subjects in both groups at one time had walked to work. Falls are listed as a major reason for admission to nursing homes, so it was surprising to learn that, compared to the nursing home residents (49 percent), more of the community dwellers (62 percent) had suffered serious injury from a fall at some time in their lives.

Gueldner and Spradley (1988), in an earlier study, found no difference between ambulatory nursing home residents and community-dwelling elders relative to weekly participation in available group activities. Fewer than half (40 percent) in each group reported that they attended group activities (such as church and craft classes) weekly.

## IMPLICATIONS FOR PRACTICE

Although simplistic and somewhat preliminary in nature, these findings document the need for continued diversity and community presence within the human–environmental field process of elders who live in nursing homes. Increasing the options available within the mutual human–environmental field process is a special need for those who have limited contact with friends and relatives. All nursing measures developed within the Rogerian conceptual system involve alterations within individuals' environment that promote (or at least allow) the fullest and most knowing participation in their unique mutual human–environmental process.

The remainder of this discussion will be directed toward the design of a nursing plan that will provide a broad menu of options and increased community presence within the nursing home environment.

## INCREASING THE PRESENCE OF HUMAN AND OTHER
## LIFE FORMS WITHIN THE ENVIRONMENTAL FIELD

When the human-environmental field lacks the personal intimacy that exists between family members or close friends, an individual's field pattern manifestations include loneliness or isolation. Individuals who live in nursing homes seem especially prone to believe that their environment lacks persons who are important to them. Following the Rogerian perspective, this feeling of loneliness or estrangement from the larger community may be overcome by altering personhood patterns within their environment.

For instance, it may be possible to add other beings—human and other life forms such as pets and plants—to the environment of a nursing home resident who feels isolated or lonely. In the Rogerian system, it is not always necessary to put the physical body of another being into the immediate environment in order to bring about the desired change. In these high-tech times, the sense of human presence may be facilitated through a variety of indirect imaging measures. For instance, an individual may be able to image a meaningful human presence by viewing audio or video tapes of family or friends. Placing familiar photographs or memorabilia in the environment, or playing favorite music, may suggest the presence of persons with whom the individual shared special moments in the past. Meaningful human presence may also be provided through books, newspapers, and television. Guided reminiscence offers another way to breach the feeling of loneliness and isolation by bringing meaningful memories of the past, including the persons in the memories, to the present experience. It is particularly important to facilitate pangenerational representation within the available environmental personhood for elders living in nursing homes, because their contact with children and youth tends to be noticeably limited.

There is considerable evidence that animals (Gammonley & Yates, 1991; Netting, Wilson, & New, 1987; Rosenkoetter & Bowes, 1991; Sarishinsky, 1992; Weisberg & Park, 1991) and plants (Langer & Rodin, 1976; Marino-Schorn, 1986; Riordan & Williams, 1988) can help to breach the feeling of isolation commonly reported among nursing home residents. Accordingly, an increasing number of nursing homes have made arrangements for animals of suitable temperament to visit the residents on a regular basis; some have even adopted one or more pets to live in the home permanently. One innovative

nursing home administrator, collaborating with the local humane society, volunteered the facility as an emergency animal shelter. Residents who were able cared for stray animals until new homes could
be found for the pets. Adding plants is another simple yet important
way to add diversity and community presence to the mutual human-
environmental process of nursing home residents. As with animals, it
is especially beneficial if the residents can assume some responsibility for the care of the plants (Langer & Rodin, 1976), such as watering
small plants in their rooms or helping to tend and harvest a small outdoor flower or vegetable garden.

## PROVIDING ACCESS TO THE ORDINARY TOOLS
## THAT SUPPORT INDEPENDENT LIVING

Nursing home residents should continue to have access to the everyday "tools" of daily living that are generally available within the
larger community. It was serendipitously discovered by this investigator during an early research effort that many (perhaps most) nursing home residents do not have pencils in their possession, and that
those who do have them may not have a way to keep them sharp.
There are implications to not having a pencil: one's knowing participation in the mutual process is greatly limited. An individual who
doesn't have a pencil is unable to: (1) sign his or her name, (2) endorse a check, (3) write a letter or note to another person, (4) make a
list of things he or she needs or would like to have or to do, (5) write
down a telephone number or an address, or (6) address an envelope.
This widespread societal oversight conveys to elders that they are no
longer expected to need a pencil. Nurses practicing within the Rogerian conceptual system would note and correct such limiting over-
sights in the environments of elderly individuals coming within their
care.

A summary of nursing actions that may increase diversity and
community presence within the environmental field of elders living
in nursing homes is offered in Table 8.1. The activities described are
not in themselves unique to nursing; anyone can do them. But nurses
practicing within the Rogerian system would give first priority to
these environmental concerns so that every person can participate
fully (knowingly, with maximum choice) in the mutual process that
we call life. Participation in change is maximized by providing a
larger menu of available choices.

## Table 8.1
## Strategies to Increase Continued Diversity and Sense of Community Presence in the Available Environmental Field of Nursing Home Residents

1. Encourage nursing home residents who are able (even if only barely able) to participate in excursions that involve:
   a. Dressing suitably.
   b. Exchanging money.
   c. Riding in motorized vehicles.
   d. Having day-to-day contact with the rest of society.
2. Assist ambulatory nursing home residents to access special community-based transportation services.
3. Mobilize nursing home staff and volunteers to facilitate two-way communications, through mail, between the residents and their family and friends:
   a. Encourage family members to write.
   b. Encourage and assist older adults to write and send cards and small packages.
   c. Help elders prepare or update an easy-to-read address book.
   d. Make supplies for mail communication (pens, stamps, cards, stationery) readily available.
4. Facilitate increased telephone communication between residents and their family and friends:
   a. Encourage them to use the telephone.
   b. Make telephones more accessible; encourage residents' families to have a telephone installed in their relatives' rooms, and install public telephones low enough for comfortable use by stooped or wheelchair-bound residents.
   c. See that public telephones are installed in areas that provide privacy and low levels of competing environmental noise.
   d. Be sure that residents know a number at which their family and friends can reach them.
   e. Help residents to develop a large-print, easy-to-read list of telephone numbers of their family and friends.
   f. Be sure that residents have quarters, if needed.
   g. Assist residents with dialing, if needed.
   h. Help residents obtain general devices needed to enhance their ability to use the telephone (such as large number dialing pads, volume magnifiers, and electronically programmed dialing).
5. Offer the following options within the human–environmental process:
   a. Animals.
   b. Plant care.
   c. Audio or video tape exchange with family and friends.
   d. Familiar photographs and other memorabilia.
   e. Choice of familiar music.
   f. A variety of reading materials.
   g. Guided reminiscence.
   h. "At hand" supplies commonly available within the larger community: paper, pencils, stick-on pads, transparent tape, paper clips, staplers, emery boards, magnifying glasses, and scissors.
6. Create an atmosphere within the facility that makes children feel special and welcome.

Adapted from "Environmental Interaction Patterns among Institutionalized and Non-institutionalized Older Adults," by S.H. Gueldner, G.M. Clayton, M.A. Schroeder, S. Butler, and J. Ray, 1992, *Physical and Occupational Therapy in Geriatrics, 11*(1), pp. 37–53.

## REFERENCES

Barney, J. (1984). Community presence is the key to quality care in nursing homes. *American Journal of Public Health, 64,* 265-268.

Barney, J. (1987). Community presence is the key to quality care in nursing homes. *Gerontologist, 27,* 367-369.

Barry, J., & Miller, D. (1980). The nursing home visitor: Who, when, where, and for how long? *Long Term Care and Health Services Administration Quarterly, 4,* 261-274.

Gammonley, J., & Yates, J. (1991). Pet projects: Animal-assisted therapy in nursing homes. *Journal of Gerontology Nursing, 17*(1), 12-15.

Gottesman, L., & Bourestom, N. (1974). Why nursing homes do what they do. *Gerontologist, 14*(6), 501-506.

Gueldner, S.H., Clayton, G.M., Schroeder, M.A., Butler, S., & Ray, J. (1992). Environmental interaction patterns among institutionalized older adults. *Physical and Occupational Therapy in Geriatrics, 11*(1), 37-53.

Gueldner, S.H., & Spradley, J. (1988). Outdoor walking lowers fatigue. *Journal of Gerontological Nursing, 14*(10), 2-12.

Kosberg, J. (1973). Differences in proprietary institutions caring for affluent and non-affluent elderly. *Gerontologist, 13,* 299-304.

Langer, E., & Rodin, J. (1976). The effects of choice and enhanced personal responsibility for the aged: A field experiment in an institutional setting. *Journal of Personality and Social Psychology, 34*(2), 191-198.

Marino-Schorn, J. (1986). Morale, work and leisure in retirement. *Physical and Occupational Therapy in Geriatrics, 4*(2), 49-59.

Netting, F., Wilson, C., & New, J. (1987). The human–animal bond: Implications for practice. *Social Work, 32,* 60-64.

Pfieffer, E. (1975). A short, portable mental status questionnaire for the assessment of organic brain deficit in elderly patients. *Journal of the American Geriatric Society, 23,* 433-441.

Riordan, R., & Williams, C. (1988). Gardening therapeutics for the elderly. *Activities, Adaptation and Aging, 12*(1), 103-111.

Rogers, M. (1970). *Introduction to the theoretical basis of nursing.* Philadelphia: Davis.

Rosenkoetter, M., & Bowes, D. (1991). Brutus is making rounds. *Geriatric Nurse, 12,* 227-278.

Sarishinsky, J.S. (1992). Intimacy, domesticity and pet therapy with the elderly: Expectation and experience among nursing home volunteers. *Social Science Medicine, 34,* 1324–1334.

Weisberg, J., & Park, M. (1991). Hannah Katz: Resident tabby. *Geriatric Nurse, 12*(3), 117–118.

# 9

# Viewing Polio Survivors through Violet-Tinted Glasses

*Dorothy Woods Smith*

Dr. Martha Rogers (1970), who wrote, "the science of nursing is an emergent—a new product," predicts that, by the turn of the century, the majority of nurses will work outside of the hospital, promoting health in the community. Reflecting on her vision, I began to see my work with polio survivors as representative of an emerging model for nursing practice. By describing how Rogers' nursing model is manifested in my nursing practice, I hope to illustrate a few of the many new ways in which Rogers' Science of Unitary Human Beings has inspired me to view human beings, health, and the environment.

I started meeting polio survivors in 1984, the year in which I began to study Rogers' nursing model as a graduate student at New York University. As a polio survivor myself, I was frightened by reports that had begun to circulate that new symptoms, similar to those of the original illness, were appearing in people who had recovered from polio 30 or more years earlier. This phenomenon, now identified as post-polio syndrome (PPS), is characterized by new muscle weakness in previously affected and unaffected muscles, typically accompanied by pain and fatigue. Of the 650,000 survivors of paralytic polio who live in the United States (National Center for Health Statistics, 1987), it is estimated that at least 25 percent are presently experiencing PPS (Halstead, 1991).

My nursing practice is not limited to one place; it extends to wherever there are polio survivors. It is grounded in the shared experiences of polio survivors and their families. As I participate as learner and teacher, advocate and facilitator, and liaison between polio survivors and health professionals, we are involved in a continual, mutual process of change.

The process of creating a post-polio network began when I became the liaison between polio survivors in Maine and the International Polio Network. Following a series of news stories about the late effects of polio, over 100 polio survivors wrote or called to share their individual stories, many of which had remained untold for 25 or more years. All of them were deeply touching. The shared need for information and support inspired our coming together for a statewide polio survivors' conference (now an annual event). We started a newsletter to share information and ideas and established local support groups through which people could regularly meet. Information has been communicated to polio survivors, health professionals, and the general public by publishing articles in newspapers, newsletters, and journals; making appearances on radio and television; and giving presentations at meetings and conferences. Recently, our first statewide meeting was held using Maine's "electronic highway" to reach people in remote areas through interactive television. Membership in our statewide support group, now named the Post-Polio Support Group of Maine, has grown to over 700, and polio survivors from Maine and across the country regularly call and write seeking and contributing information, guidance, and support.

Rogers' Science for Unitary, Irreducible Human Beings changed the way in which I perceive people and reality. Since being introduced to Rogers' nursing model, I see through different, violet-tinted lenses that symbolize not only New York University, but higher-frequency wave patterns. Prior to studying Rogers' nursing model, I was comfortable describing polio survivors in terms of disease, dysfunction, and losses. When discussing post-polio syndrome, the terms *second disability* and *polio victims* seemed appropriate. *Compliance* and *coping* appeared to be acceptable nursing goals. Such terms represent static, unacceptable goals for any human being, and my ongoing nursing practice with polio survivors reflects concepts increasingly congruent with Rogers' vision. For example, my nursing practice encompasses the belief that a person can be healthy without having all neuromuscular connections intact. People do not return to a previous state; they move forward and develop new patterns. Promoting knowing participation in change and the actualization of valued potentials are dynamic nursing goals. Even the term *survivors* brings questions to mind. *Thrivers* may better represent the growth experiences that many report.

My previously perceived duality of polio survivor and nurse has been transformed into an awareness of myself as a pandimensional whole. The personal and professional aspects of my life are no longer separated, and a philosophy of integration has brought great richness to my work and to my life. Viewing clients and health professionals as being in mutual process with one another, rather than in one-way relationships defined by roles, has expanded my previous awareness of integrality.

Barrett's (1983) theory of power, derived within Rogers' model from the postulate that people are capable of knowing participation in change, guides me in viewing polio survivors as people who have participated in change, initially through rehabilitation and more recently by creating or joining post-polio support groups. I recognize that they have devised creative and diverse ways of accomplishing tasks and reaching goals in order to lead meaningful and productive lives. They have been able to attain high levels of education (Bell, 1984), maintain high levels of employment and community involvement (Raymond, 1986), and remain actively involved in their own health care (Holman, 1986). Through the Post-Polio Support Group of Maine, I work with other polio survivors in mutual process to encourage and support the tradition of actively participating in change. Barrett's (1990) concept of power comprises four dimensions: (1) awareness, (2) choices, (3) freedom to act intentionally, and (4) involvement in creating change. These four aspects of power are represented in my practice as polio survivors become aware of PPS and choose how to deal with it. They are supported as they actualize their choices, and they are encouraged to be involved in change, for example, in creating partnerships with the health professionals of their choice. The theme of power as knowing participation in change has been shared with polio survivors locally and nationally through post-polio conference presentations and publications.

Phillips' (1990) theory of human field image, derived within Rogers' nursing model, has expanded my nursing practice so that it is not confined to the physical realm, nor is it subject to the limits of viewing polio survivors as biopsychosocial beings. Human beings and their environments are viewed as pandimensional energy fields. Health, which is an expectation for all human fields, is not limited to physical aspects of being. As the words *health* and *healing, whole* and *holy* are understood to come from the same source (Quinn,

1989), transcendence of "disability" (Vash, 1981) becomes a realistic and healthy possibility. Polio survivors' stories of near-death experiences, answered prayers, visions of self as whole, and walking or even flying, are not viewed as denial or fantasy to escape reality, nor are they viewed as abnormal or paranormal. Nursing modalities that pattern human energy fields are helping some polio survivors by reducing pain and fatigue and promoting a sense of health and wholeness. These strategies include the practices of meditation, prayer, guided imagery, visualization, and Therapeutic Touch (Krieger, 1981), a nursing intervention that promotes healing of human fields through mutual process.

A nursing model provides a framework in which new ideas evolve and new questions are asked. Rogers (1970) wrote, "The all-too-common perception of [human beings] as predominantly subjected to multiple negative environmental influences with pathological outcomes denies [their] unity with nature and [their] evolutionary becoming" (p. 85). Through Rogers' negentropic model, I learned to look beyond the apparent physical losses to perceive patterns of growth related to the critical experience of polio. My recent national study, in which I examined power and spirituality in polio survivors compared with people who had not had polio or any other life-threatening illness (Smith, 1992), was inspired by viewing the personal stories of polio survivors from a Rogerian perspective.

Although Rogers has not specifically discussed spirituality, several themes central to a humanist conceptualization of that phenomenon synthesized by Elkins, Hedstrom, Hughes, Leaf, and Saunders (1988) are congruent with her model. These include the perception that human beings are continually evolving and seeking meaning. They are engaged in continual, mutual process with other living things, including a transcendent dimension or Being, and they have a commitment to actualizing valued potentials in the process of becoming. Findings, indicating that polio survivors manifest the same power and greater spirituality than people who have not had polio or any other life-threatening illness, have provided the basis for ongoing explorations and discussions of spirituality with polio survivors, nurses, and other health professionals. Participating with others to promote power as knowing participation in change and to support the actualization of valued potentials are among the many ways that we as nurses participate in mutual and continuous process to promote healthy patterning in ourselves and others.

## REFERENCES

Barrett, E.A.M. (1983). An empirical investigation of Martha E. Rogers' principle of helicy: The relationship between human field motion and power. Doctoral dissertation, New York University. (University Microfilms No. 84-06,278)

Barrett, E.A.M. (Ed.). (1990). *Visions of Rogers' science-based nursing.* New York: National League for Nursing.

Bell, H.E. (1984). Polio survivors: Their quality of life. Doctoral dissertation, Columbia Pacific University. (University Microfilms No. LD00763)

Elkins, D.N., Hedstrom, L.J., Hughes, L.L., Leaf, J.A., & Saunders, C. (1988). Toward a humanistic–phenomenological spirituality. *Journal of Humanistic Psychology, 28*(4), 5-18.

Halstead, L.S. (1991). Post-polio syndrome: Definition of an elusive concept. In T.L. Munsat (Ed.), *Post-polio syndrome* (pp. 23–38). Boston: Butterworth-Heinemann.

Holman, K.G. (1986). Post-polio syndrome. *Postgraduate Medicine, 79*(8), 44–53.

Krieger, D. (1981). *The Therapeutic Touch.* Englewood Cliffs, NJ: Prentice-Hall.

National Center for Health Statistics. (1987). *National health interview survey.* Washington, DC: Author.

Phillips, J. R. (1990). Changing human potentials and future visions of nursing: A human field image perspective. In E.A.M. Barrett (Ed.), *Visions of Rogers' science-based nursing* (pp. 13–25). New York: National League for Nursing.

Quinn, J.F. (1989). On healing, wholeness, and the haelen effect. *Nursing & Health Care, 10*(10), 553–556.

Raymond, C.A. (1986). Polio survivors spurred rehabilitation advances. *Journal of the American Medical Association, 255*(11), 1403–1404.

Rogers, M.E. (1970). *An introduction to the theoretical basis of nursing.* Philadelphia: Davis.

Smith, D.W. (1992). A study of power and spirituality in polio survivors using the nursing model of Martha E. Rogers. Doctoral dissertation, New York University. (University Microfilms No. 92-22,966)

Vash, C.L. (1981). *The psychology of disability.* New York: Springer.

# 10

# Developing an Effective Pattern Appraisal to Guide Nursing Care of Children with Heart Variations and Their Families

*Nancy J. Morwessel*

As a clinical nurse specialist (CNS), I provide nursing care to children with heart variations, and to their families, by both direct and indirect client contact and by working with other nurses and professionals in the hospital and community. The practice setting is a 350-bed children's hospital in the Midwest. The clients are children with heart variations who receive inpatient and/or outpatient services, and their families.

Application of Rogers' system in my nursing practice will be described herein, along with an illustration of one way to approach pattern appraisal in pr●ctice. I wish to acknowledge Martha Rogers, Elizabeth Ann Manhart Barrett, and Richard Cowling for their contributions to my learning and to this chapter.

## MAJOR FEATURES OF THE SCIENCE OF UNITARY HUMAN BEINGS

The first step in developing an approach to practice application is to examine major features and beliefs about Rogers' system (Barrett, 1988, 1990; Rogers, 1970, 1980, 1988, 1990). Those that I find helpful for this purpose include the following:

1. Unitary human beings are irreducible, pandimensional energy fields.

147

2. Human and environmental energy fields are inseparable, pandimensional, and integral to each other.

3. Energy fields are identified by field patterns. One perceives manifestations of pattern, not the field itself. Manifestations are unique and specific to the whole.

4. Human and environmental energy fields' characteristics and manifestations are unique to each unitary human.

5. Changes in energy field patterns are specific to the unique human and environmental energy fields. Change is continuous, innovative, increasingly diverse, unpredictable, and characterized by nonrepeating rhythmicities.

6. Each unitary human being has the capacity to participate knowingly and unpredictably in field pattern change (nurses cannot predict the change or the participation).

7. Nurses also participate knowingly in the process of a client's field pattern change by mutual process.

8. The goal of nursing care is to participate with the client in changing health dynamics and direction of change as defined by the client.

## APPLICATION TO PRACTICE

Using pattern manifestation to guide nursing practice is the process of integrating pattern into the context of the individual who is the focus of care (Barrett, 1990; Cowling, 1990). Since pattern manifestations are constantly changing, nurses need to focus on the relative present (while considering the relative past and future).

All phenomena are unitary and provide information about human and environmental field patterns. Nursing care is the process of a nurse's and a client's knowing participation in pattern changes related to health as defined by the client. All data must be considered in a unitary context. This includes knowledge from other sciences as well as nursing knowledge. The nurse cannot separate his or her own relative present (this client) from relative past and future (other clients' life experiences).

A nurse is integral with the client's environmental field and inseparable from it (even when the nurse is not "doing" anything). The nurse is not external to the client, and the client is not external to the nurse. The client is integral with the environmental field, which includes the nurse. One example of this concept is relevant to the nurse–client "relationship." Think of the label of the "overinvolved" nurse. This nurse often gets the advice, "Don't get so involved," and "Stay detached." What are the real issues in this situation?

Is it possible for a nurse to be involved with a client in a minimal, moderate, or very close "relationship?" What is desirable? How does a nurse decide? Is the issue, instead, the mutual process between client and nurse? Is there a partnership? Who is making decisions about change for the client, and who is defining health? Are the desired changes, in reality, mutually agreed on by client and nurse? Nurses often talk about developing a nurse–client relationship, and they describe the value or quality of that relationship. (Who judges? What are the criteria for "good" or "bad?") Instead, the nurse can focus on the dynamic mutual process of partnership with a client.

Mutual process between the nurse and the client reveals knowledge about their individual human and environmental energy field patterns. Strategies to pattern the human and environmental fields to direct change in health and health dynamics are also revealed. Changes in patterns involve both the client and the nurse. The client may participate in changes related to his or her health behaviors. Examples of a client's participation include learning about a new medication, taking medication, changing activity level, stopping smoking, learning about a new medical treatment plan, or participating in treatments. A nurse may participate in changes related to a client's health behaviors by giving information to the client in a manner that is consistent with his or her identified learning needs. Other possibilities include forgoing personal biases, negotiating health behaviors that promote human betterment, working with each client as a unique individual with unique needs, and using nursing and other scientific knowledge in a unitary context.

## THE PATTERN APPRAISAL PROCESS

The pattern appraisal process is a method of planning and providing nursing care in order to provide a focus for nursing care (Barrett, 1990; Cowling, 1990). Therapeutic nursing care is defined as a nurse's use of nursing science or knowledge in mutual process with a client by participating in health-related changes so that the client may benefit. The nurse is not "doing to" the client; instead, the nurse acts by using nursing knowledge and pattern appraisal information, in mutual process with the client, to promote the client's definition of health. Throughout the pattern appraisal process, there is knowing participation in change of both the client and the nurse, and continuing validation and evaluation of goals, actions, and outcomes by deliberative mutual process. This work with clients is what Barrett (1990) defines as health patterning.

Using energy field pattern manifestations to guide nursing practice is one approach to practice application of Rogers' system. This approach is outlined briefly and illustrated with a case study later in the chapter.

## Pattern Appraisal

Pattern appraisal is the process of acquiring information and knowledge about phenomena that manifest human and environmental field patterns in a unitary context, capturing the client's experience, perception, and expression (Barrett, 1988, 1990; Cowling, 1990). A client's experience occurs in the relative present; this moment in time is neither processed or interpreted. A client's perception is reflected by processing or attempting to make order of experience. A client's expression is reflected by the integration of experience and perception (Cowling, 1990).

It is important to recognize that the information about a client's "disease" or treatment is almost always known to the nurse and to the client. This information is in the client's and the nurse's experience, and is, therefore, integral with the process of perceiving and expressing patterns that define health and desired changes.

Pattern appraisal includes knowledge of the state of well-being: position, mobility, activity, sleep, breathing, comfort, eating, and drinking. Introspective insights related to the past, present, and future emerge from both the client and the nurse. These insights may arise from thoughts, feelings, awareness, and sensory information.

## Pattern Profile

A pattern profile is developed from the nurse's mutual process with client and family (Cowling, 1990). Information from the pattern appraisal is used to identify the foci of nursing care. The acquisition of pattern appraisal information is accomplished by the nurse through multiple levels of awareness, which involve observing, asking, sensing, listening, and knowing. Major life themes and issues are identified from the appraisal process.

The pattern profile puts pattern appraisal information into a format that both the client and the nurse can understand. It is developed from the mutual process with the client and his or her family, and it captures the experience, perception, and expression of both the client and the nurse. This is quite different from a traditional "nursing care plan," which is understandable only to the nurse. The profile format can be in single words, short phrases, symbols, or pictures. It is specific to the client, unitary, and not particulate in nature, and it reflects pandimensionality. It demonstrates that human and environmental energy fields are integral and that patterns continuously evolve and change.

The pattern profile reflects major life themes and dominant issues in a unitary human's life; they encompass the relative present, past, and future. Pattern information is specific to the individual human being appraised. Generalizing pattern information or appraisal, for more than one individual should, therefore, be discouraged even if there are similarities in pattern characteristics. Although there may be common aspects or trends in human and environmental field patterns, pattern manifestations are relevant only when received in the context of a unique unitary human being (Rogers, 1970, 1990).

Standardized plans for nursing care are not appropriate, even as a basis for later individualization. The individualization should always be first, with the nurse later adding knowledge of her or his experience with other clients. The nurse's perspective and knowledge must be shared with the present client if they are to be used as a basis for decision making and initiation of nursing care.

### Deliberative Mutual Patterning

Deliberative mutual patterning is accomplished by sharing knowledge gained from the pattern appraisal from both the client's and the nurse's view (Barrett, 1988, 1990). It involves placing the meaning of pattern knowledge within the context of the client's health goals. Deliberative mutual patterning is a participatory process in which the nurse and the client determine how to pattern the human and environmental fields in order to promote the client's definition of health. Nursing strategies are developed that reflect the nature of the pattern change desired by the client.

Deliberative mutual patterning is continuous. It begins with the onset of pattern appraisal and continues throughout the time when the nurse and client are in mutual process and nursing care is being formulated and carried out. Deliberative mutual patterning is the essence of evaluation of both nursing care and the process of pattern appraisal. Both the nurse and the client are integral and equally important contributors to the process, and both participate deliberately or intentionally in the patterning.

The key to mutual patterning is power, defined as the capacity to participate knowingly in change (Barrett, 1990). Power involves the client's and the nurse's knowing participation. The changes are in and with the client and in and with the nurse. The changes concern both the nurse and the client and they evolve from the mutual patterning.

## A SPECIALTY NURSING PRACTICE: CHILDREN WITH HEART VARIATIONS AND THEIR FAMILIES

This section describes the practice application of nurses using Rogers' system in an acute, tertiary care setting. The client in the case application had complex health needs and received intensive medical and surgical treatment that frequently changed. The nurse's role in this setting was focused on the client as a unitary human being.

Interpreting physical appraisal data; understanding present medications, medical and surgical treatments, and future plans; interfacing with many physicians in more than one specialty; and incorporating knowledge of multiple health care professionals' plans and priorities are all a way of life for a nurse in this setting. Establishing a nursing identity that reaches far beyond coordinating everyone else's professional care is a major nursing goal for nurses in these environments.

As a clinical nurse specialist, I give direct care to clients and I work with nurses who provide both inpatient and outpatient care to clients. Together, we have explored this example of practice application of Rogers' Science of Unitary Human Beings. Nurses in intensive care, general care, and outpatient care delivery settings are enthusiastically participating in developing ways of using Rogers' science in daily practice.

As I began to use the Science of Unitary Human Beings in my practice, I reflected on specific client populations that have complex needs. I selected the population of infants who, in the first three months of life, acquire a medical diagnosis of "congenital heart disease." The physical manifestations of the infants' energy field are an index of the pattern of the field. Most often, the physical manifestations identify underlying difficulties with the infants' cardiac, pulmonary, and nutritional status. These infants require medical and surgical intervention in their first year of life and are recipients of nursing care related to these treatments.

## CASE APPLICATION: SARAH

A nurse's view of a client is the unitary perspective, using knowledge from nursing and other sciences. The first step is to ". . . take a creative leap to identify the configurations of the rhythmical flow in person-environmental process" as a starting point for inquiry (Smith, 1988, p. 94).

Sarah is an infant born to parents who have two older children, ages 14 and 16. They had not planned to have another child; they were surprised with Sarah. At two weeks of age, Sarah began to have symptoms of congestive heart failure and was given the medical diagnosis of having a congenital heart disease (ventricular septal defect). By four weeks of age, she was taking diuretics, and by six weeks of age, when she continued to show poor growth and inadequate feeding, she was placed on a high calorie formula.

Sarah had an increased risk of infection. Her metabolic rate was high, as was her pulmonary blood flow, and her nutritional needs were not being met. She was born in the winter, when there is a high incidence of respiratory viruses. To protect her, Sarah's family kept her home almost all the time, away from nonfamily members, and she remained free from infection.

In February, at three months of age, Sarah was admitted to the hospital for open heart surgery. The surgeon gave her a 90 percent chance of survival. Her parents were told that Sarah was expected to remain in the intensive care unit for four days and that her total hospital stay would be about eight days.

Sarah had a rocky course the first two days after surgery but she was doing well by day five. Her parents were happy that her respiratory status had improved markedly after surgery. Her breathing pattern was slower and less labored. On day six, Sarah had a fever, increasing respiratory distress, and a frequent cough. That evening, she was diagnosed with respiratory syncytial virus (RSV) pneumonia. On day seven, she became progressively worse and required mechanical ventilation. By day ten, she was on maximum support and was gravely ill.

Sarah's pneumonia gradually stabilized, and she began to improve. By day 14, she was weaned off mechanical support, and sedation and narcotics began. On day 19, she was transferred from intensive care to a general care unit. Throughout day 27, Sarah remained very irritable. Her sleep pattern was brief and irregular. Her oral intake was extremely poor and she occasionally would vomit. There was a sustained increase in her respiratory rate and her efforts to breathe, and she had a frequent cough. Sarah remained on enteral feedings and nasal oxygen throughout this time. Her weight, however, continued to slowly decrease.

Sarah's father was an accountant, and pressure on him to return to work increased. By then, it was March and April, his busiest time of year. Sarah's two siblings began to experience difficulties in school and to exhibit behavioral changes that the parents attributed to worry and lack of time spent with them. The parents' usual schedule was for Dad to go to work, come to the hospital for lunch, go back to work, come to the hospital early in the evening, and then go home. Mom stayed at the hospital, except for time at home in the evening while Dad was at the hospital.

## PATTERN APPRAISAL

I had known Sarah and her family since she was first diagnosed with a heart variation at two weeks of age. I left on vacation on day five of her hospitalization and returned on day 21. When I returned, Sarah's parents shared the following information with me.

The experience of Sarah and her family included concerns about the relative past, present, and future. They had expected that, after surgery, they would not have to worry any more. Sarah's heart would be "fixed," they would have a "normal child," and they would lead a "normal life." They expected to be home, where they felt safe, after about eight days of hospitalization. Instead, Sarah's family had new worries and were facing a new illness. The complications were unexpected, and they felt out of control. They had expected Sarah to be healthier after surgery; instead, she was sicker than she had been before the surgery.

Sarah's parents described her as being very different. She was irritable whether she was alone or with others. Quite often, they could not console her, and she appeared withdrawn in their presence. They did not know how to help her or what they could do to see her smile and be happy.

Her parents were concerned about her length of hospitalization and the outcome of her surgery. How long would it be before she would get better? Would there be another new problem? There was no one treatment available to "fix" Sarah this time; there was no clear plan, and no progress was seen. Would Sarah get better, or would she die? What would she be like if she made it through this ordeal?

They described their feelings of anger, disappointment, fear, and utter exhaustion. They talked about their frustration with the lack of success and what they perceived as failures. They felt that they were not able to meet Sarah's needs and were sad and fearful about the changes in her temperament and mood. They worried about their other children, whom they felt were being neglected. Dad's job, changes in the pattern of Mom and Dad's communication, and the need for "down time" to gather energy and strength were other major issues that worried them. The parents spoke frequently to each other, especially during the day, sharing their fears, hopes, and strategies, and their worries about each other.

Sarah's and her parents' expression of human and environmental field patterns demonstrated their perceptions of desired health changes and actions toward change. They took what they described as a "good patient" role and spoke to very few people about their feelings. Doctors and nurses were questioned about treatment plans and how long it would be before Sarah would be better. Sarah's parents appeared tired, anxious, and worried. Their posture was rigid; at times, they were tearful, and they reported not getting enough sleep. They were suspicious of new treatments and the initiation of changes in the current ones. Why decrease her breathing treatments when she is not better? How will enteral feedings help? They anticipated failure and new difficulties and wondered if the lack of progress meant that Sarah was getting worse. They were seeking answers. What is the daily goal, and when will it be established? How will it be carried out?

Development of new routines and evolution of parent and nurse activities continued. "Good" times and "bad" times were seen. Sarah's parents began to identify differences in her pattern manifestations when environmental or treatment changes were made. They shared this information with the doctors and nurses, telling them which treatments or environmental changes were working and which ones were not. They were also trying to pattern her room space so that it was unique, comfortable, and convenient.

## PATTERN PROFILE

Using the information from the pattern appraisal, Sarah's parents, her primary nurse, and I set out to identify and clarify desired health care changes. Through mutual process, we developed a pattern profile. I asked Sarah's parents to develop their main goals for Sarah and for themselves at this point in time. Sarah's primary nurse and I would do the same. We could write, draw, diagram, or use any method to describe, in words, what our present goals were. The lists of desired health changes are shown in Tables 10.1 and 10.2. We felt that the lists identified our priorities.

We all found it very interesting that "home" was at the beginning of one list and at the end of the other. Sarah's primary nurse explained that she saw the list as a step-by-step process in working toward the goal "home." Sarah's parents explained that going home seemed to be a low priority to the doctors and nurses, so they continued to remind everyone that this was of primary importance to them.

This is only one small example of the processing and communicating that take place when the clients' and nurses' perspectives are made clear. Everyone shared some measure of frustration about the lack of a clear plan. Everyone wanted Sarah to be less irritable, but it seemed to be a bigger concern for the nurses (Sarah's mother felt that she would be better if they could only go home). The nurses were concerned with the toll this experience was taking on the parents. The parents felt that they could cope if only they had an end point to work toward. The nurses wanted the parents to talk to them about their feelings. The parents wanted to be able to talk to each other. Lunchtime together at the hospital was very important to them: they could review the doctors' visits and Sarah's progress, and share their feelings. Sarah's mother wanted her to eat more by mouth; the nurses wanted her to start gaining weight before concentrating on oral feedings.

During the process of learning about past events and the participants' relative present, I shared my thoughts and observations with Sarah's parents and the health professionals involved in her care. It

### Table 10.1
### Goals of Parents

| |
|---|
| Home |
| Plan for each day, then home |
| Meet basic needs for family members |
| Sarah calmer, sleeping |
| Sarah feeding well by mouth |
| Sarah happy |

### Table 10.2
### Goals of Nurses

Clear plan for medical and nutritional care
Sarah calmer, sleeping, responsive, happier
Parents communicating needs to the nurses
Sarah gaining weight and meeting nutritional needs
Sarah taking more formula by mouth
Home

appeared that a major source of frustration was an inability to put into place an effective, step-by-step plan that would deal with Sarah's identified health needs and meet her parents' desired goals and outcome. Sarah's parents were receptive to the suggestion that they work with her caregivers to establish this plan. More than anything, they wanted to do "something" to help Sarah. It was very difficult for them to see that there were no clear answers to the questions and issues concerning her care. Sarah's primary nurse described her need to know that she was helping Sarah and her parents. This need was especially acute when Sarah did not seem to make progress. Further acknowledgment of values and attitudes followed. We agreed to stop looking for a "quick fix" and deal with the relative present. Through mutual process and much communication, caring, and laughter, we created together a drawing that described Sarah and her parents' pattern profile (see Table 10.3).

### DELIBERATIVE MUTUAL PATTERNING: DEVELOPING STRATEGIES TO MAKE DESIRED HEALTH CHANGES

Using the information from the pattern appraisal and the pattern profile, Sarah's parents and nurses developed a description of strategies to meet desired health changes. Communication among Sarah's parents, her nurses, the dietician, and all physicians involved in her care would be encouraged and facilitated. They would discuss Sarah's current health needs, define immediate goals and treatment plans, and develop short-term and long-term plans.

For example, one of the goals identified was: To encourage oral feedings and to go home as soon as possible. The plan included a change from continuous enteral feedings to oral feedings, and provided for intermittent enteral bolus feedings when oral intake was less than a predetermined goal. This approach encouraged immediate

## Table 10.3
## Pattern Profile

| HOME | | | | |
|---|---|---|---|---|
| | EATING WELL | | HAPPY | |
| | GAINING WEIGHT | | SLEEPING AT TIMES | |
| MOM STAY WITH CHILD | DAD TO WORK | MOM HOME IN EVENING EVERY 2 DAYS | EVERY 2 DAYS MOM & DAD TOGETHER IN EVENING | DAD LUNCH AT HOSPITAL |
| IDENTIFY PLAN: MD, NURSES, & PARENTS FOR TREATMENT DAY BY DAY | | | GOALS FOR TREATMENT: OFF OXYGEN, COUGHING LESS, EAT BY MOUTH, HOME | |

Note: The parents and nurses decided there was not one correct place to start in this image because all the important information was there.

intermittent oral feeding, supplied adequate calories, and looked toward the way Sarah's mother would feed Sarah at home.

Sarah's parents identified their schedule and discussed with the nurses some aspects of daily care they wanted to provide for Sarah. A collaborative decision was made by the nurses and the parents on how Sarah's care would be provided, and a schedule for daily care, including treatments, feeding, and medications was drawn up. A "Do Not Disturb" time was acknowledged and respected by all parties concerned.

Changes in Sarah's human and environmental pattern manifestations were monitored to find the strategies that would best promote comfort and calm and bring pleasure instead of distress to Sarah. For example, Sarah's state of well-being was integral with light, sound, motion, nonnutritive sucking, colors, shapes, toys, and people. Sarah's parents kept track of the intensity, duration, and types of environmental conditions that were most helpful. The plan for all caretakers (family, nurses) was derived from this information. The nurses, using their knowledge of human field pattern manifestations associated with sleep deprivation and the intensive care experience, minimized treatment that was noisy or unpleasant.

Sarah's parents and nurses agreed to share with each other their feelings about this experience. A commitment was made to stop guessing about the future and to try to make today better. Sarah's parents could choose to participate or not participate in her physical care, without pressure. For example, they also needed sleep, and they were free to choose not to feed Sarah at night. To improve the consistency of pattern appraisal and nursing care and to strengthen the nature of the mutual process among themselves, Sarah's parents, and Sarah, the nurses worked toward minimizing the number of different nurses providing care.

As the days passed until Sarah was discharged, this plan worked better than anyone had anticipated. Among the conclusions summarized by the nurses and Sarah's parents were:

- The nurses felt more comfortable with the parents' reticence as they focused on meeting the family's identified needs.
- The parents felt more comfortable communicating with the nurses when they identified their role as experts about the nursing care of their child.
- The physicians were eager to leave the management of treatments and feedings to the nurses, parents, and dietician.
- The physicians felt that they were communicating more with the family; they no longer felt pressured to address questions that could not be answered, such as "When will she go home?"
- Everyone viewed "going home" as the present and future goal.

Pattern information and desired health changes identified in this plan were not different from those in the previously developed, traditional "nursing care plan," but the focus and strategies were quite different when using the Rogerian practice methodology.

On day 31, Sarah was discharged. She left the hospital on oral feedings with supplemental enteral feedings as needed. Five weeks later, her parents described Sarah as happy, feeling well, and not requiring any enteral feedings.

## SUMMARY

Using energy field pattern manifestations to guide nursing practice is useful in inpatient acute care and ambulatory settings. Health patterning provides a means for nurses to identify, develop, and expand nursing practice for the nurses' purpose of participating in health-related changes so that people may benefit.

Integrating into daily thinking the theory of power as knowing participation in change is important to the application of Rogers' system in practice. The nurse no longer feels the need to know everything in order to help the client. Instead, the nurse and client pool their knowledge and values in order to mutually process the relative present, past, and future and to make decisions about health-related changes. The nurse will not "do to" the client; instead, the nurse will walk with the client throughout the process.

Both client and nurse recognize each other's values, beliefs, perspective, and knowledge in identifying goals and evaluating change. The nurse's role is enhanced as the client's participation increases. Most of us had a particular coach, teacher, manager, or mentor who is memorable because he or she helped us *do* instead of *doing* for us. Human beings who are involved in a process and can individualize their learning learn far more than those who are told what to do or what to believe. There will be times when a client prefers to let the nurse make a decision or develop a plan. This, however, will result from the client's decision; it will not be the nurse's standard operating procedure.

In my vision of the future, the nursing profession will direct attention away from the nurse as the initiator of nursing care and toward a nurse–client partnership in both initiating and receiving the process. Instead of the traditional nursing process, nurse care plan, nursing intervention, and nursing evaluation, nurses will focus on the client as a unitary human being whose unique needs and perspective are integral to all phases of the "nursing process," not afterthoughts when the plan has been developed.

Nurses will celebrate the use of their knowledge-based power for establishing mutual process with clients and for assisting clients with health-related changes, instead of "taking charge" and assuming responsibility for the changes. Providing client-centered nursing care in a high-technology, acute care environment is possible, necessary, and valuable to the client and the nurse. It calls us to the human being and person who is the focus of nursing care.

## REFERENCES

Barrett, E.A.M. (1988). Using Rogers' Science of Unitary Human Beings in nursing practice. *Nursing Science Quarterly, 1,* 50–51.

Barrett, E.A.M. (1990). Rogers' science-based nursing practice. In E.A.M. Barrett (Ed.), *Visions of Rogers' science-based nursing* (pp. 31–44). New York: National League for Nursing.

Cowling, W.R. (1990). A template for unitary pattern-based practice. In E.A.M. Barrett (Ed.), *Visions of Rogers' science-based nursing* (pp. 45–65). New York: National League for Nursing.

Rogers, M.E. (1970). *An introduction to the theoretical basis of nursing.* Philadelphia: Davis.

Rogers, M.E. (1980). Nursing: A science of unitary man. In J. Riehl & C. Roy (Eds.), *Conceptual models for nursing practice* (2nd ed.) (pp. 329–337). New York: Appleton-Century-Crofts.

Rogers, M.E. (1987). Rogers' Science of Unitary Human Beings. In R.R. Parse (Ed.), *Nursing science: Major paradigms, theories, and critiques* (pp. 139–146). Philadelphia: Saunders.

Rogers, M.E. (1988). Nursing science and art: A prospective. *Nursing Science Quarterly, 1,* 99–102.

Rogers, M.E. (1990). Nursing: Science of Unitary, Irreducible, Human Beings: Update 1990. In E.A.M. Barrett (Ed.), *Visions of Rogers' science-based nursing* (pp. 5–11). New York: National League for Nursing.

Smith, M.J. (1988). Perspectives of wholeness: The lens makes a difference. *Nursing Science Quarterly, 1,* 94–95.

# 11

# The Science of Unitary Human Beings as a Foundation for Nursing Practice with Persons Experiencing Life Patterning Difficulties: Transforming Theory into Motion

*Bela Horvath*

In their quest to understand the powerful forces and subtle complexities of human emotion and behavior, nurses have traditionally relied on psychiatric or psychoanalytic frameworks as interpretive bases in caring for persons experiencing life-patterning difficulties. In these models, extreme variances in feeling, thought, or behavior are generally seen as being pathological in nature and attributable to disturbances in either neurotransmitter functioning or "unconscious" processes. Despite the fact that most nursing theories endorse the belief that human beings are whole, multifaceted entities (Meleis, 1985), many nurses continue to provide service with a reductionistic view of mental health that particulates the mind, body, and spirit.

For example, at a recent major psychiatric nursing conference advertised under the slogan "Decade of the Brain" (Nursing Transitions, 1991), a bias toward a neuropathological approach to emotional health was clearly evident. Presentations with titles such as "The Broken Brain: Psychobiology of Major Mental Disorders," "Mending Shattered Minds," "Multiple Personality Disorders," "Wonder Drugs for the Mind," and "Advances in Brain Imaging" made it apparent that many practitioners of nursing seem resigned to perpetuation of an obei-sance to non-nursing, disease-oriented treatment ideologies.

In contrast, Rogers' Science of Unitary Human Beings provides an innovative, expansive framework to guide the nurse in creatively caring for persons experiencing life-patterning difficulties. In the Rogerian view, human beings are unique, irreducible energy fields in mutual process with the environmental field, evolving through a con-tinual, increasingly complex process of change known as patterning (Rogers, 1990, 1992). Deeply felt emotional experiences emerge as manifestations of patterning. As such, they defy the causal notion of molecular constructs (such as brain synapses) or segmented levels of consciousness as perceived by nineteenth- and twentieth-century psychoanalysts. Similarly, life-patterning strategies in Rogerian sci-ence are designed to encompass a broad range of environmental field modalities that are beyond the 45-minute therapy session or experi-mental trials of catecholamine-pumping "nerve" pills. As Rogers (1992) noted, hopeful attitudes, humor, and "upbeat moods" are more therapeutic than drugs (p. 33).

Although the Science of Unitary Beings is conceived as a unified whole, explorations of specific aspects of the model, namely the Prin-ciples of Homeodynamics and Manifestations of Field Patterning, will be discussed as they pertain to various theoretical issues and to prac-tical approaches to health patterning. Health patterning is described as the process of assisting people in their knowing participation in change (Barrett, 1990).

## THE PRINCIPLE OF INTEGRALITY

The continuous mutual and environmental field process, known as integrality (Rogers, 1992), provides a key to understanding human feelings, thoughts, and actions. The challenge to understand integral-ity invites a look at behavioral human field manifestations as emerg-ing from an evolving, unitary, ever-changing process, rather than from a reductionistic, diagnostic perspective. In the unitary perspec-tive, a "diagnosis" or "symptom" is not seen as some facet of emo-tional disease that is treated solely with medication and/or psychotherapy. Instead, it depicts a holographic "snapshot" of a broader configuration of events, experiences, traditions, beliefs, and feelings that synthesizes the relative past, present, and future.

For example, behaviors commonly characterized as obsessive–compulsive, phobic, or self-destructive may be viewed in the Rog-erian system as manifestations of hurtful patterning experiences such as child/adolescent abuse, shame-provoking traumas, or feelings of guilt, inadequacy, anger, and loneliness that have not been acknowledged. These and other behavioral manifestations are seen as unique, creative forms of expression that represent a desire to modulate feelings of distress.

The Principle of Integrality holds that human and environmental fields are in mutual process. Integral to this process is power, defined as the capacity for knowingly participating in change and making choices (Barrett, 1990). Practice implications consistent with power-oriented field patterning suggest the exploration of relevant experiences with an emphasis on enhanced awareness of feelings and thoughts, choices, awareness attuned to change, and the integration of knowledge.

Environmental field patterning modalities such as music, art, meditative exercises, pets, and work/play activities are among the choices of modalities that may potentiate feeling awareness and actualization in unitary human beings (Barrett, 1990). These modalities may yield an immediacy and directness in promoting well-being that surpass the use of only verbal therapeutic interchanges.

In addition, the utilization of naturalistic settings for patterning sessions opens up new alternatives for nurses and clients who feel more comfortable in everyday locales than in cramped office spaces: Sessions on park benches or in cafés, leisurely strolls down a pleasant avenue, or refreshing, informative "field trips" are among a few of the alternatives available to nurses and clients who prefer a more relaxed approach to health patterning.

Nurses using Rogers' model are encouraged to be active participants in the process of health patterning—sharing their knowledge, experiences, and humanness, and communicating a genuine sense of confidence in their professional abilities. Nurses need not feel conceptually confined to arbitrary boundaries of space, time, or anachronistic methodologies. The "id," the "ego," the "superego," "transference," "countertransference," or similar psychoanalytic icons have limited usefulness in an increasingly complex, accelerating world of fiberoptic networks, cocaine addiction epidemics, and self-help support groups ranging from alcoholism to zoophilia.

## THE PRINCIPLE OF RESONANCY

Resonancy refers to the continuous change from lower- to higher-frequency wave patterns in human and environmental fields (Rogers, 1992). Persons experiencing difficulties in dealing with the vicissitudes of life, however, may generate wave frequency patterns that assume prolonged cycles of lower, higher, or other rhythmic activity. For example, the human field manifestation of depression is seen as correlating with lower-frequency rhythms. Getting "high" is a common term that cogently describes the wave frequency patterns of many individuals in their quest for drug-induced states of heightened awareness. So-called "manic-depressive" or "bipolar" disorders may be viewed as a human field manifestation reflecting an intense, alternating variation of wave pattern formation.

Human field wave patterns are more meaningfully viewed as being integral with environmental field wave patterns. If, for example, early patterning experiences indicated a stringent enforcement of parental rules and traditions to the detriment of individuality and objectivity, one might later experience some degree of unitary "turbulence" during the passage from lower to higher wave frequency patterns. This is often seen in adolescent or young adult years as evolving unitary human beings begin to discover and act according to their own needs, values, and preferences. Often, this change dismays their parents, who are committed to perpetuating the frequency levels of their own wave patterns.

As environmental wave patterns evolve and accelerate, change occurs, thus giving way to new realities, opportunities, and/or difficulties in living. For some persons, however, this continuous change process is simultaneously feared and avoided. A perceived inability to achieve harmonic consonance with these new resonating patterns is often experienced through feelings of intense sadness, of loneliness, and of being compelled. Such persons manifest characteristics that suggest a pervasive wave pattern that may feel "out of sync" with their environment throughout protracted periods of their lives.

Recognizing the significance of the dynamic process of human and environmental wave patterns is critical for nurses practicing in the Rogerian model, since the directives for healing are enfolded in the mutual process rather than in the individual. As Rawnsley (1985) concluded, healing is motion—specifically, motion toward field harmonization. Its purpose is to "tune in to the basic harmony of a specific human experience relative to a larger contextual pattern of environmental change" (p. 28). This may be accomplished through the creative use of human field patterning. Exploration of reality, the sharing of knowledge, creative imagery, acceptance, and encouragement are various approaches to unitary healing that are consistent with this approach.

Finally, as Malinski (1986) wrote, nurses need to become attuned to their own rhythms in the practice of nursing. A firm belief in their own ability to heal, as well as in their sense of individuality and uniqueness as facilitators of change, is a fundamental asset in human field patterning.

## THE PRINCIPLE OF HELICY

Helicy—the continuous, innovative, unpredictable, increasing diversity of human and environmental field patterns (Rogers, 1992)—reminds us that life is an adventure to be embraced through new experiences, emergent awareness, risk taking, and evolving patterns. The inherent implications of helicy are invigorating for nurses engaged in unitary patterning, prompting a spirit of excitement and achievement, and a sense of "letting go." These concepts are integral to the facilitation of human field motion, and they reflect an attitudinal shift toward actualization and fulfillment. Helicy denotes individualism, choices, and freedom from attachments and outcomes, and it allows for the inevitability of human error. As songwriter Billy Joel (1985) compassionately states in a song about teenage suicide, "You're supposed to make mistakes."

## THE MANIFESTATIONS OF FIELD PATTERNING

Rogers (1992) postulated that the manifestations of field patterning assume a path of faster motion, shorter rhythms, and greater diversity. Unitary patterning practices may assume a similar course as manifested by short-term, action-oriented sessions predicated on change, movement, and the enjoyment of life through productive endeavors. In traditional terms, the goal is to economically, efficiently, and safely get people out of "treatment" and into "the world" as soon as possible.

In many ways, the essential nature of the principles of homeodynamics may be expressed through music rather than by words. An excerpt from the final scene of Richard Wagner's (1983) opera *Siegfried,* shown in Figure 11.1, is one of the countless musical examples that convey the confluent nature of human and environmental fields in the mutual process and depict the continuity, accelerated change, increasing diversity, and unpredictability of field patterning. Music may also be seen (and heard) as a metaphor for the dynamic process of unitary patterning. (The reader is invited to listen to this

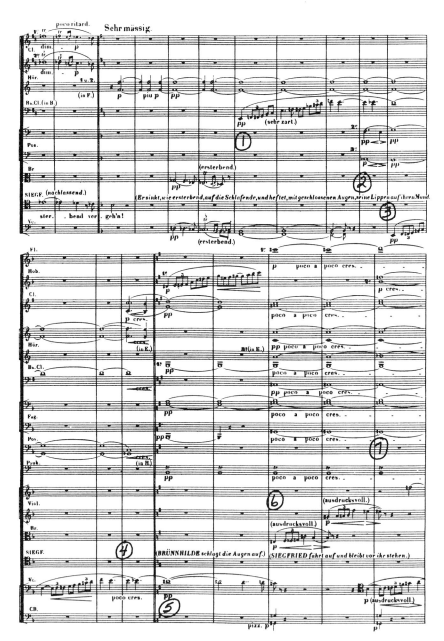

Figure 11.1
Excerpt from final scene of Richard Wagner's opera, *Siegfried*.

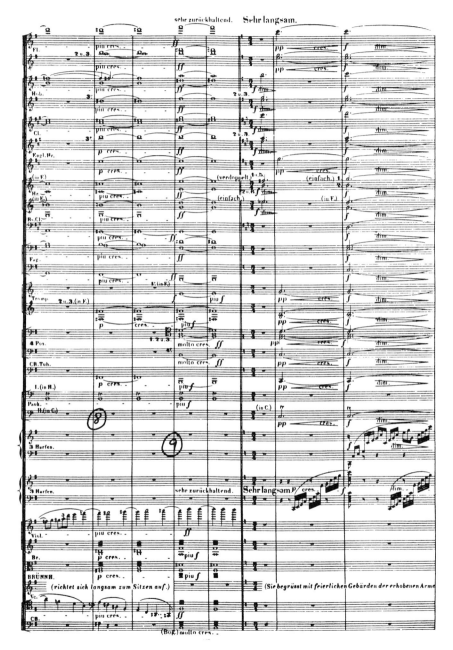

**Figure 11.1    (continued)**

example from any of the commercially available recordings of the opera.)

In this excerpt, Wagner uses one motif, immersed in constantly shifting harmonies and an expanding orchestration, to express the awakening, from a kiss by Siegfried, of the mythological Walkure, Brunnhilde, after a long slumber. Immediately after Siegfried's opening musical soliloquy in Act 3, Scene 3, the motif of this awakening begins with the bass clarinet at ①, in the tonality of $B^\flat$. At ②, the melody of the clarinet blends with the nearly imperceptible modulation through $B^\flat$ minor to C major at ③, where the same melody is repeated (now transposed in C) by the lower strings.

At ④, the final notes of the melody are used to create another modulation through C minor, this time resting momentarily on an $E^\flat$, which becomes part of the new, diminished-sounding tonality of the B-9th at ⑤, as well as the starting note of yet another statement of the motif by the oboes. Two measures later, at ⑥, Wagner creates an entirely new, anticipatory mood, using the final note of the melody to top off an inverted $D^\flat$-7th chord, again repeating the melody, but in shortened fragments. At ⑦, he modulates again to a tonality of a G-7th, shifts to an inverted B-7th chord at ⑧, using more common harmonic threads, and finally rests on a root-position B-7th chord at ⑨, purposely avoiding a final cadence.

If, for a moment, the motif of this section can be imagined to be a musical metaphor of a unitary human being, it is possible to envision the continual, increasingly diverse movement and exhilaration achievable through the harmonic interpolation of environmental field potentials. The following case studies may exemplify these possibilities.

## CASE STUDY 1: RAYMOND

Raymond was a 52-year-old male who had an intense fear of leaving his apartment, which was located on the Upper West Side of Manhattan. By most accounts, Raymond had not ventured out of his building in four years, although he occasionally (albeit reluctantly) went to the lobby to pick up his mail. He was unemployed and had been referred to a local community mental health center by his wife, who took care of most of their domestic affairs. Over the years, Raymond had seen a number of therapists and psychiatrists. He was taking a maintenance dose of a major tranquilizer medication. Raymond justified his seclusion through a long-standing delusional fear he had developed over the possibility of running into a man he had identified seven years before as a mugger.

My initial contact with Raymond was at the request of the mental health center, which wanted to establish a relationship with him in the hope that he would eventually choose to join its day program. A phone call was made to his wife, and an appointment was set up for me to begin home therapy health patterning sessions with Raymond. The short-term goal of having Raymond get out of his building and into the street was established.

When I met Raymond and his wife, I assumed my usual casual, friendly demeanor. I commented on their comfortable apartment and explored Raymond's fears only to the point of gaining an understanding of them. After listening to him, it occurred to me to share with him a story about my own fear of elevators, which developed after being stuck in a World Trade Center elevator for two hours. I told him how tiring it had been for me to climb stairs all day and how I had finally begun to feel ridiculous about allowing my fears to control my life. I laughed at my own folly. Raymond was deeply absorbed in listening, and then he laughed. I sensed that he could identify not only with my sense of fear, but with the interminable amount of energy invested in keeping his fears alive. I thought that he was ready to move on.

"Let's get together Thursday," I suggested. "We'll go out for pizza or something." He asked if I would stay with him for the entire outing and take him home. I agreed. We shook hands, and I left. My visit with Raymond had lasted 25 minutes.

When we met on Thursday, Raymond seemed nervous, yet brimming with anticipation. We walked through the building lobby, exited through the front door, and went to "Tony's Pizza." From there, we went to the day program. The following week, I took him for a haircut. He could not remember the last time he had gone to a professional barber.

From a Rogerian perspective, Raymond's visit to "Tony's Pizza" may be seen as a behavioral manifestation of increasingly diverse, motion-oriented, accelerating, unpredictable human field patterning as explained through helicy. Generating this process was Raymond's capacity to participate in changing his day-to-day routine. The process of deliberative mutual patterning began with an emphasis on pattern recognition and attunement.

On several occasions, Raymond came to the program by himself, but he eventually chose not to attend on a regular basis. He implied that he felt uncomfortable among "crazy people" and would rather just go out where he wanted to. In touch with his own sense of power, he was free to choose according to his desires.

Although his next step was unforeseeable, it really didn't seem to matter. Health patterning had helped Raymond to "come out of his shell" and into the flow of life in the Upper West Side, New York City, March 1988.

## CASE STUDY 2: JULIE

Julie, a 36-year-old psychotherapist, had been admitted to a psychiatric inpatient unit for the latest in a long series of hospitalizations for self-mutilative behavior. Julie had been in psychiatric treatment for years and had an unusually congenial relationship with her psychiatrist. Yet, despite multiple trials of various psychotropic medications, her symptoms had persisted.

Although my role was that of a nursing administrator, I had clinical input into treatment decisions. I decided to get involved in Julie's care regime. I wanted to find the "missing answers" to Julie's problem in a timely manner and was curious as to why, over the years, her "treatment" had not been more effective.

Being aware of my own rhythmic patterning, I was determined to proceed in an expeditious manner. I introduced myself to Julie and said, "Do you want to get better? If you do, let's fix this right now." Understandably, she looked at me as though I were out of my mind. My intentions were clear. I was confident that, through mutual process, Julie and I had the capacity to participate knowingly in change. I had the desire to do so; I was hopeful that she did.

Since power is predicated on knowledge (Barrett, 1990), it seemed critical to gain a better understanding of Julie's patterning relative to her current difficulties. The pattern of her mutilative behavior was clear. On weekends, she would isolate herself at home and cut her arms with razors or scissors. Julie often considered suicide but admitted that her love for her cat prevented her from doing so. I suspected that her difficulties were related to early patterning experiences.

I asked her to tell me about the first time she cut herself in such a fashion. She told me that she was not aware of when or where it first happened. I told her that I knew it was difficult for her but it was important that she recall the initial episode. She realized that it had occurred when she was eleven. While playing in the street, she had picked up a razor blade from the gutter and cut herself. I knew the concomitant environmental dynamics of this incident were critical at this point, and I asked her where her parents had been at the time.

Suddenly, Julie froze and stared blankly. She had the kind of numb, vacant look on her face that would usually prompt a therapist to run for more medication or whisk the patient away to the "quiet room." I stayed with her, realizing that I had resonated with something very painful for her. She looked at me as though I had uncovered some deep, dark, secret memory of a terrifying legacy, shrouded from her immediate awareness through years of shame, confusion, and hurt. Now, in the relative present, through pandimensional transcendence and imagery, Julie was experiencing a new reality from the relative past (Rogers, 1992, p. 32).

I asked Julie to describe what she was feeling and remembering. What ensued was a disconnected, yet graphic description of a childhood filled with pervasive feelings of abandonment, neglect, and anger. I asked Julie to write a letter to her parents expressing some of those feelings. She vehemently refused at first, but finally she agreed.

The next day, Julie showed me two pages torn out of a notebook. Huge letters were carved on it in red ink, almost as though she had mutilated the notebook. The writing was unintelligible. I asked her to keep on writing and to concentrate on what she was feeling. I implied to her that I knew she was capable of doing it. She continued writing over the next few days. Soon the sentences were longer, less fragmented, and more expressive. The flow of her writing was likened to a metaphorical manifestation of the patterning process. Writing gave Julie the power to participate in change.

On the unit, it was characteristic of Julie to openly express her affinity for certain staff members and her dislike of others. Although this was perceived by some as an unhealthy "personality trait," it provided an opportunity to capitalize on a relationship with one of her favorite staff members, a nurse named Linda. Linda and I worked together on a plan that would help Julie to verbally express her feelings instead of acting on them. I knew this would help Julie increase her feelings of integrality with others, heighten her awareness and understanding of human encounters, and shift her focus from engaging in destructive rituals to promoting fulfilling and creative endeavors.

It was helpful to envision Julie's journey into wellness as a voyage on a small sailing ship in a tumultuous storm. Looking into the relative future beyond the immediate dilemma, far in the distance and behind the fury of the high seas, we could see calmer waters and serene surroundings. By increasing awareness of the mutuality of human and environmental fields, it was possible to ride in concert with the course of the waves, eventually drifting toward a safer, more tranquil space.

Julie was discharged several days later and, at my recommendation, continued seeing Linda for patterning sessions in coffee shops. I received a letter from Julie shortly thereafter, thanking me for my efforts and letting me know it was the most productive hospitalization experience that she had ever had. She returned to her job as a therapist, began to spend more time out of her apartment on weekends and traveling, and became aware of personal issues that had remained unexplored. She continued to knowingly participate in change by having health patterning sessions with Linda. Her self-mutilation abated, and Julie's life became more serene and enjoyable in her movement toward well-being.

## CASE STUDY 3:  STEVE

Steve was a young, gifted musician who suffered from pervasive anxiety, fits of anger, and a propensity for getting involved in ultimately destructive relationships. He spent most of the time in his apartment, sulking, ordering in Chinese food, and watching X-rated movies. He made a meager living playing at weddings and teaching music privately. Yet, Steve was also an extremely creative composer, songwriter, instrument maker, and cook.

He seemed tormented by his sense of what he perceived as being "entrapped" by the legacy of his parents and brother, all of whom he thought were "losers." He was angry at their inability to live harmoniously, and he had tremendous resentment about his father's inadequacies. He saw his own problems as an extension of theirs and saw no way out of their intrusion in his life. He did not feel free to act intentionally. This was manifested in lower power choices and lower power involvement in creating change.

Steve and I initially met for breakfast at a diner. When we discussed his parents, he often became so irritated that he nearly propelled our coffee cups into the air every time he banged the table with his fists. I felt it necessary to help Steve see himself as a human being who had the capacity to participate in the evolution of his life on terms of his own choice. I shared some simple affirmations with him. He would jot them down on a napkin, just as fast as I could think of them, and read them back to himself. The observable manifestations of his energy field would remarkably change after he did this: he seemed relieved and relaxed, and a big grin would often flash across his broad, bearded face.

We met several times in the diner, and then Steve invited me over to his house to continue our patterning sessions. There, I had the opportunity to experience the pattern of his environment and to gain more insight into his human field pattern. I began to appreciate his love of music, invention, and antique memorabilia. Not meeting at the diner also allowed Steve to save some money and gave me the chance to enjoy some of his Italian pasta specialties.

We expanded the sessions to include his girlfriend and often recorded them on a cassette at his request, for future review. We made only tentative plans for future meetings, since our schedules often changed, but we made sure never to leave an issue "hanging" when we met. Our sessions routinely lasted one and one-half to two hours and focused on personal choices, knowingly participating in change, feelings, and career development.

We met on an average of twice a month, according to Steve's desires, over the course of approximately seven months. During this period, Steve began to manifest behaviors that illuminated his potential for actualization. The changes in his life were characterized by a succession of lower- to higher-frequency choices and creative endeavors. Steve's participation in family affairs became leaner and more fulfilling. He transformed a hurtful relationship with his girlfriend into one of mutual respect and caring, launched a nightclub act, and wrote a music instruction book that was eventually published. He became a calmer, more relaxed person, and began to study meditation.

Health patterning is predicated on a personal belief that we can help to change people's lives for the better. It requires a vision of what life may be like, a belief in the human potential to create that kind of life, and knowledge of "the way life is." Many people ask me where I had my "formal" psychiatric training. Most of them are surprised when I admit that I never had any, and they're even more astounded when I proclaim that I never needed it. When they ask why, I just tell them about the principles of homeodynamics. That's just the way life is.

## REFERENCES

Barrett, E.A.M. (1990). Health Patterning with clients in a private practice environment. In E.A.M. Barrett (Ed.), *Visions of Rogers science-based nursing* (pp. 105–115). New York: National League for Nursing.

Joel, B. (1985). "You're only human: Second wind." *Billy Joel Greatest Hits, Volume I and Volume II* CBS Records C240121 New York.

Malinski, V.M. (1986). *Explorations on Martha Rogers science of Unitary human beings.* Norwalk, CT: Appleton-Century-Crofts.

Meleis, A.I. (1985). *Theoretical nursing: Development and progress.* Philadelphia: J.B. Lippincott.

Nursing Transitions. (1991). *Advances in Psychiatric-Mental Health Nursing 91': The Decade of the Brain* (Conference) Hilton Head, S.C.

Rawnsley, M.M. (1985). H-E-A-L-T-H: A Rogerian perspective. *Journal of Holistic Nursing, 3*(1).

Rogers, M.E. (1990). *Nursing: Science of unitary irreducible human beings: Update 1990.* In E.A.M. Barrett (Ed.), *Visions of Rogers science-based nursing* (pp. 5–11). New York: National League for Nursing.

Rogers, M.E. (1992). Nursing science and the space age. *Nursing Science Quarterly, 5*(1) 27–34.

Wagner, R. (1983). *Siegfried.* New York: Dover Press.

# 12

# The Rogerian Abstract System and Chinese Healing Theories: Applications to Nursing Practice

*Martha Hains Bramlett*
*Jiafang Chen*

Chinese healing traditions have been evolving for over two thousand years within a culture and philosophy markedly different from the culture and philosophy that have provided the background for the evolution of Western health care. Rather than following the path of mind-body duality with an inherent division of the person into parts, Chinese theories stress the unity and integrality of human beings within the greater universe. Noting the philosophical similarities between Chinese healing modalities and Rogers' Science of Unitary Human Beings, this chapter explores the potential uses of Rogers' Science of Unitary Human Beings (1986, 1990, 1992, 1993) as a base for nursing practice in China. Similarly, Chinese healing traditions are examined for their potential utility within the Science of Unitary Human Beings.

## ROGERS' SCIENCE OF UNITARY HUMAN BEINGS

Rogers' Science of Unitary Human Beings (1986, 1990, 1992, 1993) is based on the concepts of energy fields, openness, pattern, and

The authors would like to acknowledge the critique of Sarah H. Gueldner, DSN, FAAN, Professor and Director of the Center for Nursing Research at the Medical University of South Carolina.

pandimensionality. Rogers proposes that the universe consists of energy fields and, more specifically, that both human beings and the environment are energy fields. Energy fields are open and are therefore in constant mutual process. These fields are recognized by their patterns; each is perceived as a single wave pattern. The universe of open energy fields is pandimensional in nature, distinguished by neither spatial nor linear characteristics. Rather, the universe is acausal and nonlinear in nature, and it has infinite dimensions to be explored. Since human beings are pandimensional energy fields, they must be considered as unitary beings and different from the sum of their parts.

Rogers (1986, 1990, 1992) proposed three homeodynamic principles: (1) Resonancy, (2) Helicy, and (3) Integrality. These principles describe the relationships among the four primary postulates, as well as the nature of unitary human beings. According to the Principle of Resonancy, change is proposed to be continuous and to occur in the direction of lower to higher frequencies. Thus, human and environmental fields change dynamically and constantly and attain higher frequency patterns. Human and environmental energy fields, as described in the Principle of Helicy, are innovative and unpredictable, manifesting increasingly complex and diverse patterns that are characterized by nonrecurring rhythmicities. The Principle of Integrality proposes that energy fields, both human and environmental, are in constant mutual process. Thus, neither human nor environmental fields can be considered in isolation from other energy fields.

## THE UNIVERSE AND HUMAN BEINGS
## IN CHINESE HEALING

Chinese healing traditions have evolved within the context of Chinese culture and philosophy, which differs markedly from traditional Western beliefs about the healing process. In order to understand Chinese theories of healing, one must have some cognizance of the Chinese view of the universe. The Chinese traditionally believe that the health and well-being of the individual are inextricably tied to the greater universe. Believing that human life is inseparably linked to all other life—animals and plants, as well as the non-live earth of soil, rocks, and water—human beings are seen as one phase of existence (Hume, 1940). Health, or the lack of health, is considered to be a balance or imbalance of the living forces of the universe. Hume (1940) explained, "The life of man, in all its phases, is inseparably linked with every other form of life" (p. 5).

Philosophically, this linkage or inseparability is congruent with the Rogerian Principle of Integrality. Both Chinese healing and the Science of Unitary Human Beings propose the unitary nature of the universe and the integral nature of human beings in the universe. The proposal is especially apparent in the Chinese viewpoint of health as a dynamic balance with the universe rather than a condition of illness versus wellness, as seen in Western medicine. As in the Rogerian abstract system, the Chinese perception of health considers the whole or unitary individual in the context of his or her environment rather than limiting the field of vision to dysfunction or particulate parts of the person.

## CHINESE HEALING THEORIES

Basic to Chinese healing theories are five concepts: (1) Yin-Yang, (2) Five Elements (Wu Xing), (3) Vital Substances (Zang Xiang), (4) Qi (Chi), and (5) Essence (Jing) (Hume, 1940; Maciocia, 1989; Wong & Wu, 1936). Of these concepts, Yin-Yang is probably the most familiar in Western cultures.

### Yin-Yang

Yin-Yang is based on the simultaneous opposition and unity of two cosmic forces in the universe. According to Chinese philosophy, all primal matter was originally divided into two aspects with the "grosser and heavier part" (Yin) (Hume, 1940, p. 17) precipitating to form the earth and the "finer, lighter part" (Yang) (p. 17) forming the heavens (Hume, 1940; Wong & Wu, 1936). Yin and Yang represent opposite complementary qualities or stages in the process of change and transformation of all things (Xie & Huang, 1988).

The symbol for Yin literally means the dark side of the hill (Maciocia, 1989). Yin represents the passive, darker elements and phenomena. Although the categorization as Yin or Yang is relative, constituents of Yin traditionally include darkness, femaleness, earth, water, and inside (Hume, 1940; Maciocia, 1989) (see Table 12.1).

Literally translated, Yang means the sunny side of the hill. Yang represents elements symbolizing warmth, light, strength, and life. Concepts generally considered as Yang include maleness, light,

### Table 12.1
### Categorizations as Yin and Yang

| Yin | Yang |
| --- | --- |
| Female | Male |
| Darkness | Light |
| Rest | Movement |
| Earth | Heaven |
| Water | Fire |
| Cold | Warm |
| Produces form | Produces energy |
| Right | Left |
| North | South |

movement, and heaven. (Hume, 1940; Maciocia, 1989; Xie & Huang, 1988) (see Table 12.1).

Yin and Yang have four aspects that describe the manner in which they are interrelated: (1) opposition, (2) interdependence, (3) mutual consumption, and (4) intertransformation. All of these aspects can be seen in the traditional symbol of Yin and Yang (Hume, 1940; Maciocia, 1989; Xie & Huang, 1988) (see Figure 12.1).

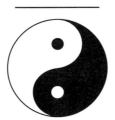

### Figure 12.1
### Symbol for Yin and Yang

The aspect of opposition describes the relative nature of Yin and Yang. Anything is categorized as Yin or Yang only as it is related to something else. Nothing is considered to be totally Yin or Yang. As demonstrated by Figure 12.1, within Yin there is a seed of Yang, and within Yang there is a seed of Yin (Hume, 1940; Maciocia, 1989; Xie & Huang, 1988).

Interdependence refers to the concept that neither Yin nor Yang can exist without the other. The opposite forces of Yin and Yang exist within everything; they are mutually exclusive, yet they are interdependent. Mutual consumption refers to the dynamic nature of Yin and Yang. With either Yin or Yang is out of balance, the other is influenced and changes proportion in an effort to achieve balance. Intertransformation also describes the dynamic and constantly changing nature of Yin and Yang. Yin transforms into Yang as Yang transforms into Yin. (Hume, 1940; Maciocia, 1989; Xie & Huang, 1988). Thus, the principle of Yin and Yang reflects the integral and relative nature of a universe marked by dynamic constant change to maintain balance and harmony as it evolves.

The four aspects of Yin and Yang are quite similar, in their representations of the dynamic nature of the world, to the homeodynamic principles. Like the Principles of Integrality and Helicy, Yin and Yang represent continuous dynamic change marked by constant interplay and mutuality of fields. The aspects of Yin and Yang do not suggest the trend toward increasing diversity and frequency that is proposed by the Science of Unitary Human Beings. Yin-Yang represents the dynamic nature of change; Rogers' Science of Unitary Human Beings further proposes the direction of the evolutionary process.

### Five Elements (Wu Xing)

The five elements (Wu Xing) are: (1) water, (2) fire, (3) wood, (4) metal, and (5) earth. They are representative of the five types of resonances or qualities in the universe. Literally translated, Wu means five and Xing means movement, process, to go, or to conduct behavior (Maciocia, 1989). Thus, the five elements can also be considered five processes, qualities, phases of a cycle, or inherent capabilities for change (Maciocia, 1989). Each of the five elements has basic qualities, as illustrated by the following quote from Shang Shu (c. 659–627 B.C.):

> Water moistens downward, fire flares
> upwards, wood can be bent and
> straightened, metal can be molded and
> can harden, earth permits sowing,
> growing and reaping. That which soaks
> and descends (water) is salty. That
> which blazes upwards (fire) is bitter,
> that which can be bent and straightened
> (wood) is sour, that which can be molded
> and become hard (metal) is pungent,
> That which permits sowing and reaping
> (earth) is sweet.
>
> (Cited in [Practical Chinese
> Medicine], 1975, p. 32)

Thus, the elements symbolize five different inherent qualities and states of natural phenomena. The elements also symbolize all phenomena in the universe that have similar resonance characteristics. For example, they symbolize corresponding directions of movements of natural phenomena as well as stages of a seasonal cycle. Each season is associated with an aspect of the cycle of life, and each of the elements corresponds to a body organ. The Chinese conception of organs differs from the meaning used by Western medicine. In Chinese healing, each organ is a system incorporating the anatomical aspects, the interrelationships between organs, and the corresponding natural phenomena. The main function of the organs within Chinese healing theories is to facilitate the production and movement of vital substances such as Qi and Essence (see below). Selected correspondences of the five elements are presented in Table 12.2 (Hume, 1940; Maciocia, 1989; Xie & Huang, 1988).

*The Five Elements' Interrelationships.* The interrelationships of the five elements, as well as their corresponding phenomena, are described by five sequences:

1. The cosmological sequence.
2. The generating sequence.
3. The controlling sequence.
4. The overacting sequence.
5. The insulting sequence.

## Table 12.2
## Correspondences of the Five Elements

| Correspondences | Water | Wood | Fire | Earth | Metal |
|---|---|---|---|---|---|
| Basic Quality | Moistens Downward | Sour | Flares Upward | Sowing, Growing, Reaping | Pungent |
| Movement | Downward | Expansive-Outward | Upward | Neutrality/ Stability | Contractive-Inward |
| Season | Winter | Spring | Summer | Late Season | Autumn |
| Stage of Development | Storage | Birth | Growth | Transformation | Harvest |
| Yin Organs | Kidneys | Liver | Heart | Spleen | Lungs |
| Emotions | Fear | Anger | Joy | Pensiveness | Sadness |
| Sounds | Groaning | Shouting | Laughing | Singing | Crying |
| Yin-Yang | Utmost Yin | Lesser Yang | Utmost Yang | Center | Lesser Yin |
| Direction | North | East | South | Center | West |

Adapted from *The Foundations of Chinese Medicine*, by Giovanni Maciocia. 1989. New York: Churchill Livingstone.

These sequences evolved from many centuries of observations, by ancient Chinese, of the relationships among natural phenomena. The Chinese identified in the functional systems of the human body relationships and characteristics similar to those observed in nature. They applied these characteristics of the natural environment to the human body's functional systems. For example, plants cannot grow without water. The characteristic of plants is wood since many plants are woody in their nature. Therefore, water generates wood. A basic necessity for fire is a flammable substance such as wood. Therefore, wood generates fire. After a fire, especially when grasslands and forests are burned, there is good earth for farming. Therefore, fire generates earth. Metal is acquired from earth or rock. Therefore, earth generates metal. A well can be dug by using metal tools; a river can be channeled for irrigation by using metal tools. Therefore, metal generates water. These relationships are extended to the human body's functional systems, and each functional system has an identity of an element (Yin & Zhang, 1991). This cycle is continuous.

There is a sequence of control among the five elements. It is interpreted that wood—or plants, generally—take their nutrition from earth or soil. Therefore, wood controls earth. When water becomes a flood, earth can be used to stop flooding. Therefore, earth controls water. Water is used to put out fires. Therefore, water controls fire. In order to make tools, metal must first be melted using fire. Thus, fire controls metal. The tools made by different kinds of metal can be used to cut wood or other plants. Thus metal controls wood (Yin & Zhang, 1991). When these relationships are applied to the human body's functional systems, the same sequences apply.

The cosmological sequence emphasizes the importance of water as the basis of the sequence. The corresponding organ is the kidney, and this emphasizes the importance of the kidneys as the grounding or basis for all other organs. The generating sequence describes the manner in which each element generates or creates another. As illustrated in Figure 12.2, water generates wood; wood generates fire; fire generates earth; earth generates metal; metal generates water. If the names of the corresponding organs are substituted for the elements, then kidney generates liver; liver generates heart; heart generates spleen; spleen generates lung; lung generates kidney. The purpose of the controlling sequence is to maintain balance among the elements. As illustrated in Figure 12.2, water controls fire, which controls metal, which controls wood,

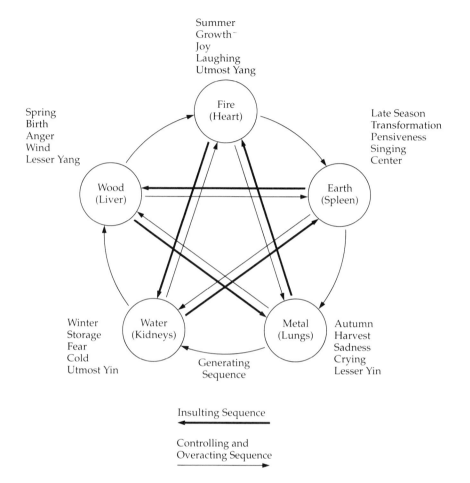

**Figure 12.2**
**Five Element Sequences with Correspondences**

which controls earth, which controls water. Concurrently, the kidneys control the heart, the heart controls the lungs, the lungs control the liver, the liver controls the spleen, and the spleen controls the kidneys. Thus, between the generating sequence and the controlling sequence, the balance of the universe is maintained at both the macro and micro levels. The overacting and insulting sequences deal with relationships among the elements when balance is lost.

The overacting sequence follows the same pattern as the controlling sequence but allows one element to overact or to overcontrol the target element. The insulting sequence operates in the reverse direction of the overacting sequence, allowing suppression of the various elements (Maciocia, 1989; Wong and Wu, 1936; Xie & Huang, 1988).

Thus, each element brings its correspondences with it to the sequences. These correspondences represent the Chinese belief of similarity of resonances (and, therefore, characteristics) within each set of correspondences. Through the correspondences, the sequences are extrapolated to the greater universe, thus explaining the balance of the cosmos (Maciocia, 1989; Xie & Huang, 1988).

*The Five Elements and the Science of Unitary Human Beings.* An immediate area of incongruity with the Science of Unitary Human Beings is the causality presented as one element controls another. Although the concept of one element controlling another is causal on the surface, this apparent causality may be an artifact of the difficult process of translating from Chinese into English. Rather than suggesting causation, the intent of the sequences of the elements is to demonstrate the nature of the balance of the individual human being, as well as the universe. Through the five elements and their correspondences, Chinese healing demonstrates the integrality of the universe—the belief that all within the universe, while different, is also the same. The Science of Unitary Human Beings proposes that all in the universe is composed of energy fields—distinguishable one from the other by pattern, but still energy fields. Chinese healing theories would seem to take this idea a step further, proposing that the five elements represent groupings of elements with similar resonances and patterns—again, different in pattern but ultimately the same.

### Vital Substances

Chinese medicine views the functioning of human beings as involving the interrelationships of four vital substances: (1) Qi, (2) Blood, (3) Essence, and (4) Body fluids. Qi, the basis of all the vital substances, manifests itself in varying degrees of condensation or materiality (Maciocia, 1989).

*Qi (Chi).* Qi (a concept with no literal English translation) refers to the energy that makes up all aspects of the universe. Qi has been alternately referred to as vital force, ether, or life force. The Chinese symbol incorporates the symbols for steam and rice indicating that Qi is a subtle or rarefied substance (steam) which is derived from a material or coarse substance (rice). Qi is given several attributes. Qi is proposed as the substance that composes the entire universe. As Qi comes together or condenses, it forms the more material aspects, such as matter; as Qi disperses, it forms the more immaterial aspects such as the heavens or the mind (shen). Wang Cheng (27-97 A.D.) described this process:

> Qi produces the human body just as water
> becomes ice. As water freezes into ice,
> so Qi coagulates to form the human body.
> When ice melts, it becomes water. When a
> person dies, he or she becomes spirit
> (shen) again. It is called spirit, just
> as melted ice changes its name to water.
> (Cited in Wing Tsit Chan, 1969, p. 300)

Thus, all that is consists of Qi in some state of rarefication or condensation. Furthermore, Chinese philosophy proposes that Qi can neither be created nor destroyed but only transformed. This is illustrated by Zhang Zai (1020-1077 A.D.) in his description of birth and death.

> Every birth is a condensation, every death a dispersal. Birth is not a gain, death not a loss . . . when condensed, Qi becomes a living being, when dispersed, it is the substration of mutations.
> (Cited in Fung Yu Lan, 1966, p. 280)

Qi is proposed to be a continuous form of matter, with the characteristics of the matter determined by the state of condensation of Qi. Lei Zi (300 B.C.) stated: "The purer lighter tending upwards, made the heaven, the grosses and heavier, tending downwards, made the earth." (Cited in Needham, 1956, p. 372).

Qi takes six forms in order to carry out its various functions:

1. Original Qi (Yang Qi).
2. Food Qi (Gu Qi).
3. Gathering Qi (Zung Qi).
4. True Qi (Zhen Qi).
5. Nutritive Qi (Ying Qi).
6. Defensive Qi (Wei Qi).

Original Qi (Yang Qi) provides the vitality and dynamic nature of all visceral functions. It is closely related to essence and is sometimes considered to be essence in the form of Qi. Original Qi is nourished by postheaven essence (Maciocia, 1989; Xie & Huang, 1988).

Food Qi (Gu Qi) or food energy is a coarse form of Qi that represents the first stage in the transformation of food into energy (Qi). This relatively direct relationship provides the base for the close association between food and health, as well as for the use of herbal medicine in Chinese healing modalities (Maciocia, 1989; Xie & Huang, 1988).

Gathering Qi (Zung Qi)—also known as ancestral Qi, original Qi, genetic Qi, or pectoral Qi—consists of food Qi combined with air. Stored in the belly, it nourishes the heart and lungs and provides the dynamic force needed for respiration and speech. Thus, if one's voice is weak, gathering Qi may be depleted or weak (Maciocia, 1989; Xie & Huang, 1988).

True Qi (Zhen Qi) is composed of the combination of the individual's unborn vital energy and the energy acquired from air and food. This combined energy represents the last stage in the refinement and transformation of Qi and serves as the dynamic force underlying all vital functions (Maciocia, 1989; Xie & Huang, 1988).

True Qi can take the form of either nutritive Qi or defensive Qi. Nutritive Qi (Ying Qi), also referred to as constructive Qi, flows with blood through the vessels or channels, providing nourishment and dynamic force to all the organs (Maciocia, 1989; Xie & Huang, 1988).

Defensive Qi (Wei Qi), a coarser form of Qi than nutritive Qi, circulates outside the conduits or channels permeating skin and muscles. Defensive Qi protects the body from pathogens, such as wind, cold, and damp, thus providing the individual with resistance. Furthermore, defensive Qi serves to regulate body temperature (Maciocia, 1989; Xie & Huang, 1988).

*Qi and the Science of Unitary Human Beings.* The concept of Qi bears a strong resemblance to the Rogerian concept of energy fields. Qi, within Chinese theories, and energy fields, within the Rogerian abstract system, are proposed as the material of which the cosmos is made. The descriptions of how Qi and energy fields comprise the universe differ slightly, but it is difficult to determine whether this is a true theoretical difference or only an artifact of translation. Within the Science of Unitary Human Beings, human beings and the environment are composed of energy fields that are distinguishable one from the other by pattern. Thus, various fields manifest themselves in patterns differing infinitely in amplitude, frequency, and wave form. Qi, the Chinese building block, similarly presents a variety of manifestations in a range of rarefication or condensation. Possibly, rarefication and condensation are alternate ways of expressing wave form pattern.

## Essence (Jing)

One aspect of Qi is essence or refined essence. Essence is something derived from a process of refinement or distillation. Three contexts of essence are identified in Chinese medicine: (1) Pre-Heaven Essence (the essence one is born with), (2) Post-Heaven Essence (the essence acquired from food, air, and so on), and (3) The Essence (or Kidney Essence) (Maciocia, 1989; Xie & Huang, 1988).

*Pre-Heaven Essence (Congenital Essence).* Pre-Heaven Essence is acquired by the individual at conception. It originates with the blending of the sexual energies of man and woman. Since pre-heaven essence is essentially inherited from parents, it can be influenced only with difficulty in adult life (Maciocia, 1989; Xie & Huang, 1988).

*Post-Heaven Essence (Acquired Essence).* Post-Heaven Essence is refined and extracted from food and fluid after birth. Post-heaven essence, acquired after birth, is substantially influenced by digestion and is closely related to the energies that modulate the functioning of the stomach and spleen (Maciocia, 1989; Xie & Huang, 1988).

*The Essence (Kidney Essence).* The Essence is derived from Pre- and Post-Heaven Essence. Pre-Heaven Essence contributes the person's hereditary constitution. Post-heaven essence serves the role of replenishing the essence. It derives the name Kidney Essence since it is thought to reside in the kidney; however, the fluid nature of essence suggests that it constantly circulates throughout the body.

*Essence versus Qi.* Although Essence and Qi are very similar, there are some noteworthy differences. Essence is fluid-like; Qi is energy-like. Essence is replenished with difficulty; Qi is easily replenished. Essence follows long cycles (seven or eight years); Qi follows shorter cycles (yearly or shorter). Essence changes slowly; Qi changes quickly. These differences are of critical importance in the context of therapeutic modalities (Maciocia, 1989).

*Essence and the Science of Unitary Human Beings.* Essence, an aspect or manifestation of Qi, provides a description of the individual's acquisition and utilization of Qi or energy. The nature of Essence also has implications for the process of altering energy or Qi. As such,

Essence can be compared to energy fields within the Science of Unitary Human Beings. However, congruity between the two abstract systems is somewhat lacking in this area. Rogers describes human beings as energy fields, but the means by which such energy fields come into being is not addressed. Nor does Rogers address the patterns of energy utilization or the flow evidenced in Chinese healing theories—an apparent point of divergence, or at least of inconsistency, between the Science of Unitary Human Beings and Chinese healing theories.

## Blood and Body Fluids

*Blood.*    Blood is seen in Chinese healing as a condensed form of Qi (Maciocia, 1989). The production of Blood is accomplished by the transformation of food essence or nutrients in the spleen and stomach, facilitated by the vital Essence of the kidney. Blood, nourished by food essence, originates from congenital essence (Maciocia, 1989; Xie & Huang, 1988). Blood, flowing with Qi throughout the body, nourishes the body. Blood moistens the body tissues and provides the harbor or foundation within which the mind flourishes (Maciocia, 1989; Xie & Huang, 1988). Qi is essential in the formation of blood and provides the energy that moves blood. Qi maintains the blood within vessel walls and is itself nourished by blood (Maciocia, 1989; Wong and Wu, 1936).

*Body Fluids (Jin Ye).*    Body fluids, derived from the same source as blood, encompass all liquids within the living organism and provide a general term for referring to saliva, tears, and urine, as well as liquid nutrients (Maciocia, 1989; Xie & Huang, 1988). Body fluids are purified and separated by the spleen, lungs, kidneys, and small intestine. Impure fluids are transformed into urine and eliminated (Maciocia, 1989).

Two types of body fluids exist within Chinese healing theories: (1) Jin and (2) Ye. Jin are composed of the thin, clear fluids that are distributed primarily over the exterior of the body. Serving to moisten and nourish skin and muscles, these fluids include tears, sweat, mucous, and saliva (Maciocia, 1989; Xie & Huang, 1988). Ye include thick, turbid fluids that are stored in body cavities. Rather than circulate with Qi, they lubricate areas such as the joints, spine, and brain.

*Body Fluids and Qi.*    Qi transforms and transports body fluids, thus preventing their undesirable accumulation. Simultaneously, Qi contains the body fluids within the appropriate spaces. Conversely, the body fluids contribute to the nourishment of Qi. If body fluids are deficient, Qi also becomes deficient (Maciocia, 1989; Xie & Huang, 1988).

*Blood, Body Fluids, and the Science of Unitary Human Beings.*   That the Chinese characters for these substances translate into the English words *blood* and *body fluids* is truly unfortunate. These English words conjure up images of Western physiology's red corpuscles, mucous, and saliva; they represent a particulate view of human beings that is conceptually incongruent with the Science of Unitary Human Beings. However, these translations may not fully capture the Chinese meaning of these concepts. Blood and body fluids represent more condensed forms of Qi within Chinese healing. As such, they may represent both the red fluid coursing through the arteries and the flow of Qi. One must ask whether viewing only the blood or body fluid is particulate, or whether the blood is a pattern manifestation of the whole. Rogerian scholars deal with similar conflicts when they debate what is a manifestation of pattern of the whole versus what is particulate (Cowling, 1991). Chinese healing theories may provide a model for dealing with such duality of meaning.

## CHINESE THERAPEUTIC MODALITIES

Chinese healing modalities have evolved over time in accord with supporting theoretical and philosophical bases. These modalities strongly emphasize the promotion of well-being. Chinese therapeutics have been developed as ways to help the individual maintain a balance of Qi, as well as a balance with the universe. An ancient Chinese proverb reads:

> The superior doctor prevents sickness; the mediocre doctor attends to impending sickness; the inferior doctor treats actual sickness (Hume, 1940, p. 60).

Although this may sound like illness prevention in Western modality, it is important to remember that, in Chinese philosophy, illness is defined as imbalance of Qi, the life force. Examples of modalities to maintain or reestablish balance include acupuncture, Taijiquan, and Qigong. These modalities are intended to facilitate the establishment of patterns of harmony and balance.

## Acupuncture

The goal of acupuncture is to access the channels through which true Qi circulates, in order to manipulate flow and to achieve harmonious and balanced flow. The practice of acupuncture dates back to as early as the twenty-first century B.C. Using sharp objects initially and needles more recently, the acupuncturists pricked certain areas to achieve cures for various ailments. Specifically, the areas pricked fell along meridians or channels through which Qi flows. Twelve meridians, symmetrically distributed bilaterally over the body, are currently recognized. Each meridian has numerous acupuncture points (Lo & Tsui, 1984). By needling these points, the flow of Qi is manipulated to restore balance and harmony, thereby facilitating health and well-being.

## Taijiquan

Taijiquan, a martial art, is directed at supporting and balancing Qi. It is practiced by individuals of all ages, including the very young and the very old. Consistent with the principles of Yin and Yang, it emphasizes the interplay of softness and dynamism of movement (Ying-hua & Yueh-liang, 1988). Historically, the regimen included 88 forms; however, over time, an alternate 24-form version has been developed. In Taijiquan, the individual focuses on the movement and the center, feeling the energy flow through the body. Postures are natural and relaxed, and the mind is tranquil yet alert. Various exercises are designed to facilitate the flow of Qi through the body (*Traditional Chinese Fitness Exercises,* 1984). Taijiquan has been proposed as a modality useful in positively influencing Pre-Heaven Essence, thus supporting one basic constitutional makeup (Maciocia, 1989). It is often practiced simultaneously with Qigong.

## Qigong

Qigong is a set of exercises proposed for the old and middle-aged. Primarily focusing on breathing, Qigong also involves a set of movements. It is intended to be an outside exercise performed in the morning in an environment of sun and fresh air, preferably near water. Qigong is purported to be beneficial for the entire body, effectively preventing and curing disease as well as facilitating health. Qigong is reputed to facilitate recovery of the ill, to strengthen the weak, and to prolong the life of the healthy (Guoquan, 1989). Indeed, the practice of Qigong is considered to be one way to positively influence pre-heaven essence (Maciocia, 1989). To successfully practice Qigong, the individual must eliminate distracting thoughts, concentrating on the exercise, and allow the mind to lead the exercise. Thus, the mind is joined with the Qi or vital energy. Breathing must be gentle, even, and slow, marked by deep abdominal inhalation and exhalation. The individual should relax every part of the body, proceed through the exercises with correct posture and rhythm, and alternate relaxation with tension. Names of Qigong exercises are highly descriptive: "White Crane Spreads Wings," "Horse-Ride Breathing," and "Golden Rooster Stands on One Leg" reflect the intrinsic tie of the practice of Qigong to the greater universe (Guoquan, 1989).

Qigong differs from Taijiquan in that Qigong emphasizes the breathing as a means of replenishing Qi. Concentration is needed to maintain a focus of attention on the breathing and movement, and Qigong is targeted to middle and older adult populations. Only with age does the individual develop the maturity to maintain the necessary concentration. This is highly congruent with the Rogerian view of unitary human change. However, it should be noted that the Chinese utilize chronological aging as a marker for development. This is incongruent with the nonlinearity inherent in the Science of Unitary Human Beings.

## CHINESE HEALING THEORIES AND THE SCIENCE OF UNITARY HUMAN BEINGS

Chinese healing theories and Rogers' Science of Unitary Human Beings have areas of congruence and noncongruence. Furthermore, each provides proposed relationships not addressed by the other. The concept of Qi bears strong resemblance to the concept of energy fields. Just as the universe is composed of energy fields (human and environmental) according to the Science of Unitary Human Beings, the universe is composed of Qi within the Chinese abstract system. Within Rogers' abstract system, energy fields are identified by pattern perceived as a single wave form. Pattern is an abstraction, which cannot be seen in and of itself. Rather, manifestations of pattern are perceived (Rogers, 1986, 1992). Similarly, Qi is not perceived in and of itself. Rather, it is the manifestations of Qi that are observable.

Rogers' principles of homeodynamics also reflect some congruence with Chinese healing theories. The Principle of Integrality, which describes the continuous mutual process between human and environmental energy fields, is highly congruent with Chinese healing theories. In the concept of Qi and in the correspondences and interrelatedness of the five elements, traditional Chinese healing is grounded within a world-view that accepts the integral and unitary nature of the universe.

Chinese healing theories also imply congruency with the Principle of Helicy. Rogers (1986, 1990, 1992, 1993) proposed that human development is characterized by increasing complexity and diversity and that change is continuous and unpredictable. The concept of Yin-Yang describes the dynamic and constantly changing balance inherent in the universe. Specifically, the concept of Yin and Yang portrays a dynamic balance and harmony marked by constant change. The consistencies between Chinese healing theories and the Principle of Helicy can also be seen in specific therapeutic modalities. The suggested restriction of the use of Qigong to adults of middle and old age would indicate that the increasing complexity of age allows the practice of Qigong to be of greater benefit.

## ROGERIAN HEALING MODALITIES AND CHINESE HEALING THEORIES

Noninvasive health patterning modalities utilized within the Rogerian science are congruent with Chinese healing theories and may have potential for use within Chinese medicine. Therapeutic Touch is a therapy based on awareness of human energy fields through the mutual process of fields (touch) (Krieger, 1975). This modulation, aimed at achieving harmonious flow of energy, can be compared in some respects to the therapy of acupuncture so common in Chinese healing. Therapeutic Touch could perhaps provide a noninvasive alternative for Chinese medicine. Simultaneously, acupuncture could provide a complementary modality to be used in addition to Therapeutic Touch. Such potential mutual benefits are worthy of further investigation.

Relaxation and imagery modalities also exhibit congruence with Chinese healing theories. Relaxation and imagery are both intended as means by which individuals can center and change their energy fields (Krieger, 1981). The turning into the field and "concentration on being" utilized in relaxation and imagery is very similar to the concentration and direction of thought utilized in the practice of Qigong. This similarity would suggest a potential for utilization of relaxation and imagery within Chinese healing theories. Furthermore, Qigong and other Chinese exercise modalities may provide healing techniques consistent with the Rogerian abstract system.

Only in their extensive emphasis on body organs do Chinese healing theories seem to diverge from the world-view undergirding the Science of Unitary Human Beings. Yet, this divergence may be only an artifact of translation. As previously discussed, the five elements have corresponding body organs. However, Maciocia (1989) cautions that, when studying Chinese healing theories, the Western interpretation of body organs must be disregarded. Within Chinese healing theories, body organs exist as complex systems integral with the corresponding emotions, colors, climate, and season. Thus, the heart is integral with summer, the color red, growth, birds, the tongue, joy, and laughing, among other correspondences. If one suspends one's Western perception of body and adopts the Chinese perception of organs as integral with the universe, then the perspective of organs is unitary rather than particulate. Indeed, the theoretical model for Chinese healing may even provide a model by which Rogerian scholars can articulate pattern manifestations of the more condensed aspects of the human field while avoiding the hazard of seemingly particulate conceptualization. Following this line of thinking, body organs may be seen as condensed forms of energy (Qi) within the human field. Similarly, condensations and rarefications of the human field could be conceptualized as manifestations of pattern. By demonstrating the dynamic and integral nature of organs, such a model could open portholes for investigation into phenomena now avoided because of their apparent particulate nature.

Although care must be taken to avoid mixing these two abstract conceptual systems, each does provide models for the other. By closer examination of Chinese healing theories, insight into the controversies of the Science of Unitary Human Beings may be gained.

## REFERENCES

Cowling, R. (1991). Presentation and discussion at the fall meeting of Region 7 of the Society of Rogerian Scholars, Pigeon Forge, TN.

Fung Yu Lan. (1966). *A short history of Chinese philosophy.* New York: Macmillan.

Guoquan, Y. (1989). Characteristics of three-bath qigong. In Lui Yu Xian (Ed.), *Three-Bath Qigong.* Hong Kong: Hai Feng Publishing Co.

Hume, E.H. (1940). *The Chinese Way in medicine*. Baltimore: The Johns Hopkins University Press.

Krieger, D. (1975). Therapeutic Touch: The imprimatur of nursing. *American Journal of Nursing, 5*, 784–787.

Krieger, D. (1981). *Foundations for holistic health nursing practices: The renaissance nurse*. Philadelphia: Lippincott.

Lo, C.K., & Tsui, S.K. (1984). *Acupuncture in clinical practice*. Hong Kong: The Commercial Press.

Maciocia, G. (1989). *The foundations of Chinese medicine*. New York: Churchill Livingstone.

Needham, J. (1956). *Science and civilization in China, Vol. 2*. Cambridge, England: Cambridge University Press.

*Practical Chinese medicine*. (1975). Shi Yong Zhong Yi Xuen. Beijing Publishing House: Beijing.

Rogers, M.E. (1986). Science of Unitary Human Beings. In V.M. Malinski (Ed.), *Explorations on Martha Rogers' Science of Unitary Human Beings* (pp. 3–8). Norwalk, CT: Appleton-Century-Crofts.

Rogers, M.E. (1990). Nursing: Science of Unitary, Irreducible, Human Beings: Update 1990. In E.A. Barrett (Ed.), *Visions of Rogers' science-based nursing* (pp. 5–11). New York: National League for Nursing.

Rogers, M.E. (1992). Glossary update. *Rogerian Nursing Science News, 4*(3), 7.

Rogers, M.E. (1993). An interview with Martha Rogers: Surfing in the year 3001. *South Carolina Surfer, 1*(4), 1, 9.

*Traditional Chinese fitness exercises* (1984). Beijing: New World Press.

Wing Tsit Chan. (1969). *A source book of Chinese philosophy*. Princeton: Princeton University Press.

Wong, K.C., & Wu, L. (1936). *History of Chinese medicine* (2nd ed.). Shanghai: National Quarantine Service.

Xie, Z., & Huang, X. (Eds.). (1988). *Beijing Medical College dictionary of traditional Chinese medicine*. Hong Kong: The Commercial Press.

Yin, H., & Zhang, B. (1991). *The fundamental theory of Chinese medicine* (2nd ed.). Beijing: People's Health Press.

Ying-hua, W., & Yueh-liang, M. (1988). *Wu style Taichichuan: Forms, concepts, and application of the original style*. Hong Kong: Shanghai Book Co.

# 13

# Unitary Human Football Players

*Nancey E. M. France*

Football is a macho, no-pain/no-gain sport played at middle schools, high schools, and universities across the country. Winning each game is definitely a goal shared by players and coaches. Although striving for a win is an expectation, the process of winning may become a hindering experience.

The football environment is very volatile during practice and at game time. Completed plays are praised and applauded. Missed plays are openly admonished and chastised. Injuries bring about despair and pain. Consequently, moods and emotions rush like a roller coaster from the extremes of exhilaration and jubilation to frustration, gloom, and intolerance. One incorrect play or one screaming coach can quickly send out a ripple that engulfs the entire team. Yet, certain tactics prevail among coaches teaching the sport, in order to secure the outcome of winning.

This chapter reflects how Rogerian science has guided my practice with a university football team. This nursing practice is most assuredly nontraditional and is creating new images of nursing for the present and the future. Rogers (1990) stated: "The purpose of nurses is to promote health and well-being for all persons wherever they are. The art of nursing is the creative use of the science of nursing for human betterment" (p. 5).

## FOOTBALL AS EXPLORED THROUGH ROGERIAN SCIENCE

The football team consists of 90 to 120 male players and seven or eight coaches. The majority of the players are young men who are in the same developmental stage, vacillating between adolescence and young adulthood. Most of these players have played high school football; a few are beginning their experience as walk-ons. A great number of individuals are recruited and awarded scholarships to play at the university level. The scholarships pay for a majority of their educational expenses in return for the individuals' playing football for the university as long as they are eligible. These young men choose to play football because they like the sport and/or it pays for their college education. Everyone's objective early in the season is to have a winning season.

Coaches remain coaches based on their success each year. Success is usually marked by a higher number of wins than of losses. Little attention is given to how those wins are achieved. The main objective of the head coach and his assistants is to have a winning season. A winning season brings fame and fortune to the school by increasing ticket sales, booster support, recruitment of students and future players, and renewed coaching contracts.

Although all interested individuals share the desire for a winning season, each player brings his own expectations and past experiences to the team. The team, as an energy field, may be viewed two ways:

1. It may be regarded as a group field, a single, indivisible team-as-group field where players and coaches are one in mutual process with the environmental field.

2. Everything other than the team can be regarded as its environment (Rogers, 1990, p. 8).

An example of the team-as-group field occurs during the game, when there is a home team and a visitor/opponent.

When focusing on the players and coaches as individuals, the individual energy fields are integral with the environmental field, which includes the team (Rogers, 1990, p. 9). Each team player is a unique energy field in mutual process with the environmental field. Players and coaches are continuously in mutual process with their environmental fields, which encompass the team. Each individual player is an energy field different from the sum of parts, and the team-as-group field is different from the sum of parts; thus, the team is a very dynamic field. Rogers stated, "Regardless of the group identified, the group field is irreducible and indivisible to itself and integral with its own environmental field. . . . The principles of homeodynamics postulate the nature of group field change just as they postulate the nature of individual field change" (p. 8).

Whereas the expectation of winning the game is shared, the players' expectations of the *process* of winning may differ from the coaches' expectations. Everyone anticipates a certain protocol for practice: a profusion of sweat and repetitive drills to enhance each player's ability to transfer the Xs and Os from paper to the field. In preparing for practice, coaches watch films and sketch out plays that they hope will lead to first downs, field goals, and touchdowns. Players study and memorize the plays for implementation on the field. Coaches then scrutinize and analyze the quality of the plays.

Although practice and games involve much hard work and physical pain, the past experiences of learning the sport seem to prejudice the temperament of practice and game time. When most coaches coach football, they imitate the manner in which they were coached. If, as players, they were subjected to strategies that achieved results through tactics that were sarcastic or demeaning in nature, they probably will use the same strategies. Conventional strategies for winning, therefore, reflect familiar patterns from the relative past that were deemed to be successful in preventing mistakes. Examples include screaming criticism, either from across the field or while nose-to-nose with a player; cursing; offering sarcastic and cynical remarks; and inducing fear to gain respect. Consequently, this pattern of being does not allow or encourage the style of each individual player to emerge and reflect further actualization of unitary wholeness.

"The life process is homeodynamic" and we are always in mutual process (Rogers, 1970, p. 96). The human and environmental fields are continually participating with one another *whether knowingly or unknowingly.* The team-as-group field can unknowingly be a participant as certain pattern manifestations are revealed and become a major dynamic impetus within the mutual process. Although the pattern identifies the team and reflects its wholeness, the ambience of mutual process within the environmental field blinds players to this wholeness. Through the use of conventional strategies, therefore, the coaches have *unknowingly* patterned the mutual process with the team-as-group field.

What happens to the team as a manifestation of environmental field and team-as-group field when such strategies are implemented? In contrast to their recognition as unitary human beings, players are treated as pawns capable only of sensation and emotion. Recall the developmental status of these players. Self-esteem, esteem for others, motivation, and the desire to win take precedence over all else. Fear of failure and resentment may also emerge. Chronic injuries flare up and new injuries happen, but everyone still wants to win.

Another conventional strategy is employed with the team-as-group field. The team, as a single, indivisible field, is incited (or incites itself) to win against the opponent. Prior to game time, chanting may ensue: "Kill 'em," "Rip their heads off," "Tackle to hurt them bad enough to leave the game." This conventional strategy is an example of *knowingly* participating in deliberative mutual patterning. The intent is to enhance the team to become "fired up" and win.

When one appraises a football team within the framework of Rogers' Science of Unitary Human Beings, the energy seems chaotic. It must be remembered, however, that even in what appears to be chaos, energy fields evolve.

As an energy field, the human is an open system in continuous mutual process with the environmental energy field. Being aware of this universal life energy or the energy fields, the human can recognize alterations in the pattern of the human and environmental fields. Therefore, it is postulated that any change of the rhythmic pattern of one field is manifested in the pattern of the other field. In addition to discovering alterations in pattern, it is postulated that the human energy field can knowingly participate in the mutual process with the environmental field according to a vision of wholeness and unity. The new pattern emerges through the mutual process of energy fields (France, 1992, p. 8).

## EVOLUTION OF THE PRACTICE AS GUIDED BY ROGERIAN SCIENCE

The Therapeutic Touch (TT) process, developed by Krieger and Kunz (Krieger, 1979), is recommended by Rogers' (1970) as a nursing modality that can be used in the Science of Unitary Human Beings. Therapeutic Touch facilitates the flow of universal life energy to promote healing. It is an alternative, noninvasive method of healing that patterns the energy field of unitary human beings.

For the past four years, TT has been the primary modality of my nursing practice with a university football team. Rogers' Science of Unitary Human Beings has guided not only the use of TT and holistic treatment for football injuries, but also the implementation of strategies used in the mutual process with the team and coaches.

More than four years ago, when I embarked on this practice, I approached the head coach about doing TT for players with injuries.

He patiently and carefully listened to my explanation of the TT process and its scientific base. When I finished, being a new and exuberant head coach, he asked, "Will this help us win?" I explained to him that TT could decrease the healing time of injuries, which translated into the players' returning to the game sooner. Injuries are the most debilitating predicament for a team and the team, as a whole, would be at a better advantage if injuries healed faster. He liked the concept and granted me permission to begin. He told me that he would inform the head trainer that I would be working with the players and that I would explain the process to him.

Head trainers are similar to physicians. They "own" the players and have sole control over their injuries. Needless to say, the head trainer (nicknamed "Doc") was a little annoyed with the whole situation. He let me know immediately that he and the head coach had an agreement—he wouldn't call the plays, and the head coach wouldn't diagnose and treat injuries. I then explained to Doc that my work would not interfere at all with his work. I would use TT in addition to his treatments, and I would accommodate his routine. He smiled, told me that injuries were treated every morning at 7:00 A.M., and gave me the practice and game schedules.

Doc pretty much let me fumble along in the first few weeks of the season. People would ask him what I was doing, and he would answer, "Oh, it's some nursing energy thing. If you want to know anything about it, you'll have to ask her."

People in show business talk about their "big break." I got my own big break (not literally). At a game away from home, the star running back was injured. I immediately began treating him from a distance, and he was in first thing Monday morning to see me. He was a senior. It was his last year to play, and he didn't want an injury interfering with his last season. The team physician, who is an orthopedic surgeon, diagnosed the injury as a completely separated shoulder. The medical treatment for this type of injury is to immobilize the shoulder via a sling, and wait for six weeks.

I treated this player with TT twice a day. In addition, I taught him how to use visualization and other forms of imagery, and we monitored his diet. Ten days after treatment began, he walked into the training room and said to Doc, "Look what I can do." He took his sling off and showed how he had complete range of motion *without pain.* Doc looked at the player, then at me, and said, "Oh, my! It works."

That afternoon, the team physician came to practice. After the player exhibited his abilities, the team physician asked Doc, "What's going on here? What did you do to him?" Doc nonchalantly replied, "We've been doing TT [with] him."

"What in the world is TT?"

"Oh, don't you know? It has to do with physics and energy fields." Doc was now the expert and one of the biggest fans of my practice. He also requested that a file on TT research (Heidt, 1981; Keller & Bzdek, 1986; Quinn, 1984; Wright, 1987) be kept in his office. In that way, he had scientific reading material handy for skeptics who wandered into his training room.

The following week, I was very busy in the training room. Players who weren't newly injured brought their old injuries to me for treatment. Some just wanted to experience TT. Other athletes (other than football players) asked Doc if they could be treated. He said, "No. This is football season, and the head coach said that football players have top priority."

Doc was more helpful to me now. He triaged players to me. Imagine my surprise when I heard him say to the quarterback one morning, "Sit down and get your energy field assessed. You need to have this touch treatment." And so, TT came to be known in the training room as touch treatment.

I became much more involved with game time. Instead of just showing up when the game started, I was to be there one and a half hours prior to game time. I not only treated injuries and aches and pains of players, but the coaches wanted to be treated for anxiety. During TT treatments, I would explain to the players how TT helped to ground their energy so their anxiety would not get out of control. These players would then relate their experiences to others who would then come by just to try it once. They usually came back for more, phrasing their request and referred to as "Juice me up."

When I felt it was safe, I introduced healing at a distance. Doc didn't even blink an eye. An assistant trainer was assigned the task of signaling the injuries to me from the field. The head coach wanted me to be on the sidelines, but I decided that was too risky in such a conservative culture. (I sit in the front row in the stands, which allows me to be closer to the players when they are on the sidelines.)

During practice, I became attuned to the rhythms and patterns of the individuals and of the team as a whole, and I appraised them within the context of field performance. I observed that players and coaches used touch only when someone correctly completed a play or scored a touchdown. During missed plays, if touch was used, it was employed by coaches in shoving the player or in grabbing a face mask to make a point. During these circumstances, most players would not touch each other, speak to each other, or have eye contact with each other. When winning, everyone was in harmony. When losing, everyone was in disharmony. When this emerged during game time, winning became much more arduous but usually succumbed to losing.

I shared with the head coach my observations and appraisals on how the players needed to be aware of how they are participating in continuous mutual process with one another. I suggested using the caring aspects of touch throughout the game and particularly during the distressing times. An appropriate time to initiate touch is at the beginning of a play. This reminds the players that, as a team, they are one and are continually in mutual process with each other. I had also observed how the pattern of the Defense was more passionate in nature than the patterns of the Offense and the Special Teams. Their energy seemed more dynamic and bombarded everyone. I suggested to the coach that the Defense huddle in a circle, holding hands. The physical act of touching would serve as a reminder of how their energy fields are one. The coach implemented my suggestion during the next practice, and it has become the new pattern for the Defense.

The Offense is not of the same passionate nature as the Defense. It took me three years of assessing the rhythms and patterns of the Offense to discover a new pattern for them. Instead of huddling, the Offense now lines up in front of the quarterback with the center literally in the center of the line and bending forward. As the quarterback is relaying the play, he has both hands on the helmet of the center and has eye contact with each of the other players. This actually was the quarterback's own unique pattern. I explored with him how this pattern was manifested in the mutual process of the Offense. By sharing and implementing my knowledge of Rogerian science, I am increasing the team's awareness of the integrality of life and how that is manifested in all that they do.

I discovered that I had increased the awareness of others as well. The assistant trainer, who signals injuries from the field, asked me if there was something he could do on the field that might help. I taught him the beginning steps of TT. He was amazed at what he felt with his hands. He now clears or unruffles the energy field of the injured player before the injury is examined by the trainer or the physician. Prior to game time, the two of us review who is playing with an injury and plan our strategy. For example, the quarterback had a nagging ankle injury that flared up during practice. Although I had been treating the ankle, because of its chronicity, I suspected that he would experience trouble with it during the game. I advised the assistant trainer to unruffle the field each time the quarterback came off the football field to the sideline. The quarterback experienced no discomfort with his ankle and was able to play the entire game.

The practice was firmly established with the players and the trainers. The coaching staff was just beginning to follow suit when there was a big midyear turnover in coaches after the end of the season. The advent of spring football brought the same chaos of energy and disharmony I had observed four years earlier. My approach this time was to increase the coaches' awareness of mutual process and energy fields.

I observed every practice during the 15 days of spring football. I became attuned to the rhythms and patterns of the coaches and players and of the team as a whole, appraising them within the context of the mutual process between human and environmental energy fields. I then took the head coach to lunch and shared my observations and appraisals with him.

This time, I presented my appraisal strictly within the framework of Rogerian science. I shared with him the four postulates and the principles of homeodynamics—specifically, the Principle of Integrality.

I presented the role of coach within Rogers' conceptual framework and the practice trends as described by Malinski (1986). Although Malinski described practice trends within the role of the nurse, these trends have far greater implications. Through Rogerian science and Malinski's practice trends, coaches can knowingly participate in the mutual process of the team-as-environmental field. Through this process, they can enhance relationship and mutuality. The process of winning, therefore, encompasses:

1. Enhanced power of all individuals of the team.
2. Accepting diversity as the norm.
3. Becoming attuned to patterning.
4. Recognizing and using wave modalities such as touch, music, movement, and encouraging phrases as integral to the patterning process.
5. Viewing change as increasing diversity.

6. Accepting the integral mutual process of life. (Malinski, 1986, pp. 28–30)

We discussed the wave modalities of touch, music, movement, and encouragement. I emphasized the need for touch during disappointment and frustration; the need for coaches to actively participate in pre-game warm-up and in the demonstration of plays; and the need for encouragement at all times by all players and coaches.

When I finished, the coach looked at me and said, "How do I do this? I don't know how to do this. I'll need a lot of help in doing this." He then grinned and asked, "Will this help us to win?" I acknowledged the importance of the score, of counting and adding up the points. But I advised, "Remember what Einstein said. 'Not everything that matters can be counted. And not everything that can be counted, matters.'"

## SUMMARY

Through TT and Rogers' Science of Unitary Human Beings, players and coaches are learning the value of how to knowingly participate with one another as individuals and as a team. With this unitary approach to football, and when combining TT with traditional Western medicine practices, I have seen a decrease in pain, anxiety, and healing time of musculoskeletal injuries. I have seen an increase in the development of "team-oriented" relationships and of knowing participation between coaches and players, players and players, and coaches and coaches.

Research questions are created through this practice. Specific to TT, how does TT, when combined with traditional Western medicine practices, facilitate healing and decrease the healing time of acute football injuries as compared to the use of traditional Western medicine practices? Specific to Rogerian Science, how does TT and the presence of a nurse pattern the environment of any sport as compared to the traditional paternalistic sports environment?

As Malinski stated:

The Science of Unitary Human Beings presents a new worldview for nursing, one that requires a quantum leap from what we think we know to speculations about what might be. It suggests that total openness of experience, allowing us to reframe obstacles as opportunities. The dynamic, ever-changing dance of patterning with unitary human beings and their environments challenges us to find creative, innovative methods of practice. (1986, p. 30)

## REFERENCES

France, N. (1992). A phenomenological inquiry on the child's lived experience of perceiving the human energy field using therapeutic touch (doctoral dissertation, University of Colorado Health Sciences Center, 1991). *Dissertation Abstracts International, 52*(12), 6315-B.

Heidt, P. (1981). Effect of therapeutic touch on the anxiety level of hospitalized patients. *Nursing Research, 30*(1), 32–37.

Keller, E., & Bzdek, V. (1986). Effects of therapeutic touch on tension headache pain. *Nursing Research, 35*(2), 101–106.

Krieger, D. (1979). *The therapeutic touch: How to use your hands to help or heal.* Englewood Cliffs: Prentice-Hall.

Malinski, V. (1986). Nursing practice within the Science of Unitary Human Beings. In V. Malinski (Ed.), *Explorations on Martha Rogers' Science of Unitary Human Beings* (pp. 25–32). Norwalk: Appleton-Century-Crofts.

Quinn, J. (1984). Therapeutic touch as an energy exchange: Testing the theory. *Advances in Nursing Science, 6*(2), 42–49.

Rogers, M. (1970). *An introduction to the theoretical basis of nursing.* Philadelphia: F.A. Davis.

Rogers, M. (1990). Nursing: Science of Unitary, Irreducible Human Beings: Update 1990. In E.A.M. Barrett (Ed.), *Visions of Rogers' science-based nursing* (pp. 5–11). New York: National League for Nursing.

Wright, S. (1987). The use of therapeutic touch in the management of pain. In *Nursing Clinics of North America, 22*(3), 705–714.

# 14

# Rhythms of Living: A Rogerian Approach to Counseling

*Linda K. Tuyn*

Elizabeth Barrett (1992) was on target in her keynote address at the Fourth Rogerian Conference when she asserted that a revolution in health care is taking place. Indeed, an interdisciplinary revolution is under way. Renegades from several disciplines are alive, well, and practicing in the field quaintly referred to as "psychotherapy," challenging many of the traditional pathology-oriented assumptions of that field. The approach they are defining is called solution-focused (de Shazer, 1985, 1991) or solution-oriented therapy (O'Hanlon & Weiner-Davis, 1989). I was first introduced to these ideas and methods as the only nurse participating in a three-day intensive workshop for therapists. During breaks, I kept hearing psychologists, social workers, and psychiatrists murmuring, "Isn't this different? powerful? unique?" I kept thinking, "Isn't this *nursing?*" The approach seemed especially congruent with Rogerian nursing science. It allows the nurse to be both pragmatic and creative in assisting clients to fulfill their intentions, and it emphasizes client strengths and resources over pathology. In addition, it is based on the concepts of continuous change, mutable "realities," and unlimited possibilities.

In short, solution-oriented therapy puts forth a world-view similar to that of the Science of Unitary Human Beings and offers specific counseling methods that make Rogerian-based practice more helpful to clients. As Barrett (1990) stated, "In Rogerian nursing science, practice modalities concern human life patterning and reflect the wholeness of the unitary person in continuous innovative change with the universe" (p. 35). New modalities must be examined and tested for their "goodness of fit" with the most current knowledge in Rogerian science. Rawnsley (1985) has been helpful with ideas on designing pandimensional healing modalities consistent with Rogerian science that have some similarities to therapies previously used within a three-dimensional framework. However, Barrett (1990) pointed out that modalities that may be appropriate for patterning of human and environmental fields must also evolve from a new worldview consistent with the Science of Unitary Human Beings.

The purpose of this chapter is to articulate one of many possible answers to a question posed by Rogers (1992): "How can nurses best demonstrate imagination and ingenuity in helping people design ways to fulfill their different rhythmic patterns?" (p. 33). The first section will attempt to show "goodness of fit" of the solution-oriented approach with Rogerian nursing science by exploring their philosophical common ground and logical nursing implications. The second section will illustrate the phases of the Rogerian practice methodology as defined by Barrett (1988) through case examples using specific modalities. The application to practice will show how this approach is useful in a variety of counseling situations that extend beyond traditional mental health settings; it can apply in any situation where nurses and clients participate in creating solutions to human concerns.

## PHILOSOPHICAL COMMON GROUND: ROGERIAN AND SOLUTION-ORIENTED ASSUMPTIONS

Philosophically, the Science of Unitary Human Beings and solution-oriented therapy share common ground regarding at least four essential concepts: change, field uniqueness, rhythms and patterns, and power.

### Change

Rogerian and solution thinkers agree that change is inevitable and continuous (Barrett, 1990; de Shazer, 1991; Fisch, Weakland, & Segal, 1989; Furman & Ahola, 1992; Malinski, 1986; O'Hanlon & Weiner-Davis, 1989; Rogers, 1992). Barrett (1988) maintained that continuous change is the unifying concept in the practice application of Rogerian nursing science. As nurses, we are often helping clients deal with unwanted changes in their lives. We must, however, also be skilled at helping people recognize and use potentially helpful changes that may be going unnoticed. Constructionist philosophy teaches that we tend to dismiss that which is right in front of us (de Shazer, 1991), and practitioners of "solution talk" maintain that change does not exist for any useful purpose until someone notices it (Furman & Ahola, 1992). People and their environments are often changing in ways that can help them get through a difficult time, increase their competence and confidence, and achieve their goals. Attending to these changes is fully congruent with Rogerian nursing science.

## Field Uniqueness

All energy fields are unique in terms of field patterning and the human being's experience of the relative present (Malinski, 1986). O'Hanlon (1990) coined a wonderfully paradoxical phrase, "Everyone is an exception," to state this in solution-oriented terms. Change is continuous, and all human and environmental fields are unique. We live in a world of unlimited possibilities for synergistic evolution and for constructing solutions to human dilemmas.

## Rhythms and Patterns

One of the Rogerian concepts most useful in clinical practice deals with human and environmental rhythms; that is, rhythmic phenomena characterize all of life and represent a manifestation of unique field patterning (Malinski, 1986; Rogers, 1992). Put simply, people live their lives in rhythms and patterns that are continuously manifest in their day-to-day situations. Change theorists and solution-focused therapists emphasize that attention to patterns and rhythms provides many clues in helping people move toward their goals (de Shazer, 1985; O'Hanlon & Weiner-Davis, 1989; Watzlawick, Weakland, & Fisch, 1974; Zeig & Gilligan, 1990).

## Power

This author believes that an important purpose of nurse–client mutual process is to create a context in which clients experience power and confidence while working toward their goals. Rogerian and solution-oriented thinkers agree that people are resourceful and resilient in solving dilemmas, surviving difficulties, and creating satisfying lives for themselves. Our central challenge in nursing is to support that process. Therefore, a person's ability to change and to participate knowingly in change (Barrett's (1988) definition of power) must never be underestimated. Indeed, clients can actually be harmed by the use of pathological labels and frameworks that underestimate their abilities.

### Clinical Implications of Philosophical Assumptions

How do we use these philosophical assumptions in our nursing practice? Accepting the concepts of continuous change and field uniqueness requires us to let go of many of the expectations and generalizations we assign to our clients. Specifically, we must set aside our assumptions of what a person will be like based on his or her disease label, and how that person should feel, think, and act based on our own view of "good health." O'Hanlon (1990) noted that we must beware of "hardening of the categories" as we get to know our clients and their situations. It is also time to lay to rest the deadening concepts of "resistance" and "noncompliance" in our clients. Use of these words usually means consumers are not seeing their situations from the professional's point of view. Furman & Ahola (1992) found it more useful to consider that the client may be expressing "discontent with the [therapeutic] agenda" set up by the practitioner. "Resistance" and "noncompliance" may be better descriptives of clinicians who stubbornly insist that clients should fit their clinical frameworks and reality maps.

Another practice implication involves carefully observing and attuning to the unique strengths and resources of each client, or what O'Hanlon & Weiner-Davis (1989) refer to as the utilization approach. This simply means learning who this person is by recognition of his or her unique pattern manifestations and abilities, and using whatever is happening in the human and environmental fields to promote change in the desired direction. An example of the utilization approach is the use of guided imagery exercises in the classroom to promote learning (Tuyn, 1994). In a classroom situation, most students are in a state of reverie at one time or another; it is part of the mutual, simultaneous process involving the people present, the information shared, and their internal reflection on their relationship to process and content. Instead of fighting this tendency to "daydream," instructors can use the naturally hypnotic atmosphere of the classroom in designing brief, guided imagery exercises to encourage dialogue and enhance critical thinking. The discussion on modalities will offer nurse–client examples of the utilization approach. Additional cases are described elsewhere (Tuyn, 1992).

Finally, attention to rhythms of living may offer the most valuable clues for helping people make changes in the directions they choose. Rhythms are present in all of life, from the smallest subatomic scale to the movements of the heavens. They cannot be predicted or controlled, but we can observe them, formulate possibilities and plan actions accordingly. Regarding the human field, we recognize rhythms in many obvious ways: in all the body's systems, in eating and sleeping activities, in the ebb and flow of relationships, and in symptomatic or distressing experiences, to name but a few. There are three major points to note about human and environmental rhythms:

1. They are not things; they are processes that unfold in the ways we live our lives.
2. Many of our rhythms of living are habitual and exist out of our awareness for much of the time.
3. Symptomatic or distressing experiences alternate with periods of no or fewer symptoms or distress.

This last point is particularly relevant in counseling. For example, binging and vomiting can easily be seen as rhythmic; the important information may be the fact that these behaviors alternate with symptom-free periods as well. Someone who experiences depression usually has some "better days" that can be explored; the insomniac has nights of a bit more sleep; the parent notes a day when the children played well without fighting. Noting patterns of living, particularly paying attention to what is happening when life is going well or better, is perhaps the most useful aspect of the Rogerian and solution-oriented approaches. Appraisal from a Rogerian perspective is directed toward rhythms of living as possibly the most relevant data about clients; solution-oriented modalities involve finding creative and often enjoyable ways to change distressing rhythms and use or amplify the ones that work well for clients. Rogerian nurses familiar with the outstanding work of Kunz (1991) will recall that she also talks about the importance of noting patterns or rhythms—rhythms of pain, rhythms of resentment—and the role this plays in promoting health.

## PRACTICE MODALITIES WITH CASE EXAMPLES

Barrett (1988) articulated the essentials of the Rogerian practice methodology when she defined the two major phases as pattern manifestation appraisal and deliberative mutual patterning. In the first phase, nurse and client engage in "the continuous process of identifying manifestations of the human and environmental fields that relate to current health events" (Barrett, 1988, p. 50). Nurse and client are engaged in relevant learning about the client's experiences and beliefs regarding possibilities for change, rhythms of living, and power. In the second phase, "The nurse with the client patterns the environmental field to promote harmony to health events" (Barrett, 1990, p. 50). Nurse and client may engage in a variety of activities that are consistent with the Rogerian view of the unitary nature of human and environmental fields as they are continuously changing. As Barrett (1988) pointed out, and as the following examples will illustrate, these two phases are nonlinear and do not necessarily occur in sequence.

Four basic modalities derived from a variety of solution-oriented approaches are congruent with Rogerian nursing science and consistent with Barrett's phases:

1. Clarifying client intentions using language that supports the idea that desired changes will occur.
2. Highlighting strengths and distress-free periods.
3. Suggesting a relationship between perception and patterning.
4. Directly addressing clients' rhythms of living.

However, the language used previously to describe these "techniques" was drawn more from solution-oriented therapy than from the Rogerian model (Tuyn, 1992). The careful reader will find that some of the language is inconsistent with Rogers and tends to reflect years of "systems" and "strategic" thinking in the "psychotherapy" field. An attempt is made here to clarify the language differences and use terms more congruent with the Rogerian model.

### Clarifying Client Intentions Using the Language of Change

As a participant in an interdisciplinary peer-supervision group for therapists, I am always amazed when therapists struggle to answer these questions: What is the goal of the therapy for this client? What did the client initially say he or she wanted to get out of therapy? Therapy tends to meander when neither the client nor the therapist is clear about the criteria for success. Like Rogerians, solution-focused therapists do not look for a hypothetical, linear, cause-and-effect relationship between people and their concerns. de Shazer and his associates are most emphatic in their focus on solutions, stating that "all the therapist and client need to know is: 'How will we know when the problem is solved?'" (de Shazer et al., 1986, p. 210). During pattern manifestation appraisal, there are two key questions to explore with clients:

1. What are they looking for in the way of improvement?
2. What will be an early sign that things are on the desired track?

As Rawnsley (1985) pointed out, the way we define and use language can evolve from a three-dimensional behavior to a pandimensional healing pattern. Barrett (1990) maintained that meaningful dialogue is a very important health patterning modality. One way in which the nurse encourages meaningful dialogue, and thereby uses language to promote change, is by introducing "videotalk"—asking the client to project into a future time when the situation will have changed in a satisfactory way.

Videotalk requires people to describe their lives and what will determine successful therapy in action terms (O'Hanlon and Weiner-Davis, 1989). In other words, what would we actually see and hear on a video recording if we were to follow a client around with a camera once his "self-esteem" has improved, or her "depression" has lifted? Using questions like "What will you be doing *when* you're feeling better, and what *will* others notice about you?" subtly communicates the expectation that success will occur. When clients clearly state actions that to them represent success ("I'll enroll in junior college"; "I'll use time out with my kids instead of screaming at them"), the counselor can then explore what the client needs to do to accomplish these actions and how any potential difficulties might be overcome.

Another way to use solution language to learn client intentions and identify actions for attaining them is to project into a future time when the concern will have been worked out, and get as clear a picture as possible of what would be found there. For example, our family was formed through adoption; my husband and I are Caucasian, and our children are Korean American, ages one and three. I went through a brief but trying period of getting "into a tizz" over how they will ever "resolve" whatever issues they may have regarding adoption and our interracial family. (Another use of change-promoting language is stating difficulties in everyday, nonpathologizing terms such as "in a tizz" or "getting worked up" rather than "anxiety," "depression," or "panic," thereby avoiding attaching a pathological label to the person's experience.) After a few days, I reminded myself to "practice what I teach" and decided to project into a future time when the concern will have been worked out. I "saw" our family twenty-some years down the road and asked, "What will I see my children doing that will tell me they feel good about themselves and have 'resolved' issues related to how our family came to be?" Among several answers that came immediately to mind when the situation was considered from this perspective were two important ones: (1) they will be engaged in activities and interests that give them fulfillment and joy, and (2) they will have enduring and satisfying friendships. The next questions were: "What can I do now to promote that type of future? What are we already doing in this direction as parents and as a family that we want to continue and/or enhance?" When clients explore the possibilities that arise from questions such as this last one, it becomes clear that possible solutions, as well as the criteria for success, make the most sense and are most likely to work when they come from the clients themselves.

### Highlighting Strengths and Complaint-Free Periods

Clients can usually participate knowingly in change and can be the source of creative patterning. During deliberative mutual patterning, nurses can focus on strengths in order to help clients use what may already be going well for them in a way they may not have thought of before. A nurse's creativity comes through when helping clients make links among strengths, abilities, or resources they have and thereby alleviating a concern, even when the resources may have no apparent relationship to the concern. For example, a client who stated she had trouble managing anger and experienced strained friendships because of her tendency to "explode" revealed that she had been happiest years ago when she had been very active in sports. After some discussion, she became intrigued with the possibility that she might be able to manage her anger by returning to sports activities, which offer opportunities to "blow off steam." She resumed jogging that week, then regularly added competitive activities, and, within a few weeks, reported significant improvement in her relationships.

Another client sought a single consultation because of his preoccupation with and feelings of despair over a broken love relationship. He was in an intensive course of study and, during pattern manifestation appraisal, described his intentions as "getting through my summer courses, and being able to focus on other things besides the relationship." We spent the session primarily discussing the moments in his life when he had been in touch with the sparks that, for him, made life worth living. Based on the interests he expressed, the following suggestions evolved in the phase of deliberative mutual patterning:

1. That he continue an exercise program started the week before.
2. That he read some works by his favorite poet that were unfamiliar to him.
3. That he call one friend living near him and one living out of town and tell them about the breakup and what he had been going through lately.

An additional suggestion was that he might find himself talking about other things as well (which is what happened during this session).

Four months later, when I happened to see this client, he reported his situation much improved, and said that the suggestions had been particularly beneficial in helping him get perspective on his situation and move on.

### Suggesting a Relationship between Perception and Patterning

This modality was previously termed "reframing" (Tuyn, 1992), a word used frequently in solution-oriented literature (O'Hanlon & Weiner-David, 1989). However, "re-"doing anything is inconsistent with the Rogerian model; change is continuous and innovative. It is more accurate to describe this modality as exploring with clients how their perceptions relate to specific patterning concerns and offering suggestions that may lead to new points of view and ideas for action. Rogers (1987) frequently delights audiences when she points to a favorite example of how we give an observed situation different meanings: when an 18-year-old steps out onto a porch in the middle of the night to see the moon, he is "romantic"; an 80-year-old doing the same thing is "senile." In the counseling context, it is important to remember that there are many points of view and legitimate interpretations of one situation. Here are some examples.

A student advisee confided that she had been "devastated" by feeling "attacked" by her peers in a small discussion class. After hearing her story, I wondered aloud if this occurred partly because her peers respected and admired her strength and saw her as someone who could handle confrontation. She agreed this could be so and admitted that she would like them to see that she also has a vulnerable side and was hurt by some of their comments. After careful listening and a plausible suggestion that gently challenged her completely "negative" view of the event, this student generated her own ideas for bringing this up in the next class and worked it out to her satisfaction.

At times, this modality simply involves helping someone identify a helpful aspect to something that seems completely distressing (Weiner-Davis, 1990). This can help the person place the concern in a wider perspective or even cease to label it as a concern. As Cowling (1990) pointed out, perception, experience, and expression are inextricably linked. A friend, describing her fear of driving across bridges, emphasized that it worsens when she is fatigued. She thoughtfully considered the suggestion that she has "a clear barometer that tells you when you may be too tired to drive." A student who had once had a frightening encounter with a stranger on an elevator was embarrassed about the "foolish fear" she sometimes experienced under similar circumstances. She was pleased to consider the thought that, instead, this experience taught her that she probably has "a healthy gut sense regarding potential danger."

Making suggestions regarding perception and patterning is definitely an art in the nurse–client process. It is not about minimizing people's pain and difficulty; rather, in an attempt to support clients' efforts to move forward, we respectfully acknowledge their interpretations, then open up room for other possibilities. In short, it is a way of saying, "Yes, I see that it could be that; I wonder, could it also be this?" and then supporting the client's choice to accept, reject, or ponder the new suggestion. Offering these suggestions also illustrates the nonlinear, nonsequential nature of the two phases of Rogerian practice methodology, noting that nurse and client are continuously engaged in the processes of appraisal and patterning.

## Directly Addressing Clients' Rhythms of Living

Strategic therapists have, for many years, focused on helping people change distressing "patterns" (Fisch et al., 1989; Haley, 1984), and solution-oriented therapists are greatly influenced by Milton Erickson's creative work with people and their "patterns" (O'Hanlon, 1987; O'Hanlon & Hexum, 1990). It is a long tradition of nursing, dating back to Nightingale, to be meticulously observant of the helpful, healthy rhythms of living and to plan care that uses and amplifies these rhythms. Both solution-oriented and Rogerian approaches seek to maximize patterning that contributes to intentionality of goal attainment and enjoyment of life, and to limit the intensity of distressing rhythms.

A simple and effective suggestion that shines a light on helpful rhythms might sound something like this: "Over the next week, notice everything that is happening in your life and that you would like to have continue. Write it all down, so you can describe it to me in detail the next time we meet." O'Hanlon and Weiner-Davis (1989) and Furman and Ahola (1992) elaborated on this and many similar actions that serve the dual purpose of uncovering valuable information for possible solutions and directing attention to what is going well. Another beneficial patterning approach is to simply talk with someone about something he or she enjoys or cares about. For example, I was asked to be adviser to a student who was not meeting program objectives related to therapeutic communication, collaborating with others, and so on. We spent our first meeting chiefly discussing his deep love for animals and his years of experience caring for them. It became clear that his ability to work with people could surely improve by tapping his capacity for compassion and attunement to other living beings. This was accomplished in part through using metaphors and analogy, but primarily by identifying and acknowledging what he already could do well.

One of the most challenging and enjoyable projects to tackle with a client is helping him or her find a way to limit the intensity of a distressing rhythm. Together, we try to identify a small change that can throw a "monkey wrench" into the habitual course of the concern and turn things toward the stated intention. Cases where this modality was used to help one client to stop binging and another to manage anxiety are described elsewhere (Tuyn, 1992). In the following examples, this patterning approach was applied to improving intrafamily relationships.

A married couple wished to do something about their frequent, nonproductive arguments over managing the family finances. They were both intrigued by de Shazer's (1985) maxim that when the usual "response" to a distressing situation does not work, try anything as long as it is not the usual response. The wife reported that a simple discussion that seemed like it was on a new topic began to veer in the direction of their usual fight. Suddenly, she turned to her husband and said, "At this point, dear, I think there's only one thing we can do." He worriedly asked her what that could be, and she answered, "The Freddie!" and began to do that singularly ridiculous dance from the 1960s. The husband took but a moment to make the choice to join in, and soon they were both laughing. The "Freddie" is now their code word for "This is going nowhere—let's change direction."

Many teenagers enthusiastically take to a suggestion that they do something unexpected to change a relationship that seems to be "in a rut." One college-age woman who reported almost constant struggles with her father took him completely by surprise when she asked him out for dinner and a movie—her treat. In the other direction, parents who forcefully disapproved of their teen daughter's relationship with an older, married, teenage man so unnerved her by their sudden insistence on inviting the man and his wife to dinner "so we can all get to know each other better" that the daughter swiftly broke off the relationship. Yet another example is an adult woman who always felt "on the defensive" when talking on the telephone with her mother. She found that wearing Groucho Marx-style nose and glasses while on the phone (and not telling her mother) provided enough of a change that she could stay detached and amused in a way that felt good to her.

These examples of patterning modalities are not offered in the spirit of trivializing people's difficulties, and they may sound too simple to have had any lasting benefit in these people's lives. However, they illustrate two important points regarding change and health patterning. First, people have remarkable, creative capacities to shift out of nonproductive patterns without necessarily spending years in therapy examining their childhoods, "experiencing" old traumas, or looking for insights into a hypothetical "cause" of their problems. This is, no doubt, useful work for some, but depth psychotherapy is often not the most appropriate or power-enhancing model to apply to people and their concerns. Second, we go back to the assumptions regarding continuous change and mutual field process: a very small change is manifest throughout the entire field and can direct patterning toward the desired outcome. Most people's life experiences support the conclusions that small changes can lead to bigger changes, and a new idea leads to more ideas.

One case example has taught me a great deal about the power of this approach. An older man whom I will call Martin sought counseling because of his anger and despair over his marital relationship. He had a history of significant childhood trauma, which he told me about during pattern manifestation appraisal "because I want you to know this about me, but I am done with it and want to talk about the present." His wife refused to join him for counseling, although she was a central figure in a stressful matter the family had been trying to work out on their own for several years. Martin was angry with her, yet his goals reflected his desire to get on with life and find some way to enjoy the rest of their time together. After three sessions over two months, he called to say their lives were going much better and he didn't think further meetings were necessary. Martin added that the suggestion to focus on what he enjoys about his wife, instead of trying to change her, had been particularly helpful. Three months after this conversation, his wife died unexpectedly.

After the funeral, he told me, "I was at peace and she was at peace—these were the best months of our marriage." There is no way to know how, if at all, a counseling approach emphasizing rhythms of living and strengths may have made a contribution to their final time together. However, I know that, in the role of counselor, I could have coached him in a more pathology-oriented direction by suggesting exploration of the childhood trauma or simply encouraging expression of the anger he felt toward his wife. Instead, Rogerian modalities enhanced with solution-oriented ideas with a "goodness of fit," at the very least, did not interfere with the healing that took place between these two people. Martin taught me a lesson worth learning again and again: Listen to clients, believe them, believe in them, and support the strength and beauty that yearns to unfold.

## CONCLUSION

An exploration of Rogerian concepts and solution-oriented therapy reveals congruent philosophical assumptions and leads to pragmatic, creative, and beneficial counseling modalities. Areas for further study include designing research to investigate practice applications of this approach and exploring the applicability of solution-oriented methods to health care management. The possibilities, like the human being's capacity to participate knowingly in change, are unlimited. Rogers (1992) has continued to give us encouragement by telling us that as new modalities evolve, "A helpful attitude toward change will be generated while vision and imagination grow" (p. 33). Let the call to action from leaders such as Elizabeth Barrett inspire us to take Rogerian nursing practice to a new level of service to humanity.

## REFERENCES

Barrett, E.A.M. (1988). Using Rogers' Science of Unitary Human Beings in nursing practice. *Nursing Science Quarterly, 1,* 50–51.

Barrett, E.A.M. (Ed.). (1990). *Visions of Rogers' science-based nursing.* New York: National League for Nursing.

Barrett, E.A.M. (1992, June). *Rogerian scientists, artists, revolutionaries.* Keynote address, Fourth Rogerian Conference: The Science and Art of Nursing Practice, New York University, New York.

Cowling, W.R. (1990). A template for unitary pattern-based nursing practice. In E.A.M. Barrett (Ed.), *Visions of Rogers' science based nursing* (pp. 45–65). New York: National League for Nursing.

de Shazer, S. (1985). *Keys to solutions in brief therapy.* New York: Norton.

de Shazer, S. (1991). *Putting difference to work.* New York: Norton.

de Shazer, S., Berg, I.K., Lipchik, E., Nunnally, E., Molnar, A., Gingerich, W., & Weiner-Davis, M. (1986). Brief therapy: Focused solution development. *Family Process, 25,* 207–221.

Fisch, R., Weakland, J., & Segal, L. (1989). *The tactics of change: Doing therapy briefly.* San Francisco: Jossey-Bass.

Furman, B., & Ahola, T. (1992). *Solution talk: Hosting therapeutic conversations.* New York: Norton.

Haley, J. (1984). *Ordeal therapy.* San Francisco: Jossey-Bass.

Kunz, D. (1991). *The personal aura.* Wheaton, IL: Theosophical Publishing House.

Malinski, V. (1986). *Explorations on Martha Rogers' Science of Unitary Human Beings.* Norwalk, CT: Appleton-Century-Crofts.

O'Hanlon, W. (1987). *Taproots: Underlying principles of Milton Erickson's therapy and hypnosis.* New York: Norton.

O'Hanlon, W. (1990, August). *Brief solution-oriented therapy.* Conference handout, First Annual Family Therapy Training Series, Syracuse University, Blue Mountain Lake, NY.

O'Hanlon, W., & Hexum, A. (1990). *An uncommon casebook: The complete clinical work of Milton H. Erickson.* New York: Norton.

O'Hanlon, W., & Weiner-Davis, M. (1989). *In search of solutions: A new direction in psychotherapy.* New York: Norton.

Rawnsley, M.M. (1985). H-E-A-L-T-H: A Rogerian perspective. *Journal of Holistic Nursing, 3*(1), 25–28.

Rogers, M. (1987, March). *Nursing science for the future.* Paper presented at the State University of New York, School of Nursing, Binghamton, NY.

Rogers, M. (1992). Nursing science and the space age. *Nursing Science Quarterly, 5*, 27–34.

Tuyn, L.K. (1992). Solution-oriented therapy and Rogerian nursing science: An integrated approach. *Archives of Psychiatric Nursing, 6*, 83–89.

Tuyn, L.K. (1994). Using guided imagery exercises in the classroom. *Journal of Nursing Education, 33*(4), 157–158.

Watzlawick, P., Weakland, J., & Fisch, R. (1974). *Change.* New York: Norton.

Weiner-Davis, M. (1990, November). *Solution-oriented therapy.* Workshop handout, St. Joseph's Hospital Teaching Day, Rochester, NY.

Zeig, J., & Gilligan, S. (Eds.). (1990). *Brief therapy: Myths, methods, and metaphors.* New York: Bruner/Mazel.

# 15

# Toward a Unitary View of Nursing Practice

*Martha Raile Alligood*

Never before in history has the time been more right for nursing to complete the transition to professional status. We can't achieve that goal, however, until we revolutionize nursing practice. Rogers' Science of Unitary Human Beings provides a framework and directs nurses toward a unitary view of nursing practice. The unitary view of practice can be established by completing three shifts: (1) from reductionism to holism, (2) from vocational to professional, and (3) from four to five assumptions. This chapter sets forth a unitary view of practice that can only be achieved by the completion of these three shifts.

## THE SHIFT FROM REDUCTIONISM TO HOLISM: A NEW LOOK AT THE WORLD

The first shift, from reductionism to holism, requires a new look at the world. This shift, already in progress, is most obvious in discussions of philosophy of science, theoretical knowledge development, and research methods (Gortner, 1990; Suppe & Jacox, 1985; Webster, Jacox, & Baldwin, 1981). Since nurses are currently involved in the challenging task of learning to view persons in their human wholeness, some may think of holism as a new idea. Actually, nurses were concerned with holism at the turn of the century. A review of Rogers' writings reveals more references to holism in her earlier works than in her later ones (Rogers, 1970, 1980, 1990, 1992).

Allen (1991), from her review of the holism literature, reported that the number and complexity of holistic ideas in nursing literature escalated early and remained high until the middle 1930s, when they began to decrease. In her review of the early literature, wholeness was discussed in relation to themes pertinent to the topic of this chapter: "The major thrust of holistic statements from 1900 to 1919 supported the relationship among professionalization, public health nursing, and higher education in nursing" (p. 264). Therefore, the literature of that day was replete with discussions of wholeness, but the emphasis was on the nurses themselves and their need to be professional and well-educated, not on the holism of the patient. In the next two decades, district nurses were able to use holistic ideas to engender a belief that district or public health nursing was a type of nursing set apart from other specialties. "Holism was linked to professionalism . . ." (p. 264) by these nurses, and the echo of their effectiveness can still be heard today.

These district nurses (public health nurses) were also the fulcrum for nursing's move to academia. When Rogers entered nursing (in the early 1930s), she joined the ranks of the holistic thinkers. The emphasis on holistic health, now generalized to all areas of nursing, had its roots in the holistic ideas of the district/public health nurses. Following World War II and the influx of nonprofessional workers into hospitals, nurses again used holistic ideas and the ideal of comprehensive care to distinguish their practice from others, such as LPNs and aides, in the health care arena (Allen, 1991). These early concepts of holistic health, comprehensive nursing, and professionalism were seeds that were to grow into our view of nursing practice today.

Rogers (1970) discussed reductionism in the "purple book" and concluded it was contrary to a perception of wholeness. She stated, "The subjective world of human feelings must be incorporated into so-called objective science" (p. 87). However, "between 1940 and the 1980s there is neither the volume nor depth of holistic statements that characterized the earlier part of the century" (Allen, 1991, p. 262–263). Rather, the literature of this period reflects movement of nurses into higher education and their embracing of science. During this stage, holistic ideals took a back seat to traditional mechanistic science.

The outcome of the movement from reductionism to holism has implications for all of nursing, not just research methodology and theoretical knowledge development. The day-to-day practice of nursing has been influenced more strongly by the scientific ideal of objectivity than we may think. Therefore, the shift from objectivity to subjectivity, already begun in research methods, must be embraced by nurses for nursing practice as well. In reductionism, we were on our way toward shutting down our own humanness and viewing the patient in a very mechanistic manner. This is evidenced by the values displayed in nursing settings where, at times, the focus is on machines rather than on humans. Nurses must question whether they have been socialized to practice values that sacrifice the person for the procedure. When we view persons in their wholeness, we will deliver their nursing care within that context.

This view no longer sees nursing science and nursing art separately; rather, the two merge into a science that encompasses the art of practice. Science, as we have known it traditionally, had severe limitations—especially for nurses, who are humans caring for humans. Our knowledge is never perfect at any point in time in nursing practice since there are varying amounts of information and several sets of values involved with the nursing judgments and decisions to be made. Nurses make judgments in what they propose to clients as they participate with them and facilitate their knowing participation in decisive changes. However, "Factual or theoretical studies alone cannot logically lead to a practical recommendation. A practical recommendation or valuational conclusion can be derived only when there is at least one valuation among the premises" (Myrdal, 1962, p. 1052). This quote demonstrates another truth set forth by Myrdal (1962), which nurses have only recently begun to understand: nursing requires a human science, and human science requires human premises. I believe we came to this understanding as a product of our holistic ideal; that is, our holistic heritage has served us by pointing us in the right direction. The mechanism of reductionism in traditional science became evident to nurse researchers when the reducing procedure eliminated the characteristic human integrity of the whole individual.

Rogers (1970) has said that the perception of wholeness is synergistic. Her view of unitary human beings (she prefers unitary to holistic) seeks to understand the synergistic manifestations of pattern. When we consider a person in his or her wholeness, humanness is addressed rather than omitted in a particulate manner. Therefore, we conclude that the shift from reductionism to holism leads us to a view of the world that encompasses our view of human beings and, therefore, our view of nursing practice.

## THE SHIFT FROM VOCATIONAL TO PROFESSIONAL: A NEW LOOK AT NURSING

The shift from vocational to professional is also in progress—in fact, some might think this is old news. Nursing finds itself on the threshold of recognition as a profession, but first we must launch professional practice. With the changing philosophy of science (already presented in the first shift, from reductionism to holism) there emerges a realization of problems with the nursing process as we know it. This is not new to most Rogerian scholars who have embraced simultaneous change (Parse, 1987). Many nurses, however, still labor within the traditional nursing process.

Nursing process began to be adopted in the late 1950s and early 1960s (Orlando, 1961). There was great excitement about the nursing process at that time since it brought organization to the delivery of nursing care and self-esteem to nurses regarding their practice. Experienced nurses knew how they organized their practice but they had not generally written it down; therefore, it was very personal and had not undergone the scrutiny of other practitioners. Moreover, it did not derive from theory or research findings; instead, it was based on an occupational or vocational model (Meleis, 1991). If two nurses practicing side-by-side had developed a way to organize their practices, they often didn't discuss it and saw no need to do so. They might share information about isolated procedures, but it was a vocational sharing of "know-how." With the coming of nursing process, nurses began to have a common language that facilitated sharing in practice. When nurses began to share their experiences about the process of delivering care, the focus shifted from procedures to nursing practice.

The nursing process served nurses for a period of time by organizing thinking to make decisions and providing a language to communicate with other nurses. A handicap associated with the linear process began to emerge, however. Although the nursing process facilitated the shift of focus from diseases and procedures to delivery of nursing care, the use of the process and its discussion fit a vocational, rather than a professional, model of education.

The process, as outlined in linear steps of assessment, diagnosis, planning, intervention, and evaluation, may have utility for vocational nursing, but its linear structure will not lead professional nurses where they need to go. Rather, it will lead to a particulate view of the client and will align with the functional aspect of nursing, which comes from our vocational heritage.

The linear process approach to the client is geared to episodic care and a focus on "What is wrong?" Furthermore, the process assumes that what is needed to answer that question is an at-the-moment sequence of assessment, diagnosis, goals, plan, intervention, and evaluation. This process uses a very brief cross-sectional survey of the person as the basis for prescription of nursing care and endorses the medical model of focusing on the current problem or signs and symptoms. Integrating health into the process and changing assessment to appraisal will not lead to something different. Instead, these changes will mislead nurses into thinking they are being scientific.

Our nursing textbooks are filled with this pseudo-science. Science is a method of discovery, a search for something that is not known. Many nursing textbooks, however, teach that the application of scientific principles or rationale comes *after* a decision on what needs to be done. An example of this is attaching a seemingly related statement as justification for a plan of care arrived at by intuition or some other means. I call this science-after-the-fact or pseudo-science (a better name since it isn't science at all). Verhonick (1973) understood this problem 20 years ago when she cautioned baccalaureate students at the University of Virginia about the level of development of nursing as a science: "The bedside nurse is bathing the patient and saying to herself as she washes the little finger, let's see—I believe this is north by northwest" (Verhonick, 1973). At first, I was angered by her humorous view of nursing science, but when I began to observe this pseudo-science, her words came to me. The method is functional, and it is aligned with the philosophy and process of vocational education. Ironically, Rogers (1970) had already written: "The science of nursing is prerequisite to the process of nursing" (p. 87).

Vocational schools teach functions—how to do something. Nursing has a vocational heritage, and we have brought along with us some tools that we must discard if we are to move on into professional practice. If we are to make the shift from vocation to profession, we must revolutionize nursing practice. The focus must be on the person or the human being. The environment and the person's health are only relevant or important in the context of the person. Therefore, the focus must be restored to the person and his or her life process (Rogers, 1970).

This view argues against the current discussion of caring as the central focus of the discipline (Leininger, 1991; Newman, Sime, & Corcoran-Perry, 1991). Some writers have countered the focus on caring on the basis of lack of development of the concept and its lack of relevance for nursing practice (Morse, Bottorff, Neander, & Solberg, 1991). More importantly, the emphasis on caring is vocational nursing: caring focuses on nurses and on what nurses do. We cannot put the emphasis back on nurses and what nurses do. The unitary view of practice set forth in Rogerian science clearly places the focus of nursing on the person as a human being within an environment that synthesizes his or her past, dreams for the future, relationships with people and things in the world, and health as he or she experiences it. The meaning of what nursing is emerges from this focus; therefore, the understanding of nursing is dependent on this focus. Nightingale understood this, and when we had drifted away from her idea, it was Rogers who pointed us back in the right direction.

The nature of professional practice is that it is guided by scientific theory. The idea that theory and practice are separated and need to be linked is erroneous. Such a view assumes that we begin with practice *as it is* and then try to link theory to it. This view fails to recognize that theoretical structure guides practice. Efforts at such linkages in the literature (Nicoll, 1986, 1992) were attempts to link theory to vocational practice; that will not work. Just as theory forms a structure to guide research, it also provides a structure to guide practice. Theory and practice are not different entities; rather, they are different aspects of the same phenomenon. When professional practice is structured according to a theoretical model, the very activity that the nurse does will have a therapeutic value even if it is being done in a research project.

Theory, research, and practice are not separate entities in professional practice. When we recognize what professional practice means, then we realize theory, research, and practice are best understood as overlays or transparencies superimposed on one another (Figure 15.1). Some researchers have happened onto this idea when conducting qualitative studies that involve mutual process with the client and a healing process becomes observable.

What we are coming to understand is the nature of professional practice. When we break out of the linear, vocational idea of nursing process and embrace clients as human beings in their wholeness, our

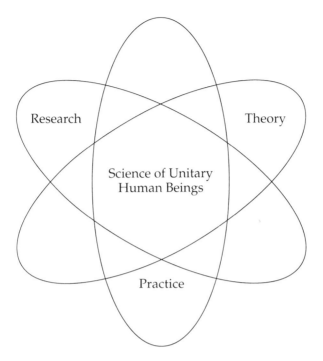

**Figure 15.1**
**Theory, Practice, and Research as Overlays**
**Rather Than Separate Entities**

practice, guided by Rogers' (1990) Science of Unitary Human Beings, is structured by providing a decision-making framework.

## THE SHIFT FROM FOUR TO FIVE ASSUMPTIONS: A NEW LOOK AT HUMAN BEINGS

The final shift builds on the ideas presented in the shift from reductionism to holism and the shift from vocation to profession. The final shift required for a unitary view of nursing practice is four assumptions back to five. In this shift, the prominence and role of Rogers' ideas of sentience will be explored.

In the first shift, it was noted that "a practical or valuational conclusion can be derived only when there is at least one valuation among the premises" (Myrdal, 1962). Therefore, this shift might be called "Why sentience is the heart of the matter." This chapter, in presenting a new view of nursing practice, suggests that the new holistic view not only includes sentience but moves sentience to a position of prominence. Sentience is an essential assumption in Rogers' Science of Unitary Human Beings.

Rogers (1970) identified five assumptions of man that formed the basis for "nursing's conceptual model" (p. 89):

1. "Man is a unified whole possessing his own integrity and manifesting characteristics that are more than and different from the sum of his parts" (p. 47).

2. "Man and environment are continuously exchanging matter and energy with one another" (p. 54).

3. "The life process evolves irreversibly and unidirectionally along the space–time continuum" (p. 59).

4. "Pattern and organization identify man and reflect his innovative wholeness" (p. 65).

5. "Man is characterized by the capacity for abstraction and imagery, language and thought, sensation and emotion" (p. 73).

Rogers further stated: "These assumptions constitute statements of fact postulated to be true and describe the life process of man as characterized by wholeness, openness, unidirectionality, pattern and organization, sentience and thought" (p. 90).

In 1970, from her five assumptions, Rogers set forth nursing's conceptual model. There were four principles: (1) reciprocy, (2) synchrony, (3) helicy, and (4) resonancy. Rogers proposed these principles of homeodynamics of the life process as hypothetical generalizations; however, a homeodynamic principle that linked sentience to the life process was conspicuously absent. By 1980, Rogers had changed her conceptual system in the following manner: instead of the five building blocks designated in her 1970 work, there were four; instead of four principles, there were three. The building blocks were energy fields, openness, pattern and organization, and four-dimensionality. The principles were resonancy, helicy, and complementarity (Rogers, 1980). Daily, Maupin, Satterly, Schnell, and Wallace (1989) have illustrated the progression of Rogers' changes in the principles over time. In 1970, sentience was included as an assumption (Rogers, 1970, pp. 67-77) and a repeated topic in the description of nursing's conceptual model (pp. 89-94); however, Rogers no longer included it soon after. Although sentience is a cornerstone of the work of many scholars in Rogerian science, its heritage or foundational basis is not clear nor is its present role or purpose in the structure of the science. The various ways sentience has been used by Rogers (and others) will be reviewed to illustrate the problem that forms the basis for proposing the shift from four assumptions back to five.

Sentience was integral to the major premise of Rogers' (1970) original ideas; in fact, it was central, prominent, and comprehensive rather than limited to the sentience chapter (pp. 67-77). This observation is illustrated by the following review. Early in the book, before the chapter on sentience, Rogers linked the human's wholeness, "a whole in which the parts are not distinguishable . . . " and his "awareness" to his being a "thinking, feeling being" (p. 41). When discussing "man's unified wholeness," Rogers cited Polanyi, saying "To represent living men as insentient is empirically false, but to regard them as thoughtful automata is logical nonsense" (p. 46). Rogers linked "perceptual evolution" and "higher sense perception" and labeled it as an "evolutionary emergent" (p. 59). "Perception of the nature of pattern" was discussed using an example of the perception of sadness as an "expression of wholeness" (p. 65).

In Rogers' (1970) chapter devoted to sentience (Chapter 10), the human being as a sentient, thinking being was presented as a basic assumption of nursing's conceptual system (p. 67). Rogers stated, "Compassionate concern for human beings gives meaning to the [nursing] effort" (p. 82). "Sentience and thought rise out of the evolving process of the human field and environment" (p. 92).

Sentience was prominent in early views of two homeodynamic principles. Rogers (1970) stated, "The Principle of Helicy postulates an ordering of man's evolutionary emergence. The rise of cognition and feelings is encompassed" (p. 100). The Principle of Resonancy postulated, "The pattern of the human field is a wave phenomenon encompassing man in his entirety. The whole of man senses, feels, perceives, and reasons" (p. 101).

The work of Rogerian scholars also builds on sentience. Barrett (1986) derived a theory of power from helicy that had dimensions of awareness, choices, freedom to act intentionally, and involvement in creating changes based on the human capacity to think, feel, and experience awareness. Sarter (1984) pointed out the link between "sentience characterized as awareness and perception" in the "correlates of patterning" (p. 97) set forth by Rogers. This linkage has implications for other work, such as Cowling's (1990) template of mutual pattern change, which includes perception and awareness, and Parker's (1989) "theory of sentience," which "proposed that 'the beyond waking state' is sentience, experienced as a higher-frequency phenomenon" (p. 5). Both support Sarter's (1984) point. More importantly, Sarter asserted that the innovative tendency toward increased diversity in helicy is sentient-based. She quoted Rogers' premise that "creativity finds expression in the changing dimensions of man's sentience and thought" (Rogers, 1970, p. 72). Sarter asked Rogers about sentience in her interviews (which are included in the appendix of her dissertation). Rogers, quoted in Sarter (1984), replied that sentience would be retained in the new book as a manifestation of pattern: "What those [reason and feelings] really are, are manifestations of pattern. It doesn't constitute a basic postulate or assumption at all" (p. 168). This gets to the very heart of this third shift. What I am proposing here is that the manifestations of pattern of the human energy field are logically dependent on the assumptions about human beings in the conceptual system that is the Science of Unitary Human Beings. Therefore, Rogers' answer assumes sentience, which she describes in the postulate of pattern (Sarter, 1984).

Sentience is prominent in my own work (Alligood, 1986, 1990, 1991, 1992). Creativity is defined as the tendency toward variety, and empathy is defined as a feeling attribute of the person–environment process. From working in Rogerian science for a number of years, I have come to understand that resonancy explains what we feel (wave frequency), helicy explains how we feel (mutual process), and integrality explains why we feel (the fields pass through each other). Therefore, sentience, which is the basis of the awareness of feeling, is basic to the science.

Not only does the work of Rogerian scholars build on the assumption of sentience, but the current nursing literature is replete with recent references that list sentience as a basic assumption in Rogers' Science of Unitary Human Beings (Biley, 1992; Chinn & Kramer, 1991; Daily et al., 1989; Falco & Lobo, 1990; Leddy & Pepper, 1993; Meleis, 1991; Quillin & Runk, 1989; Whall, 1987).

Sentience is essential in the Science of Unitary Human Beings in order for the art and the science to embrace one another. The manner in which the art and the science of nursing relate helps us understand that they are not separate; rather, our separation of them is an artificial convenience that is actually reductionistic. The art and the science are best understood as overlaid transparencies (Figure 15.2). The current return to the ontology and the "philosophy of the art of nursing" (Rhodes, 1990) can only increase our understanding of this concept. Yet, this growth of our knowledge must come from work within the science. Sentience as an assumption has been supported, in reviews of its use, by Rogers, Rogerian scholars, and current nursing literature. I conclude, therefore, that since sentience is being used within the science as though it had remained an assumption, it is an assumption.

As we move toward a unitary view of nursing practice, it is important to note difficulties in advancing knowledge development. For example, the practice of borrowing theories from other disciplines, such as chaos theory from sociology, seems to have emerged from questioning the conceptual system rather than building knowledge within it, and does not serve the purposes of the Science of Unitary Human Beings. Bloom (1987) described the current emphasis

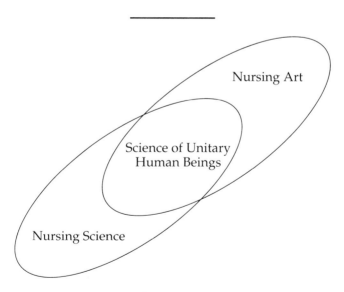

**Figure 15.2**
**Art and Science as Overlays Informing One**
**Another Than Separate Entities**

on chaos theory as ". . . a new kind of causality . . ." (p. 209). The movement ahead in Rogerian science does not require a trip through chaos. If the system is right in the first place, this is an improper procedure since changing any aspect of the system changes the whole system. Furthermore, these changes lead to confusion, as is evident with the status of sentience. Instead, it is suggested that the appeal of determinism, found in chaos theory, is better met within the Rogerian system in creative human choice (Barrett, 1986).

Rogers (1992) has continued to define unitary human beings as "manifesting characteristics that are specific to the whole" (p. 7). If unitary human beings and the environment were defined alike in nonhuman, mechanistic terms, then probability would have served us in the system with very high reliability. However, if probability is replaced with "unpredictability" (p. 29), as was done by Rogers in 1990, this supports the proposition set forth in this chapter: Recognize creative holistic humanness and restore sentience as the fifth assumption of its basis. Serious discussions of knowledge development in any system can only occur when the assumptions being made by the researchers are clearly understood.

In the shift from reductionism to holism, Rogers has proposed perception of wholeness, which has led us to look at the world in a new way. Likewise, Rogers has led in the shift from vocation to profession, which helps us look at nursing in a new way. Now it is time to restore sentience as an assumption in the Science of Unitary Human Beings so we can look at human beings in a new way.

The shifts that have been described support the movement toward a unitary view of nursing practice. Rogers (1970, 1980, 1990, 1992) has provided a world-view that affords nurses a holistic view of human beings, a unique perspective of nursing's phenomenon of concern. The movement from vocation to profession has been in progress, but practice changes have lagged. It has been proposed that vocational practice will not lead to professional practice without knowledgeable choices and changes. Finally, sentience has been reviewed, and its return to the status of an assumption in the Science of Unitary Human Beings has been proposed.

---

*Editors' Note:* Alligood's proposal to return sentience "to the status of an assumption in the Science of Unitary Human Beings" is inconsistent with Rogers' most recent writings (Martha E. Rogers, Personal Communication, October 31, 1993).

## REFERENCES

Allen, C.E. (1991). An analysis of the pragmatic consequences of holism for nursing. *Western Journal of Nursing Research, 13*, 256-272.

Alligood, M.R. (1986). The relationships of creativity, actualization, and empathy in unitary human development. In V. Malinski (Ed.), *Explorations of Martha Rogers' Science of Unitary Human Beings* (pp. 145-160). Norwalk, CT: Appleton-Century-Crofts.

Alligood, M.R. (1990). Nursing care of the elderly: Futuristic projections. In E.M. Barrett (Ed.), *Visions of Rogers' science-based nursing* (pp. 129-141). New York: National League for Nursing.

Alligood, M.R. (1991). Testing Rogers' theory of accelerating change: The relationships among creativity, actualization, and empathy in persons 18-92 years of age. *Western Journal of Nursing Research, 13*, 84-96.

Alligood, M.R. (1992). Empathy: The importance of recognizing two types. *Journal of Psychosocial Nursing, 30*, 14-17.

Barrett, E. (1986). The relationship of human field motion and power. In V. Malinski (Ed.), *Explorations on Martha Rogers' Science of Unitary Human Beings* (pp. 173-184). Norwalk, CT: Appleton-Century-Crofts.

Biley, F. (1992). The perception of time as a factor in Rogers' Science of Unitary Human Beings: A literature review. *Journal of Advanced Nursing, 17*, 1141-1145.

Bloom, A. (1987). *The closing of the American mind.* New York: Simon & Shuster.

Chinn, P., & Kramer, M. (1991). *Theory and nursing: A systematic approach* (2nd ed.). St. Louis: Mosby.

Cowling, R. (1990). A template for unitary pattern-based nursing practice. In E. Barrett (Ed.), *Visions of Rogers' science-based nursing* (pp. 45-65). New York: National League for Nursing.

Daily, J., Maupin, J., Satterly, M., Schnell, D., & Wallace, T. (1989). Martha E. Rogers' unitary human beings. In A. Marriner-Tomey (Ed.), *Nursing theorists and their work* (2nd ed.) (pp. 402-419). St. Louis: Mosby.

Falco, S., & Lobo, M. (1990). Martha E. Rogers. In Julia B. George (Ed.), *Nursing theories: The base for professional nursing practice* (3rd ed.) (pp. 211-230). Norwalk, CT: Appleton & Lange.

Gortner, S. (1990). Nursing values and science: Toward a science philosophy. *Image: Journal of Nursing Scholarship, 22*(2), 101-105.

Leddy, S., & Pepper, M. (1993). *Conceptual bases of professional nursing* (3rd ed.). Philadelphia: Lippincott.

Leininger, M. (1991). *Culture care diversity and universality: A theory of nursing.* New York: National League for Nursing.

Meleis, A. (1991). *Theoretical nursing: Development and progress* (2nd ed.). Philadelphia: Lippincott.

Morse, J., Bottorff, J., Neander, W., & Solberg, S. (1991). Comparative analysis of conceptualizations and theories of caring. *Image: Journal of Nursing Scholarship, 23*(2), 119-126.

Myrdal, G. (1962). *An American dilemma.* New York: Harper & Row.

Newman, M., Sime, A., & Corcoran-Perry, S. (1991). The focus of the discipline of nursing. *Advances in nursing science, 14*(1) 1-6.

Nicoll, L. (Ed.). (1986). *Perspectives on nursing theory.* Boston: Little, Brown.

Nicoll, L. (Ed.). (1992). *Perspectives on nursing theory* (2nd ed.). Philadelphia: Lippincott.

Orlando, I. (1961). *The dynamic nurse–patient relationship.* New York: Putnam.

Parker, K. (1989). The theory of sentience evolution: A practice-level theory of sleeping, waking, and beyond-waking patterns based on the Science of Unitary Human Beings. *Rogerian Nursing Science News, 2,* 4-6.

Parse, R. (1987). *Nursing science: Major paradigms, theories, and critiques.* Philadelphia: Saunders.

Quillin, S., & Runk, J. (1989). Martha Rogers' unitary person model. In J. Fitzpatrick & A. Whall (Eds.), *Conceptual models of nursing* (2nd ed.) (pp. 285-300). Norwalk, Ct: Appleton & Lange.

Rhodes, J. (1990). *A philosophical study of the art of nursing explored within a metatheoretical framework of philosophy of art and aesthetics.* Unpublished doctoral dissertation, University of South Carolina.

Rogers, M. (1970). *An introduction to the theoretical basis of nursing.* Philadelphia: F.A. Davis.

Rogers, M. (1980). A science of unitary man. In J.P. Riehl & C. Roy (Eds.), *Conceptual models for nursing practice* (2nd ed.) (pp. 329-337). New York: Appleton-Century-Crofts.

Rogers, M. (1990). Nursing: Science of Unitary, Irreducible, Human Beings: Update 1990. In E. Barrett (Ed.) *Visions of Rogers' science-based nursing* (pp. 5-11). New York: National League for Nursing.

Rogers, M. (1992). Nursing science and the space age. *Nursing Science Quarterly, 5,* 27-34.

Sarter, B. (1984). *The stream of becoming: A metaphysical analysis of Rogers' model of unitary man.* Unpublished doctoral dissertation, New York University.

Suppe, F., & Jacox, A. (1985). Philosophy of science and the development of nursing theory. In H. Werley & J. Fitzpatrick (Eds.), *Annual review of nursing research* (pp. 241-267). New York: Springer.

Verhonick, P. (1973). Class notes, University of Virginia.

Webster, G., Jacox, A., & Baldwin, B. (1981). Nursing theory and the ghost of the received view. In J. McCloskey & H. Grace (Eds.), *Current issues in nursing* (pp. 26-35). Boston: Blackwell Scientific Publications.

Whall, A. (1987). A critique of Rogers' framework. In R. Parse (Ed.), *Nursing science: Major paradigms, theories, and critiques* (pp. 147-158). Philadelphia: Saunders.

# 16

# Dying

*Brenda Talley*

4:30 A.M.—
a quite gentle time
to leave this life,
leaving a thousand memories
floating in the air
like downy feathers
after a pillow fight;
bringing a smile
into this soft sadness.
Slowly now, he is slipping
into the rhythms of the universe,
energy no longer intent on maintaining
this physical pattern of being
so familiar to us
who knew him by that design.
Tiring,
barely holding to old connections
but remaining still,
giving us a little time
to learn to love him
in his new way.
Dying.
Becoming.

It was late at night, and my 82-year-old uncle was dying. He had, while he still could, made the decision not to go back to the hospital for his dying. By the time we got to him, his breathing was irregular and his body temperature was poorly controlled. We did the things that people do at these times; we cried for a while and comforted each other. Soon, everyone became quiet and still as we waited for him to die. The starlight shining through the window seemed to become cold and harsh.

I started doing some of the things that nurses do—rubbing his back, holding his hands. "Talk to him," I said. "Tell him you love him." His son and daughter looked at me oddly: he had been deaf for years, and now he was in a coma.

"Do you remember," I quietly asked him, "when I was about five and you caught me jumping out of the hay loft? I always did think I should be able to fly, didn't I? Well, you threatened to spank me, and I started to cry. So you punished me by making me sit on the back porch with you while we ate ice cream. A real bear you were, a real bear."

He was deaf and very near death, but he smiled. So did his son and daughter, and the air around us seemed to relax. We began speaking of old, beautiful memories, as though we were taking softly faded patchwork quilts from an old trunk and draping them around us in love and comfort. We touched him and talked to him, and at 4:30 A.M. he stopped breathing.

# Unit III

## *DELIVERY SYSTEMS FOR ROGERIAN PRACTICE*

# 17

# Opportunities for Knowing Participation: A New Design for the Nursing Service Organization

*Cynthia Caroselli*

Writers and theorists in diverse fields have called for changes in the framework of the health care delivery system. Numerous articles have posited various models for the work environment, cost containment initiatives, and quality assurance endeavors. Some have placed the onus for revolutionizing the hospital environment squarely on the shoulders of the administrator responsible for the largest number of employees in the acute care hospital, the Chief Nurse Executive (CNE). Simultaneously, other voices decry the scarcity of research-based theory development for nursing administration practice.

My recently completed research (Caroselli, 1991) provides an opportunity for the CNE to implement a new model of practice that is powerful, participative, and derived from a Rogerian perspective. After surveying CNEs in acute care hospitals, the research demonstrated that CNEs view themselves as powerful and display attitudes characteristic of a feminist orientation. The research also established a link between feminism and a power subscale: freedom to act intentionally.

These findings have far-reaching implications for designing the nursing service organization from a Rogerian nursing science perspective. This chapter describes how these findings can be implemented in practice. The implementation plan describes changes in: philosophy; mission statement; governance; table of organization;

staff recruitment, development, and composition; and how a new organizational culture emerges that promotes the knowing participation of the nursing staff. This represents an opportunity for furthering Rogerian science by producing a practice-oriented "think tank" that, in turn, provides the locus for field testing Rogerian-based research. A spirit of inquiry is fostered that furthers both the science and art of nursing practice.

## SIGNIFICANCE

This discussion is occurring at a particularly significant time in the history of health care in this country. Despite an unprecedented number of strategic changes in organizations and experiments over the past decade, there has been relatively little stability in U.S. hospitals. Most health care organizations have become concerned about long-term survival (Taft, Minch, & Jones, 1992). In this context, it has been acknowledged that registered nurses are the most knowledgeable, most flexible, and most cost-efficient staff members. This is reflected in the increasing proportion of RNs in hospitals, delivering nursing care in a world of changing economics (Sovie, 1986). Yet, even as nursing constitutes the largest work force in the health care industry, nursing remains a subordinate group in the system (Elliott, 1990), at least in part because it is traditionally seen as women's work (Quinn, 1990).

Therefore, it becomes very clear that nursing must be granted full, unhampered, and knowing participation in the health care arena. The stakes are too high and the time is too short to permit this valuable resource to be squandered.

A future-oriented perspective will be imperative in light of the rapidity of scientific, technological, and economic change (Christman, 1991). Experience, however, can also provide direction for maximizing nursing's assets. A follow-up study of magnet hospitals provides an interesting picture of successful nursing organizations; in these hospitals, nursing not only survives, but flourishes. Nursing practice in these organizations is characterized by low turnover, increased job satisfaction, innovation, excellence in practice, and an ability to attract new nurses. These successes are felt to be due, in part, to a managerial style that is based on visibility, informal communication, timely decision making, a willingness to experiment, support for risk taking and possible failure, support for research, and a zeal for quality (Kramer & Schmalenberg, 1988). Since it is well demonstrated that this approach can produce significant results, it should be heartening to those who seek to further develop the nursing service organization by creating a new design from a Rogerian perspective. The Science of Unitary Human Beings will, I believe, promote power in the form of knowing participation in change and permit nursing administrative practice that proceeds from scientifically derived theory and research.

## THE ROGERIAN SCIENCE PERSPECTIVE

In the context of the Science of Unitary Human Beings, the nursing service of the hospital is viewed as an energy field in mutual process with its environment (Caroselli, 1990). Rogers (1990) referred to this application as a group field that is irreducible and indivisible; thus, the nursing service is integral with the organization. Further, Rogers (1990) posited that energy fields manifest continuous change in innovative and unpredictable patterns.

From a different perspective, Peters (1987) supported these ideas when he described the need for organizations to be flexible, to embrace unpredictability, and to reject a love of stability. Rogers' concept of irreducibility was echoed by Kanter (1989) and Kerfoot (1990), who advocated the development of synergies, which go beyond teamwork and are more than the sum of their parts. In discussing pandimensionality, Phillips (1991) stated that it is no longer useful to deal with polarities or opposites. This is advice well taken when applied to the nursing service, which can be seen as a community of competing constituencies.

A central issue for nursing, with respect to its role in the health care delivery system, is power. Although power has traditionally been defined in militaristic, competitive, negative terms, Barrett (1983, 1990) has provided us with a new theory of power derived from Rogers' Principle of Helicy. Barrett sees power as knowing participation in change, which is characterized by awareness, choices, freedom to act intentionally, and involvement in creating changes. These characteristics are congruent with concepts basic to feminist ideology, which seeks to amplify women's freedom and choice. Most nurses are women who have been subject to stereotypical conditioning relative to women's roles. This has had a deleterious effect on nursing in the health care delivery system. Yet, since it has also been established that nursing may be the most appropriate discipline to spearhead innovation in health care delivery, the linkage among power, feminism, and emerging nursing service designs is warranted.

From a Rogerian perspective, knowing participation is characterized by participatory management, which is itself a manifestation of open systems (Caroselli, 1990). Peter Drucker (1991), long respected as a guru of management, sees partnerships between management and workers as essential in maximizing productivity, which supports the mutuality of Barrett and Rogers. Later in this chapter, a discussion of ways in which the Rogerian perspective can be operationalized on a day-to-day basis will be presented. Efforts such as these must continue to be implemented in order to advance nursing science and practice.

## THE ROLE OF THE CHIEF NURSE EXECUTIVE

The Chief Nurse Executive (CNE), the top nursing administrator in the organization, is in an important position to direct the delivery of health care (Caroselli, 1991). As such, the CNE is pivotal to the organization as the initiator for action (Gleeson, Nestor, & Riddell, 1983), as institutional planner and decision maker (Reeves & Underly, 1983), and as the nursing constituency's representative at the policy and budget level. Nurse executives in acute care hospitals are widely influential, beyond what might be expected when comparing their numbers with nurses in direct care. Thus, they have a major role in accomplishing the organization's goals (Carroll, 1987). The nurse executive has a broad arena in which to exercise power and choice, and this exercise is wide-ranging in scope (Caroselli, 1991).

Torbert (1987) charges the leader to become a strategist and to embrace paradoxes and anomalies. The CNE experiences a life-style of paradoxes, usually managing the largest staff and administering more than half of the institution's operational budget (McClure, 1989), yet also experiencing the challenges of being a member of a woman's profession (Stivers, 1991).

If the CNE is to facilitate an environment informed by and infused with the Rogerian perspective, then the CNE's modus operandi must be one of inspiring innovation, as Simms (1991) described it. To create this new vision of nursing, the leader must define reality in a new way and become the leader-as-teacher (Senge, 1990), which is congruent with Barrett's nondominating, mutualistic theory of power.

It is essential that the CNE be a role model who clearly and accessibly provides a standard of what is possible and powerful. The CNE has both the opportunity and the responsibility to provide an emerging role model of how the powerful woman looks, sounds, and acts. There is an urgent need for this kind of role modeling; the few available models of powerful women range from Lady Macbeth and Lucretia Borgia to Linda Hamilton in *The Terminator* and Sigourney Weaver in *Aliens*. Having availed ourselves of Barrett's theory of power, formulation of a role model of power based on mutuality is the next logical step. Nursing leadership must exemplify this in ways that are clear and accessible to the nursing service and to the organization at large.

Implementing a nursing service organization based on the Rogerian perspective requires changes in the structure and fabric of the nursing service itself. The following sections of this chapter will look at ways in which this can be accomplished.

## PHILOSOPHY

The philosophy of the nursing service organization makes public and explicit the theoretical foundations that guide nursing practice in the institution. It states nursing's beliefs about central concepts, acts as a guiding system or ideology (Peters, 1987), and must emerge from the shared beliefs of the nursing constituency. It cannot be developed by one individual, such as the CNE, and must emerge from what Helgesen (1990) referred to as a web of inclusion. This emergence is particularly crucial when formulating a philosophy derived from Rogerian science. Questions considered to be important by Drucker (1991) are: "What is the task? What are we trying to accomplish? Why are we doing it?" These are answered specifically in a philosophy that states the department's beliefs about nursing, nursing practice, patients, and relationships within and external to the department.

Since nursing is seen as a women's profession, irrespective of the fact that there are growing numbers of male nurses, the philosophy must reflect feminist thought in a way that is relevant to the institution. As with other components of this plan, it is important to recognize that each institution is unique and is integral with a unique environment. Thus, there is no one, true way to implement Rogerian philosophy in practice. An evolutionary emergent appears with each implementation.

The philosophy should make clear the need to embrace change and innovation (Drucker, 1990) and should include ideas about revision as necessary. It is also important that the philosophy specify beliefs about the cooperative, mutualistic nature of administration in contradistinction to the more traditional adversarial stance (Peters, 1987).

In keeping with the notion of knowing participation, the philosophy should include statements about the responsibility of everyone in the department to assume what Drucker (1990) refers to as "information responsibility." This is operationalized as one's privilege and obligation to obtain the information necessary to perform one's job and to provide others with equally necessary information. This is true knowing participation, as opposed to simply following a policy or procedure.

Given the unique nature of each institution's environmental field, it is likely that other issues should be addressed in the philosophy. These may relate to the setting, the patient population, or other idiosyncratic variables. However, all components of the philosophy should be congruent with the overriding perspective of Rogerian science.

## MISSION STATEMENT

The mission statement further operationalizes the philosophy grounded in the Rogerian perspective. It expresses the operational values of the nursing service, and, as such, has implications for strategic planning. It makes explicit the manner in which the nursing service enacts what Drucker (1990) sees as the mission of the nonprofit organization: enacting the role of human-change agents. The mission statement should be clear, simple, and direct, focusing on what the department *really* tried to do so that the department's members can readily identify their roles (Drucker, 1990).

The mission statement should also address organizational values in making explicit the choices of nursing in the organization. This is congruent with Barrett's theory of power, which is characterized by choice. It provides a realistic appraisal of the organization's strengths and weaknesses. For instance, the nursing service can accomplish only a limited number of goals in any given year and for any given patient. Therefore, the organization must make deliberate choices regarding which goals it seeks to achieve, or, as Rogers (1970) might say, which potentials it seeks to actualize.

Manthey (1991) sees professional practice as the exercise of a nurse's autonomous decisions in the context of a responsible relationship with a patient. The relationship context may be specified in a particular care delivery model, such as primary nursing or case management. On a macro level, the mission statement might delineate the scope of these choices and further describe what the nurse–patient relationship encompasses.

The mission statement should also speak to the opportunities, competence, and commitment of the organization (Drucker, 1990). The opportunities that are presented to the organization are a function of its resources integral with its patient population. Even institutions that are severely strapped in terms of resources are able to point to strengths, as well as to unique situations that arise out of the union of case mix, staff mix, and the environment external to the institution.

The competence of the organization should be evident from an analysis of past successes and failures and should be within the awareness of all in the department. The scope of practice should specify how nursing competence in the organization is made visible. This offers the individual nurse the *choice* of delivering quality care as derived from the philosophy and mission of the organization.

Commitment is a natural extension of the valuing process and solidifies the organization's values and choices. In this way, it reifies the mission and makes it possible for an individual to identify with the organization on a personal level. This is what drove Walt Disney to build an enterprise powered by creativity. His motto, "If you can dream it, you can do it" led many Disney staffers to exceed their own expectations of productivity while experiencing high levels of job satisfaction. This is, in fact, what builds the culture of an organization.

## GOVERNANCE

The changes that are introduced cannot be merely cosmetic. Practice changes must be real, visible, and manifested in governance. The model that is most congruent with a Rogerian perspective and, more specifically, with Barrett's power theory is that of shared governance. It is based on the assumption that, given adequate information, staff will make appropriate decisions (Fagan, 1991). In other words, knowing participation is possible for all in the nursing service, if the organization is committed to participatory governance.

Operating from bylaws that have been developed by the nursing staff and approved by the hospital's board of trustees (Porter-O'Grady, 1989), nursing practice in a shared governance model is based on a council and committee structure. The staff is given the power and the authority to make decisions (del Bueno, 1991), and has an actual role to play in the governance and regulation of nursing practice and policy development. A typical structure is one in which there is a coordinating council, a clinical practice council, and an administrative council, all of which are composed of representatives of unit-based committees (Jenkins, 1991). Through these bodies, all major decisions are made and each nurse has access to knowing participation. Unlike other models, the nurse executive *shares* in the decision-making process (Porter-O'Grady, 1989), rather than owning it exclusively. This sharing provides a tangible expression of knowing participation and mutuality. Another example is self-scheduling, which requires nurse participation in contrast to the more traditional model that many nurses experience as victimization.

A further manifestation of knowing participation may be found in the establishment of "partner status." In another tangible expression of the staff members' ownership in the organization, the nurse is paid a contract wage, or "straight salary," and receives bonuses based on group performance. Paying homage to the mutuality of the group's effort, bonuses could be tied to quality assurance initiatives, length of stay trajectories, Diagnostic Related Group (DRG) gains, savings derived from decreased turnover, and so forth. Besides rewarding group performance, this plan has the advantage of increasing awareness of the need for cost containment and is beneficial to the organization at large (Lawrenz & Mayer, 1990).

Partnership status can be implemented in various forms in diverse institutions and does not necessarily have to be tied to position title. Again, the uniqueness of each institution will guide the implementation plan.

## TABLE OF ORGANIZATION

Tom Peters (1987) has stated that the successful organization, in the 1990s and beyond, will be flatter than previous models, populated by autonomous units, concerned to a great degree about quality and service, responsive to its various constituencies, and able to achieve innovation at a rapid rate. This is almost a prescription for knowing participation. The individual staff nurse uses power to make point-of-care decisions and has access to top levels of adminis-tration without having to wade through layers of managers, as in more traditional models. Further, the nurse manager of an individ-ual unit reports directly to the CNE. In addition, it may be helpful to structure the nurse manager role differently on some units, given the unique variables of some individual units (del Bueno, 1991).

As the institution moves toward full commitment to this model, inclusion of several additional roles may be helpful for the imple-mentation plan. An essential role is that of the Project Director, who serves as an internal consultant. Borrowing from clinical models, the Project Director can be viewed as a Clinical Nurse Specialist in Rogerian science, change theory, and nursing administration. This individual facilitates the values clarification necessary for group consensus building, acts as a liaison to the council and committee structure, and ensures that the staff nurse is not removed from pa-tient care by an overwhelming number of task force responsibilities. The Project Director communicates current progress and "next step" initiatives to the entire hospital community through formal and informal mechanisms.

It is crucial that the Project Director be seen as a member of the nursing staff and not as a "spy from administration." The Project Di-rector serves the needs of the entire nursing service and not just those of the persons at the top. It is conceivable that this role will be unnecessary after the new model of practice is well-established and has had the opportunity to mature. For this reason, the Project Direc-tor may be chosen from existing staff, if this is possible, or may as-sume another role within the organization after the Project Director role is no longer necessary.

Another role essential to the success of this emerging practice model is that of Research Adviser. This role is pivotal in leading the research effort that provides the locus for field testing Rogerian sci-ence. It is vital that the success of the model be made obvious in mea-surable terms, and that nurses at all levels have the opportunity to participate in nursing research. This can be accomplished by special interest groups, research committees, and research utilization task forces.

The Research Adviser also works closely with the Nursing Fi-nancial Adviser. The Financial Adviser is responsible for managing the wage and bonus database, for tracking the cost savings accrued by the new model, and for devising, in conjunction with the computer information department, a methodology that allows for knowing participation. This methodology provides the individual staff nurse with the opportunity to access budget information at any time. While preserving confidentiality, this program allows the nurse to assess the financial health of the hospital, nursing service, individual unit, and so forth, and to make informed decisions about issues presented to the council and committee structure. In this way, the staff nurse has the opportunity for both knowing participation in change and a realistic appraisal of economic imperatives, devoid of the usual mistrust of "administration." This program operates in a manner similar to an annual report that is updated on a day-to-day basis, or according to whatever time frame is relevant to the needs of the department. In this manner, knowing participation becomes a tool for cost effectiveness by deepening the individual's interest, commitment, and reward. In concert with the Project Director and the Research Adviser, the Financial Adviser must ensure that this effort remains a means to an end rather than a value in and of itself that removes the nurse from patient care (Prescott, et al. 1991).

Joint appointments with affiliating university faculty assist in the implementation of the model by increasing the pool of nurses skilled in research methodology and theory development. Other projects can include the facilitation of unique opportunities in theory development and model design for graduate students and perhaps postdoctoral fellows. These experiences benefit the organization by contributing to the research and development effort.

By virtue of integrality, and in a universe of open systems, all energy fields are in continuous mutual process, and thus every constituency (or energy field) is involved with the evolving emergent of this new model of nursing practice (Caroselli, 1990). Therefore, it is advisable that the role of Interdepartmental Liaison be included in the table of organization. This role assists the other constituencies in the hospital to understand this new model and to participate knowingly in its evolution. In some institutions, this role can be assumed by the Project Director.

## STAFF RECRUITMENT

Staff recruitment also proceeds from a Rogerian perspective and provides the potential employee with a view of knowing participation. This can be accomplished by means of the clinical passport, which provides a "snapshot" of the individual patient care unit. Data are provided in written form about the typical patient population, usual length of stay and illness trajectory, staff composition and role. The usual recruitment materials are included as well, such as an overview of the rest of the hospital, staff development and continuing education opportunities, and benefits package. In addition, information is included about specialty organizations relevant to the unit and institutional resources that supplement these special interests. Brochures from local colleges and universities imply the value placed on formal education. The clinical passport is distributed in the course of a "visiting day" during which potential staff members spend time with a senior staff nurse who discusses orientation and the preceptor/mentor program.

Included in the clinical passport is a career development questionnaire that can be used to help the potential staff member clarify values about practice, career goals, and preferences and determine how personal goals can be accomplished in the Rogerian practice model. After employment is accepted, the clinical passport becomes the basis for developing a professional portfolio of intended goals, evaluating achievement, and charting a career path. This might strike some readers as a great deal of effort expended on someone who is not yet an employee, but the time spent on determining "fit" and goal congruence is well spent when contrasted with costs associated with staff turnover.

This model is founded on concepts congruent with feminist philosophy and must acknowledge the strain of the multiple roles enacted by many nurses (Sampselle, 1990). Thus, child care must be made available to staff. While this service should be provided at competitive rates to avoid an unfavorable economic variance, the convenience and quality of a service that is available on a 24-hour, 7-day basis can be a meaningful recruitment device and may decrease staff absences.

No discussion of staff recruitment is complete without mention of basic nursing students. A student extern program can be implemented for a relatively modest cost and should be marketed to all affiliating students. Exposure to this radically different model of practice, whether as extern or affiliating student, can be a powerful draw for students as they consider their first postgraduation position.

## STAFF DEVELOPMENT

Staff development in this model proceeds from a competency-based orientation developed mutually by the nurse and a preceptor. After the orientation is completed, each nurse is paired with a mentor from within the nursing service, although not necessarily employed on the same unit or service. Matched in terms of career goals, style, and interests, the mentor and mentee map out and evaluate yearly goals, assess goal achievement, contribute information to the profit-sharing program, and develop a relationship that plays a major role in career development. It should be noted that this program is available to *all* nurses in the organization, although it is acknowledged that external resources may be needed for some individuals. It is posited that this program deepens the nurse's identification with the organization and the practice model and thus acts as a powerful retention strategy (Johnston, 1991).

Inservice education related to informatics is essential to the nurse's success within this practice model. Information technology expertise is a powerful tool in facilitating knowing participation, not only by allowing the nurse to access clinical information rapidly, but also by permitting the access of previously mentioned fiscal data. Specifics of implementation are unique to the hospital's information system and guide curriculum development in this regard.

Staff development further manifests the Rogerian perspective by providing education related to health patterning modalities (Barrett, 1990). Skill in Therapeutic Touch and imagery, for example, strengthens the repertoire of nursing care and demonstrates to both patient and provider the unique nature of nursing practice.

Given current financial trends and shortages of professional nurses, it is likely that a partners-in-care model may be incorporated into the nursing care delivery system. Based on the partnering of a professional nurse and an auxiliary worker, this approach provides a decision-making model for dividing work while minimizing the time spent by the nurse on non-nursing tasks (Manthey, 1990). This implies that *every* nurse will act in a modified leadership capacity. Therefore, staff development includes leadership theory from a Rogerian point of view, and an in-depth discussion of power from a Barrett perspective. In the spirit of knowing participation, auxiliary personnel are provided with as much information as they wish, thus avoiding an elitist, hierarchical approach.

Not all nurses will have had formal exposure to Rogerian science. Thus, orientation should include formal instruction in the conceptual system. Opportunities can be provided to streamline this process for those with previous relevant learning. Similarly, regular staff development can expand current knowledge, deepen expertise, and provide updates as the conceptual system is further refined.

## STAFF COMPOSITION

Staff composition or staff mix is quite clearly an indicant of integrality. The nursing service, in continuous mutual process with the environmental field, may assume many different configurations. The variables of setting, fiscal resources, access to a population of nurses, and case mix all have important implications for the composition of the nursing staff. Standards for staffing cannot be constructed in a vacuum, and a cookbook approach is to be avoided at all costs. The goal, however, should be the greatest number of professional nurses in direct care positions as is possible and appropriate.

## A NEW ORGANIZATIONAL CULTURE

The culture of an organization encompasses the set of shared beliefs and values most important to the organization and acts as a powerful force in shaping the institution's image. Organizational culture also acts as an agent of change and innovation (Caroselli, 1992). It is a vision of the organization's purpose and an indicant of pattern, the distinguishing characteristic of an energy field (Caroselli, 1990).

In this model, the culture of a nursing service is characterized by knowing participation and by a sense of ownership on the part of the nurse. This is very different from traditional approaches. The usual characterizations of "administration" and "the nursing office" become useless and irrelevant in the context of knowing participation and shared governance. This perspective is very attractive to the nurse who is ready and willing to assume the responsibilities of such a partnership.

Over time, and as the culture matures, staff's experience of power continues to expand, spiraling in diversity and complexity. The culture becomes a concrete operationalization of the Science of Unitary Human Beings.

## THE IMPLEMENTATION PLAN

Implementing this model of knowing participation means implementing a radically novel approach. This is indeed a formidable task.

Knowing participation begins with careful planning, which should be seen as a developmental process. It is developmental in that members of the nursing staff may be at varying levels of preparation and interest. Thus, staff may need to be educated regarding some very basic concepts related to change, planning, and the conceptual model before any values clarification or actual planning can begin.

Arikian (1991) provided some guidelines that are helpful in devising a plan. It is essential that goals be set that are consensual, realistic, and measurable, and that accountability be established, not just for the resulting organization, but also for the development and implementation of the plan. Communication must be frequent, accessible, multidirectional, and as informal as is practical. A comprehensive educational effort is required, as is the previously mentioned measurement. New policies and standards of practice will emerge, strengthened by the collective talents of knowing participation. The organizational culture experiences an evolution that is diverse and increasingly complex.

Two caveats must be mentioned. First, it is important that planning and implementation *not* be a game of outside consultants. It is essential that those who will practice in this new environment be intimately involved in creating it. Second, sufficient time must be allotted to the plan. A period of between three and five years must be allowed for this plan to come to fruition (Peters, 1987; Porter-O'Grady, 1989). As the plan moves through its various phases, annual evaluation and revision are vital to its success.

## EVOLUTIONARY EMERGENTS

This chapter has described the design and implementation of an evolutionary emergent, a nursing service based on the principle of knowing participation as derived from the Science of Unitary Human Beings. This is a beginning approach to filling the void of theory- and research-based nursing administrative practice. It represents an opportunity to further Rogerian science through the creation of a practice-oriented "think tank" that also unifies practice, education, research, and theory development—variables that have often been at odds with each other. In turn, it provides fertile ground for the field testing of Rogerian science in the setting in which nursing care is actually delivered.

This is not an easy task to accomplish, but it is an endeavor that can produce satisfying results for the nurse, the patient, and the institution. Nursing science can and does make a difference as it guides the art of nursing practice. While some may argue that health care is at too precarious a point in its history to attempt such a radical departure from traditional modes of practice, it is precisely because the stakes are so high and the risks so great that these steps must be taken. These risks are nursing's opportunity to demonstrate its value and resourcefulness as we move toward a nation where health care is accessible to all, where all patients can participate knowingly in their own care, and where nursing as a profession is truly powerful.

## REFERENCES

Arikian, V.L. (1991). Total quality management: Applications to nursing service. *Journal of Nursing Administration, 21*(6), 46-50.

Barrett, E.A.M. (1983). An empirical investigation of Martha E. Rogers' Principle of Helicy: The relationship of human field motion and power. *Dissertation Abstracts International, 45*, 615A (University Microfilms No. 8406278).

Barrett, E.A.M. (1990). Health patterning with clients in a private practice environment. In E.A.M. Barrett (Ed.), *Visions of Rogers' science-based nursing* (pp. 105-115). New York: National League for Nursing.

Caroselli, C. (1990). Visionary opportunities for knowledge development in nursing administration. In E.A.M. Barrett (Ed.), *Visions of Rogers' science-based nursing* (pp. 151-158). New York: National League for Nursing.

Caroselli, C. (1991). The relationship of power and feminism in female nurse executives in acute care hospitals. *Dissertation Abstracts International, 52*, 06B (University Microfilms No. DE9134724).

Caroselli, C. (1992). Assessing the organizational culture: A tool for professional success. *Orthopaedic Nursing, 11*(3), 56-63.

Carroll, T.L. (1987). Characteristics of nurse managers: Defining a model for management selection. *Journal of Nursing Administration, 17*, 4.

Christman, L. (1991). Knowledge growth: A challenge to administrators. *Journal of Nursing Administration, 21*, 17-19.

del Bueno, D.J. (1991). Managers: Function and form in the new organization. *Journal of Nursing Administration, 21*, 7-8, 24, 46.

Drucker, P. (1990). *Managing the nonprofit organization: Principles and practices.* New York: HarperCollins.

Drucker, P.F. (1991). The new productivity challenge. *Harvard Business Review, 69*(6), 69-79.

Elliott, E.A. (1990). The discourse of nursing: A case of silencing. *Nursing and Health Care, 10,* 539-543.

Fagan, M.J. (1991). Can unit-based shared governance thrive on its own? *Nursing Management, 22*(7), 104L-104D.

Gleeson, S., Nestor, O.W., & Riddell, A.J. (1983). Helping nurses through the management threshold. *Nursing Administration Quarterly, 7,* 11-16.

Helgesen, S. (1990). *The female advantage: Women's ways of leadership.* New York: Doubleday.

Jenkins, J.E. (1991). Professional governance: The missing link. *Nursing Management, 22*(8), 26-30.

Johnston, C.L. (1991). Retention strategies. *Journal of Nursing Administration, 26*(6), 11-19.

Kanter, R.M. (1989). *When giants learn to dance: Mastering the challenge of strategy, management, and careers in the 1990's.* New York: Simon & Schuster.

Kerfoot, K.M. (1990). From teamwork to synergy—the nurse manager in the relationship age. *Nursing Economics, 8,* 268-271.

Kramer, M., & Schmalenberg, C. (1988). Magnet hospitals: Part I, institutions of excellence. *Journal of Nursing Administration, 18*(1), 13-24.

Lawrenz, E., & Mayer, G.G. (1990). Compensation for professional practice: An incentive model. In G.G. Mayer, M.J. Madden, & E. Lawrenz (Eds.), *Patient care delivery models* (pp. 285-291). Rockville, MD: Aspen.

Manthey, M. (1990). Leadership: Accenting the positive. *Nursing Management, 21*(7), 40-42.

Manthey, M. (1991). Delivery systems and practice models: A dynamic balance. *Nursing Management, 22*(1), 28-30.

McClure, M.L. (1989). The nurse executive role: A leadership opportunity. *Journal of Nursing Administration, 13,* 108.

Peters. T. (1987). *Thriving on chaos: Handbook for a management revolution.* New York: Harper & Row.

Phillips, J.R. (1991). Human field research. *Nursing Science Quarterly, 4,* 142-143.

Porter-O'Grady, T. (1989). Shared governance: Reality or sham? *American Journal of Nursing, 89*(3), 350-351.

Prescott, P.A., Phillips, C.Y., Ryan, J.W., & Thompson, K.O. (1991). Changing how nurses spend their time. *Image: Journal of Nursing Scholarship, 23*(1), 23-28.

Quinn, J.F. (1990). On healing, wholeness, and the haelan effect. *Nursing and Health Care, 10,* 553-556.

Reeves, D.M., & Underly, N. (1983). Nurse managers and mickey mouse marketing. *Nursing Administration Quarterly, 7,* 22-27.

Rogers, M.E. (1970). *An introduction to the theoretical basis of nursing.* Philadelphia: F.A. Davis.

Rogers, M.E. (1990). Nursing: Science of Unitary Irreducible Human Beings: Update 1990. In E.A.M. Barrett (Ed.), *Visions of Rogers' science-based nursing* (pp. 5-11). New York: National League for Nursing.

Sampselle, C.M. (1990). The influence of feminist philosophy on nursing practice. *Image: The Journal of Nursing Scholarship, 22,* 243-247.

Senge. P. (1990). *The fifth discipline.* New York: Doubleday/Currency.

Simms, L.M. (1991). The professional practice of nursing administration: Integrated nursing practice. *Journal of Nursing Administration, 21,* 37-46.

Sovie, M.D. (1986). Doing things differently and better. *Nursing Economics, 4*(4), 201-205.

Stivers, C. (1991). Why can't a woman be less like a man? Women's leadership dilemma. *Journal of Nursing Administration, 21*(5), 47-51.

Taft, S.H., Minch, E.L., & Jones, P.K. (1992). Strengthening hospital nursing: Part I, The planning process. *Journal of Nursing Administration, 22*(5), 51-63.

Torbert, W.R. (1987). *Managing the corporate dream.* Homewood, IL: Irwin Publications.

# 18

# Personalized Nursing: A Science-Based Model of the Art of Nursing

*Marcia D. Andersen*
*Geoffrey A.D. Smereck*

## PERSONALIZED NURSING

People are living *and* dying simultaneously. To acknowledge this paradox is to recognize that the promotion of well-being is a more appropriate focus for nurses than the promotion of health alone. Rogers (1990) notes, "The purpose of nursing is to promote health and well-being for all persons wherever they are" (p. 6). Moreover, the American Nurses Association's Social Policy Statement agrees with this view and proposes that a nurse's responsibility is to focus on the human response to illness rather than on the illness itself (American Nurses Association, 1980). The authors recommend the promotion of well-being of people and their world be the focus for nursing in the 1990s.

### Philosophical and Theoretical Basis for Personalized Nursing

Aristotle's philosophy of ethics has something to offer modern nursing. His reasoning is sound and verified in the practice setting. The richness and coherence of his ideas and his emphasis on human

Reprinted with permission. Copyright by Chestnut House Publications. This paper originally appeared as two articles in *Nursing Science Quarterly:* 1989, Vol. 2, pp. 120–130, and 1992, Vol. 5, pp. 72–79.

fulfillment and well-being derived from the development of talents in pursuit of excellence are natural avenues for creative nursing approaches to clients (Ackrill, 1974; Griffin, 1986; Hardie, 1965; Kenny, 1965; Lear, 1988; Monan, 1968; Nagel, 1972).

Among other things, in his *Nicomachean Ethics,* Aristotle postulated that *eudaimonia* should be a transcendent goal of human activity, the vigorous seeking of which always and everywhere brings fulfillment, flourishing, happiness, and what is called well-being (Aristotle, 1984b, pp. 1734–1742; Cooper, 1975; Kraut, 1989). Since substantial literature has arisen in analysis of the Greek term *eudaimonia,* a brief account risks oversimplification. To translate it as "happiness" is too simple, though this is commonly done. A better translation is "living well in accordance with excellence." Aristotle, rejecting claims that human happiness lies in amusement, emphasized the active pursuit of excellence, within the limits applying to each individual, as the overarching human pursuit which always yields improved well-being (Aristotle, 1984b, p. 1737).

Aristotle equated human well-being with the excellent functioning of human beings. As humans devote their energy to the development of their uniquely human faculties, there is happiness as well as an improvement in well-being (Aristotle, 1984b, pp. 1734–1742).

He argued that human beings are fulfilled only by taking action toward improving themselves. The reasoning, in essence, develops from the assertion that everything that can take action has an *ergon* (what it does that makes it what it is and distinguishes it from the other acting objects and entities in the universe). What is the *ergon* of human beings, the perfecting of which will lead to *eudaimonia?* Aristotle believed that the human reasoning capacity itself, as operationalized by human beings' skills, talents, and abilities to create achievements in the pursuit of excellence, is the *ergon* of human beings. It follows that by actively working to develop personal talents, no matter what the circumstances, a person always and everywhere will enhance well-being and move steadily toward *eudaimonia.*

The congruence of Aristotle's and Rogers' human philosophies is striking. Aristotle, the founder of many sciences, nonetheless was extraempirical in the sense that he refused to be limited to an atomistic, piecemeal view of human beings. Indeed, Aristotle (1984b) in the *Physics* defined nature itself as "an inner principle of change" (p. 329). Moreover, Aristotle (1984b) in the *Physics* saw a developmental teleology at work in nature (p. 330), a purposefulness in nature that piecemeal explanations would be inadequate to explain.

Similarly, Rogers posits a universe in which change is continuous, inevitable, always novel, and developmental (M.E. Rogers, personal communication, February 16, 1989). Rogers firmly rejects a piecemeal approach to knowledge relating to human beings. Human beings, to be understood and well served by the nursing discipline, are viewed as patterned fields in continuous mutual process with their environment. They are not mere atoms or units or body parts helplessly caught in a Newtonian cause-and-effect exercise. As Rogers explained, "If you treat one's body, then you will fail. Rather, you must treat the whole person. There is no 'body,' as if that were something separate from the rest of the person" (M.E. Rogers, personal communication, February 16, 1989).

### Well-Being: The Purpose of Nursing

Achieving well-being is the goal of interest to nursing. Nursing is beset by problems, disagreements, and, perhaps most painful of all, an uncertainty as to nursing's role. Disputes are alive as to the proper, almost jurisdictional boundary separating the nurse's role and purpose from those of physicians, social workers, and other health personnel. In essence, the dispute is: What do nurses contribute directly that physicians or social workers do not? The authors claim that nurses' main goal is to improve the well-being of all people. Rogers (1983) states: "Promotion of well-being is the purpose of nursing" (p. 1). Nurses help individuals and groups achieve optimum well-being within the potential of each.

For years, nurse educators claimed that nurses focus their practices on health and illness. The authors postulate that the main focus of the Personalized Nursing practice model clarifies the nurse's role which is to assist people to improve their well-being. Rogers notes: "Change involves many potentialities, only some of which will be actualized. Nurses participate in a process of change that seems to promote well-being the best" (M.E. Rogers, personal communication, February 16, 1989).

Nursing practice is a synthesis of nursing art and nursing science. The art of nursing is the medium or vehicle for the use of the nursing knowledge generated by nursing science (Rogers, 1970). Every discipline has a scientific and philosophical knowledge base from which to derive theories, a process for action, and a series of therapeutic modalities based on the theories about how to participate in the process of change in the phenomenon of interest to a

given discipline. Further, all learned professions attempt to participate in the process of change according to the major phenomenon
central to a given field. The authors postulate:

1. The major focus of interest to medical doctors is cure of primarily physiological pathology.
2. The major focuses for psychologists are mental assessment and
   behavioral change.
3. The major focus for social workers is person–environment fit.
4. The major focus for nurses is to assist irreducible individuals,
   groups, families, communities, and society to improve their
   well-being.

### A Process for Change

Rogers (1970) believes continuous change is inevitable. Nursing's
role is to assist clients with their knowing participation in change
(Barrett, 1988, 1990). Nurses use a process where mutual "knowledgeable caring continuously evolves" (1988, p. 50) to "assist clients
with life-style changes and resolution of difficulties in living and
dying" (1990, p. 105). This helping process has two major phases:
(1) Pattern manifestation appraisal and (2) deliberative mutual patterning (Barrett, 1988, p. 50).

> Pattern manifestation appraisal is defined as "the continuous
> process of identifying manifestations of the human and envi-
> ronmental fields that relate to current health events" (Barrett,
> 1988, p. 50). Deliberative mutual patterning, the second phase,
> is defined as "the continuous process whereby the nurse with
> the client patterns the environmental field to promote harmony
> related to the health events."

### PERSONALIZED NURSING PROCESS MODEL

Personalized Nursing was developed by the authors to assist clients toward an improved sense of well-being. This process helps clients to
make desired changes in their lives. Personalized Nursing uses the two
phases of the Rogerian practice methodology as identified by Barrett
(1988). The first phase, pattern manifestation appraisal, is presented
using a heuristic called the Rainbow of Awareness (Figure 18.1). This

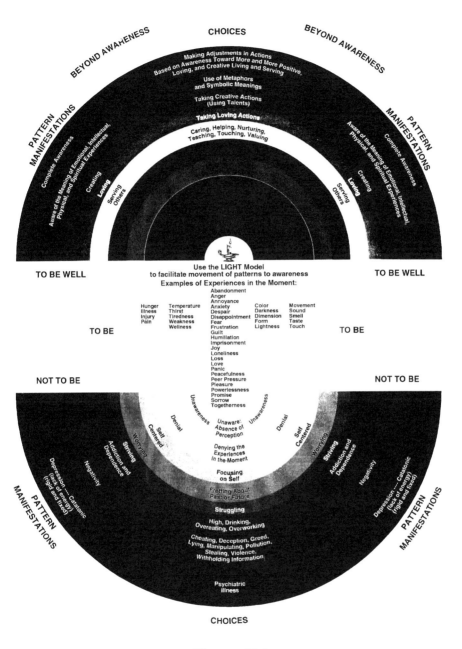

Figure 18.1
Rainbow of Awareness. In color the rainbow on top has
rings from outside in: purple, blue, dark green, green,
yellow, dark orange, orange, dark red, and red.

# LIGHT

| **Nurses and Caregivers:** | **You:** |
|---|---|
| **L**ove the Client | **L**ove Yourself |
| **I**ntend to Help | **I**dentify a Concern |
| **G**ive Care Gently | **G**ive Yourself a Goal |
| **H**elp the Client Improve Well-Being | **H**ave Confidence and Help Yourself |
| **T**each the Process | **T**ake Positive Action |

**Figure 18.2**
**Personalized Nursing LIGHT Model for**
**Personal Positive Change**

---

heuristic or teaching tool explicates pattern manifestations associated with behavior, feeling, and attitude choices (Andersen & Smereck, 1992).

The second phase, deliberative mutual patterning, is then begun. It utilizes the LIGHT model toward the goal of improved well-being (Andersen & Smereck, 1989). LIGHT facilitates understanding of the roles for both the nurses and clients in the deliberative mutual patterning process (Figure 18.2). The acronym assists both parties in role definition.

## PATTERN MANIFESTATION APPRAISAL PROCESS

Caregivers, using the Personalized Nursing well-being appraisal, assess three areas in order to facilitate clients in improving their well-being. These areas are: (1) well-being (global and current); (2) life pattern manifestations related to being, not being, and well-being; and (3) talents.

## Global Well-Being

Andrews and Withey (1976) developed a brief, valid, and reliable measure of global well-being, which they conceptualize as satisfaction with one's life to date. It asks, "How do you feel about your life as a whole?" The answers range from one to seven with one representing delighted and seven representing terrible.

They suggest asking this question early in an assessment interview and again toward the end. The second time it is asked, they reverse the scoring with one representing terrible and seven representing delighted. They suggest taking the mean between these two scores as a global well-being score representing life satisfaction.

## Current Well-Being

Currently, one measurement tool that nurses use to assess an individual's current well-being is being evaluated by the authors. It is called the well-being journal (Andersen & Smereck, 1989, p. 125). Clients are given a notebook and a pen. They are asked to make columns on the first page. They are given a carbon so that two copies of each page can be made. One copy goes to the nurse for an in-depth examination and one is to be kept by the client. The columns are: date/time; activities/actions/thoughts/situations; well-being score, physical/emotional (can be one or two columns).

A client writes down as many activities and thoughts as possible for 24–48 hours and rates his or her well-being (one through ten) during the activity (one = low and ten = high). The journal provides data on: (1) a baseline mean well-being score for 24 hours, (2) actions and pattern manifestations associated with low scores, and (3) actions and pattern manifestations associated with high scores.

The client and nurse together go over each entry and identify patterns that enhance or discourage the client's sense of well-being for use in the focal concern development process. A second appraisal is taken at some time during the deliberative mutual patterning process. By looking at changes in daily mean well-being scores, the progress of the client's well-being improvement can be measured.

## Difficulties in Achieving Well-Being

Achieving optimum global and current well-being can be difficult. Difficulties to achieving well-being are discovered in several ways.

First, clients should be asked to explain their current and global well-being measurement scores. (Why did you say "four" or "ten" on either global or current well-being scale?) Second, pattern manifestations should be appraised to find clues to disturbing patterns in the mutual process of human and environmental energy fields.

## Life Pattern Manifestations Related to Being, Not Being, and Well-Being

Daily counseling of hard-to-reach, treatment-resistant drug users in New York City, Baltimore, and Detroit provided an invaluable laboratory in which to develop a perspective about life patterning associated with well-being. Clinical experiences with over 2,000 active drug users yielded a descriptive paradigm about being, not being, and well-being. The paradigm, the Rainbow of Awareness, is used to understand the patterning represented by attitudes, experiences, behaviors, and belief systems found to be prevalent in the hard-core urban addicted population. It constitutes a description of pattern manifestations associated and not associated with well-being. The Rainbow of Awareness (Figure 18.1) was created as a heuristic, a way to frame the pattern manifestations within being, not being, and well-being.

An attempt has been made to develop a pandimensional, nonlinear description of pattern manifestation appraisal as it relates to well-being. Concepts such as "states," "levels," "good," "bad," "either," and "or" are not meant to be implied. The Rainbow of Awareness provides a useful heuristic to be used by the nurse and client to identify pattern manifestations. Additionally, it assists the client to see alternatives. When the client desires help in making deliberate changes, the Rainbow provides a tool which demonstrates how to make choices that promote different patterning.

*Being.* Being is defined as "present in the now." This definition of being is operationalized in Figure 18.3.

Many people, though completely conscious, often are not fully aware nor fully or optimally attentive to the present moment. At those times, people are not fully being. To be fully being, a person must be aware of all sense-data, feelings, and thoughts, as well as spirituality. If one or more of these awarenesses is lacking, the person is not fully being. (This definition of being is more comprehensive than Webster's (1988) dictionary definition of "to exist" (p. 476). For purposes of this chapter, it is unnecessary to solve the riddle of the

Client Is:
—Now Optimally Aware of Sense-Data
  Available to All Senses
—Now Optimally Aware of His or Her
  Feelings
—Now Optimally Aware of His or Her
  Thoughts
—Now Optimally Aware of His or Her
  Relationship or Nonrelationship with
  Higher Spiritual Power

PERSON
IS
BEING
IN
THE NOW

Client Is Not Optimally Aware of Any
One of the Above

PERSON IS
NOT BEING
IN THE NOW

**Figure 18.3**
**Definition of Being/Not Being**

ultimate nature of being. The authors note that the approaches to being of Parmenides (1965), Aristotle (1984a; 1984b), Kant (1929), and
Heidegger (1927) are radically different, even inconsistent.)

*Not Being.*     Shakespeare's (1987) Hamlet agonized over the
concept of being. He said, "To be or not to be? That is the question"
(p. 239). Hamlet went on to question whether it is better to suffer the
"slings and arrows" of outrageous fortune (the pain associated with
all the bad things that happen) or not be (die). The entire play was
built on the premise that it is painful to suffer the slings and arrows
of outrageous fortune. By trying to avoid the pain, everyone in *Hamlet* experienced not being during the play. The authors believe Shakespeare (1987) wanted the audience to see that the only way "to be"
was to suffer the slings and arrows and find new ways to move on
toward well-being.

*Well-Being.*     People living fully in the present and willing to go
beyond any pain or discomfort they experience in the now are able to
draw upon an inner source or "well" of well-being. Judy Anderson, a
nursing doctoral student at Wayne State University in September
1988, once said she views well-being as "a well of power one can
draw from to improve one's awareness state." The authors, moreover,

believe that the pattern manifestations on the colorful side of the rainbow are wells of power from which to draw genuine long-lasting well-being such as hope, loving, serving, and creating. Well-being from this perspective is defined as "being" plus dipping into one or more of the colorful "wells of power" on the Rainbow of Awareness heuristic. Conversely, not being, from the authors' perspectives, is associated with choices that are assumed to promote well-being but actually are choices within the "shadow" or dark side of the rainbow. Wells on the dark side of the rainbow are illusions and only reflections of the colorful wells. These wells contain, among others, denial, striving, and addiction, from which genuine well-being can never be drawn. These are illusionary wells, the shadows of life's true wells of power.

### The Rainbow of Awareness: A Mechanism for Pattern Manifestation Appraisal

*Reading the Rainbow.*     The Rainbow of Awareness (Figure 18.1) assists the nurse and client in pattern manifestation appraisal. For purposes of understanding, choices, as well as associated labeled pattern manifestations, are listed. The choices represent behaviors, attitudes, moods, and perceptions chosen by people. These include getting high, fretting about the past, seeking learning, taking loving actions, and many more. While directionality is intentional, the clear distinctions between patterns are not. Pattern manifestations include the characteristics of alertness with respect to the moment, as well as such characteristics as hope and complete awareness. Each color represents a different frequency range. The colorlessness of not being is represented in the lower reflection of the rainbow by black and gray. Being is represented by white in the center of the rainbow. White occurs when all the colors of light come together. Well-being in the upper reflection of the rainbow represents patterns increasing in frequency, and this increasing frequency is illustrated by vivid colors moving from red to violet.

In every pattern of being, humans (and probably other entities as well) have experiences. Examples of these experiences are listed in the center "being" part of the rainbow. People make choices when an experience occurs. They can deny experiences or see them as opportunities for learning. People often deny situations associated with discomfort. It is postulated that when people make choices in the gray and black zone of the rainbow, they are not perceiving the complete dimensionality and experience of optimum beingness. They perceive instead fewer dimensions; less joy, color, light, energy, peace, power; and perceive more heat and a sense of time as dragging. If, on the other hand, they choose to experience the moment, identify fully the feeling or experience, move beyond it to find its lesson, have hope for betterment, and take loving creative action toward a health-promoting goal, they enter a cool, peaceful, colorful, pandimensional world of love and light.

Minute by minute, each day, people experience changing conditions of being, not being, and well-being associated with their choices. The wonderful thing about awareness is that one can change where one is on the rainbow by choosing different patterns of behaviors or attitudes. Moreover, one can improve well-being by choosing to change patterns. Often, when choices in the being and well-being range are selected, the uncomfortable feelings or situations that one avoided arise. These offer an opportunity to decide differently how to handle the pain (or comfort) previously avoided, by learning from the discomfort. Long-term well-being is thereby improved.

### Addiction: A Shortcut to Well-Being

Theoretically, people can find ways to take a shortcut to another plane or dimension: to bypass "being" to get to "well-being." A shortcut represents the quickest and simplest path to overcome difficulties existing in the standard path. Figure 18.1 depicts how the rainbow is reflected in another dimension (probably many others) which are illusions like those seen in a pond or mirror. It is hypothesized that drugs are one means used to jump over the barriers of "being"—pain; slings and arrows—to reach short-term, illusionary well-being. By jumping into well-being on a different dimension, this illusion of well-being can be experienced instantly. Clinical evidence, experienced by the authors, supports the idea that drug addicts have been to the most vivid frequency patterns of the colorful rainbow. They know about letting go to the universe and metaphorical meanings. Addicts experience maximum well-being in another dimension, while most people do not.

A recovering addict, interviewed about this idea, explained:

> Addicts get well-being in another dimension. You take heroin, you get an immediate feeling everything is all right, but you know in reality it is not, it is worse. You experience the

well-being side of the rainbow, but there is no feeling of well-being and no color, so you know it is an illusion.

You take cocaine, on the other hand, and it gives you the well-being side of the rainbow just as you have it here [indicating Figure 18.1], and for one second you get the feeling and you see the colors and then everything gets even darker than it was when you started.

Cocaine and crack cocaine users will sit there and spend every cent they have to get one more second of the wonderful feelings and color in that rainbow. That is why they call taking crack cocaine "chasing the rainbow."

Addicts, under the influence of drugs, have discovered one pattern associated with drugs, but the pattern is fleeting and transitory. Most of all, it is illusionary. Going to the colorful side of the rainbow via drug use bypasses "being" and all the necessary lessons it takes to reach longer-lasting, more permanent well-being. It should be understood: the quest of the addicted person is the quest of every person.

### Talents

Talents are also assessed during the Personalized Nursing pattern manifestation appraisal process. Inside each person is an unrealized dream. Caregivers assess the client's perception of what he or she likes to do and what he or she does well. The patterning and talents provide hints and clues to the client's *ergon* and assist clients in making activity choices which may improve their well-being and begin movement toward *eudaimonia.*

After well-being, talents, and other pattern manifestations have been assessed, the client and nurse begin a deliberative mutual patterning process toward a goal of improved well-being for both.

### LIGHT MODEL: A DELIBERATIVE MUTUAL PATTERNING PROCESS

The use of the LIGHT model assists clients to experience the precious moment, "the now"; to learn from it and develop specific concerns, goals, and actions to be taken toward the goal of an improved sense of well-being. The Personalized Nursing LIGHT Model is used to assist people to become aware of concerns or discomforts; identify alternative choices; and use their talents to take action to improve their well-being.

Research has shown that by addressing well-being directly, pattern manifestations such as behaviors, attitudes, and situations change toward improved well-being (Andersen, 1986; Andersen & Braunstein, 1991; Andersen, Smereck, & Braunstein, 1991). The most efficient mechanism for improvement of a sense of well-being is for the individual to take action on his or her own behalf. The person is always, but not always knowingly, a participant in change (Rogers, 1970). Sometimes it is not possible, desirable, or probable that an individual can act to promote changes in his or her own well-being. He or she may not want to improve well-being, may not know how, may not have the resources, or may have a skewed perception of the reality surrounding the situation or action needed.

The LIGHT Model helps clarify both the nurse's and the client's roles in a process of change toward a goal of improved well-being. One track of the Personalized Nursing LIGHT Model is called Personalized Care. All actions are taken by the nurse on behalf of the person with the intent of improving the person's sense of well-being. On the other track of the Personalized Nursing LIGHT Model, the Personalized Action track, all actions are taken by the person. Both tracks are described with the acronym LIGHT (Figure 18.2).

## Personalized Care: LIGHT Model Process

As readers review the Personalized *Care* LIGHT nursing process model, it should be noted that all the actions are taken by the nurse. This model is especially useful in situations where the client is not able or willing to care for himself or herself. There is often improvement in short-term well-being.

Many clients have no hope of improved health status or cure for their illness. However, an improvement in their fundamental sense of well-being is a reasonable and acceptable goal.

*L: LOVE the Client.*    The model, as with so many models involving improvement of the human condition, starts with love. The authors have found unconditional love—the sincere valuing of another human being without any expectation of any return—to be the initial focus.

In practice, nurses cannot improve the well-being of their clients unless they love their clients unconditionally. That is, they must not only ignore superficial, demographic considerations (race, age, gender, religion, national origin, socioeconomic status, and education), but also believe them to be irrelevant. Communication of unconditional love to the client bypasses the artificial hierarchies and rigidities, the unfortunate tendency of narrowly defining the person. All of these inhibit and hamper what should be an ennobling joint participation by nurse and person in the continuous process of innovative change (M.E. Rogers, personal communication, February 16, 1989). A nurse needs to request a transfer to a different client if unable to feel unconditional love for the client.

*I: INTEND to Help.*   While it is often assumed that nurses intend to help improve well-being, their attitudes and actions do not always communicate this intention. The following are important for communicating the intention to help:

1. Prior to using the LIGHT Model, nurses need to believe improvement in well-being is possible. For many conditions like chemical dependency and cancer, nurses must develop philosophical stances that improvement in the condition (healing or "cure" or at least improvement in well-being) is possible.
2. The reason for the nurse's being in mutual process with the client must be to help the client improve his or her sense of well-being. When using the LIGHT Model, reasons such as a power trip for the nurse, a need for intimacy or closeness on the part of the nurse, a need to feel helpful on the part of the nurse, a need to finance a vacation are not legitimate reasons for therapeutic modalities with clients.
3. Nurses must communicate that they truly intend to assist the client to improve his or her sense of well-being. A thorough study of the process of neurolinguistic programming (Bandler & Grinder, 1982), a communication theory, assists nurses to communicate effectively their intentions.

*G: GIVE Care Gently.*   Giving nursing care gently implies a soft touch, genuine kindness, and what Rogers (1970) suggests as a natural energy process. Although personnel in other disciplines can love clients, intend to help, and give care gently, the key to this model's uniqueness to nursing is that nurses focus on irreducible persons and their environments (Rogers, 1970), and that the nature of nursing service is thus different.

Nursing care occurs when the gentle care given is aimed at improving the client's well-being. The uniqueness of nursing care is:

(1) the focus is on providing care to the whole person, who is integral with his or her environment and (2) the focus is on participation in improving the person's perceived well-being.

As Rogers (1970) suggests, nurses assist all persons in patterning their human–environmental energy fields in creative, individualized ways that promote well-being.

*H: HELP the Client Improve Well-Being.* The H in the LIGHT Model represents the word *help,* a complex verb composed of assistance being offered and received. The process of offering help to facilitate its being accepted includes:

1. *T*ouching or reaching the client.
2. *A*ssessing need.
3. *P*lanning action.

Receiving help includes:

1. Being touched or reached by the helper.
2. Useful assistance being received toward a goal the receiver values.

Receiving help promotes a feeling of being valued and cared about by another. This is the first step of loving one's self. Helping is a process which is truly mutual. By helping another, the helper facilitates his or her own actualization. If the helper is not open and willing to be changed or touched by the bonding with the client in the helping process, helping cannot occur. The H in the Personalized Care LIGHT Model is an action performed by the nurse.

*T: TEACH the Process.* Once the client has experienced an improvement in well-being, the Personalized Action LIGHT Process can be taught to the client so that he or she can take action to improve his or her own well-being.

### The Personalized Action LIGHT Process

A nursing care approach called Personalized Action can also be outlined by the acronym LIGHT (see Figure 18.2). The actions in the Personalized Action LIGHT process are taken by the client, however, not the nurse. The nurse is a facilitator toward actions taken by the client.

It is postulated that the use of this process by clients will be associated with an improvement in the client's sense of well-being.

Over time, extended use of this process results in long-term improvement in well-being and progress toward actualization or *eudaimonia.*

### Assumptions

Prior to proceeding with the use of this practice model, the following assumptions must be met:

1. The client must have a sincere desire to improve his or her own sense of well-being.
2. The client must have a reliable and valid perception of the situation related to his or her concern.

### Personalized Action

*L: LOVE Yourself.*    For Personalized Action to occur, the clients must have a genuine fondness for themselves. The first step toward actualization is to believe in one's own worth. People can recognize and accept the worth of their unique individual talents. Nurses, using a talent assessment, can recognize a strength and point out something the client does well. The step prior to loving oneself is being loved and valued by another.

*I: IDENTIFY a Concern.*    The principle of resonancy as developed by Rogers (1970) as part of the Science of Unitary Human Beings may be useful in understanding focal concerns or worries from the relative past that manifest themselves in the relative present. Human and environmental fields are identified by wave patterns manifesting continuous change from lower-frequency wave patterns to high-frequency wave patterns (Rogers, 1981).

Using this principle as a basis, it is suggested that life patterning becomes more complex with time. Adjustment to or acceptance of life's increasing complexities could be associated with alterations in one's sense of well-being and focal concerns. The concerns hamper optimum well-being due to identifiable human and environmental patterns related to life's increasing complexities. Personalized Action considers a client's identified focal concerns as manifestations of an unsatisfactory sense of well-being. A nurse, using Personalized Action, assists clients to identify the main concerns or worries which stand between themselves and their optimum sense of long-term well-being.

*G: GIVE Yourself a Goal.*    Rogers' (1981) Principle of Helicy explains the nature of giving oneself a goal and having confidence to act. The nature and direction of human and environmental change is continuously innovative, unpredictable, and characterized by increasing diversity of field patterns emerging out of the continuous mutual processes between human and environmental fields and is manifested by nonrepeating rhythmicities (Rogers, 1981, 1988).

This principle underlies the client's setting a goal and having confidence to act. The changes required to improve one's current sense of well-being related to the identified focal concern will always be new to the individual. Even if the concern has appeared in the past, the concern is new again because of the constantly increasing diversity of one's human–environmental field patterning. Making new changes may be stressful and require self-confidence prior to taking action. The nurse's role is to assist in goal development, explain the need for new actions, and encourage self-confidence.

*H: HAVE Confidence and Help Yourself.*    Change is inevitable and ever-present (Rogers, 1981). The changes one experiences are increasingly complex, and the manifestations exhibited as human and environmental patterns become more and more diverse.

With Rogers' Science of Unitary Human Beings, the authors believe that throughout life, more and more confidence is required to make and act upon goals to achieve optimum well-being since the actions required are more and more diverse. Optimum well-being is not static; it moves toward actualization with each time a challenge (focal concern) is met and acted upon.

*T: TAKE Positive Action.*    Rogers' (1986) Principle of Integrality postulates that human and environmental fields are in continuous mutual process. This principle illustrates the fact that when action is taken, human field patterns and environmental field patterns will both change, and movement toward optimum well-being is achieved. Things will never be the same again. Individuals must let go of the status quo in both their human and environmental field patterns and the current process between the two. Action or inaction (deliberate or not) is the important final step of the Personalized Action process. For "not acting" to qualify as the final step of the process, it must be deliberate, not passive. Any action or inaction is accompanied by natural consequences. Although action or deliberate inaction on the part of the client must occur to complete the Personalized Action process, the ramifications should be examined prior to implementation whenever possible. When this is done, the most efficient road toward long-term well-being can be chosen.

### Actualization

Well-being manifests itself in part as a sense or feeling of happiness, satisfaction, and peace. Aristotle (1984b, pp. 1735–1741) states happiness is not to be found in mere amusement, but in activity, including intellectual activity, that brings people closer to excellence or virtue. Short-term well-being includes well-being in the next clock hour or hours. Long-term well-being is a lifetime of progress toward an ongoing pursuit of excellence or actualization (Maslow, 1982; C. Rogers, 1961). Actualization is a process characterized by movement toward a happier, smarter state than was present prior to the experience of stress or pain. While striving toward that goal, if the processes of helping others and gaining knowledge are translated into actions, movement toward actualization is more rapid.

## NURSING AS A PROCESS FOR SERVING OTHERS

The Rainbow of Awareness (Figure 18.1) illustrates that serving others and helping them improve their well-being (Rogers, 1990) is in itself a pattern associated with well-being. Nursing scholars are developing processes to be used by people to serve others. By looking at the Rainbow of Awareness, one may see how magnificent, how uplifting and inspiring the challenge of nursing truly is. The art of nursing is directed toward a goal of well-being and improvement for humankind and the planet.

Nurses serve by focusing on people and their worlds (Rogers, 1990), the ill, the addicted, the unhappy, the unconscious. By serving, nurses dip into one of the true wells of power. When serving others, nurses also engage in improving their own well-being. This is especially true if they understand that challenge always represents a lesson for themselves.

Nurses are cautioned, while helping others, to avoid making choices for themselves associated with not being. When strife occurs on the job, nurses must remember to experience the pain, learn from it, and identify a pleasant pictured possible goal. One must also remember that denying pain or engaging in worry or struggle is associated with pattern manifestations on the not-being end of the rainbow.

Nursing's challenge is to promote being and well-being in people and their worlds by using the modalities of nursing. Nurses assist people to identify and participate knowingly (Rogers, 1970) in change as they suffer the slings and arrows of outrageous fortune. Moreover, nurses assist people to understand the joy, sorrow, pleasure, and pain they experience on their way to long-lasting well-being. The modalities of nursing are the modalities of assisting others to choose actions on the colorful side of the rainbow and to encourage people to dip into wells of power to move toward an improved sense of well-being. The modalities of nursing were long thought to be psychiatric, medical–surgical, pediatric, and others. Now, the modalities of nursing are known to be love, touch, caring, use of metaphors, or any modality which promotes change toward an increasing sense of well-being for people in their worlds.

### Field Testing

Several research studies have been conducted evaluating the efficacy of the Personalized Nursing LIGHT Model with substance abusers. The model has been implemented successfully with women in prison (Andersen & Braunstein, 1991) and with drug users brought into urban hospital emergency rooms in three states (Andersen, 1986; Andersen, Smereck, & Braunstein, 1991). In 1991, a three-state, federally funded study demonstrated significant behavior changes associated with the use of the model and the improvement of well-being (Andersen, Smereck, & Braunstein 1993; Smereck, Andersen, & Braunstein, 1992).

*LIGHT Model: An Effective Intervention Model Associated with Change in High-Risk Behaviors among Drug Users.*   Two thousand thirty-three hospital emergency room clients, who were current, active injecting drug users (IDUs), were voluntary participants in a pre-test, post-test research project utilizing the Personalized Nursing LIGHT Model as a counseling approach to decrease high-risk AIDS behaviors. The LIGHT Model works by directly improving well-being and thereby indirectly decreasing high-risk behaviors associated with AIDS. Addicts from urban emergency rooms in three cities (Detroit, Michigan; Brooklyn, New York; and Baltimore, Maryland) were treated with teams consisting of nurses and indigenous outreach workers.

Post-test data were gathered on 995 of the clients who received the Personalized Nursing LIGHT Model teaching and counseling modality. In a post-test, at least three months after the initial interview, these IDUs reported a significant increase in well-being ($t$ (530) = $-11.77$; $p < .001$) and significant reductions in frequency of IV heroin use ($z = -18.4$; $p < .001$), IV cocaine use ($z = -16.0$; $p < .001$), and IV speedball use ($z = -14.3$; $p < .001$), as well as significant decreases in sharing of cookers (a type of drug-using equipment) ($z = -13.8$; $p < .001$), and other high-risk behaviors associated with AIDS acquisition and transmission. At a second post-test, six months after the initial review, these results were unchanged.

*LIGHT Model: Randomized Clinical Trail with IVDUs.*    Currently, a randomized clinical trial, funded by the federal National Institute on Drug Abuse, is under way to test the efficacy of the LIGHT Model with hard-to-reach, active street drug addicts who are out-of-treatment and high-risk for AIDS acquisition and transmission. To date, 762 clients have been counseled.

## CONCLUSION

Personalized Nursing, based on the work of Aristotle (1984b) and Rogers (1970), provides a sensitive caring process to be used to foster the imaginative facilitation of improvement of well-being of individuals and the nurses who care for them.

Donahue (1985) states:

> Nursing has long been defined as both an art and a science. The primary emphasis, however, has been on the scientific aspects of nursing with little consideration given to its state as an art. Nursing is a fine art. According to Florence Nightingale, it is the finest of fine arts! Nursing is not merely a technique, but a process that incorporates the elements of soul, mind, imagination, the sensitive spirit, and the intelligent understanding that provides the very foundation for effective nursing care. (p. 469)

## REFERENCES

Ackrill, J.L. (1974). Aristotle on *eudaimonia*. *Proceedings of the British Academy, 60,* 339–359.

American Nurses Association (1980). *Nursing: A social policy statement.* Kansas City, MO: Author.

Andersen, M.D. (1986). Personalized nursing: An intervention model for use with drug-dependent women in an emergency room. *International Journal of Addictions, 21*(1), 105–122.

Andersen, M.D., & Braunstein, M.S. (1991). Conceptions of therapy: Personalized Nursing LIGHT Model with chemically dependent female offenders. In T. Mieczkowski (Ed.), *Drugs, crime, and social policy: Research, issues, and concerns* (pp. 250–262). Needham Heights, MA: Allyn & Bacon.

Andersen, M.D., & Smereck, G.A.D. (1989). Personalized Nursing LIGHT Model. *Nursing Science Quarterly, 2,* 120–130.

Andersen, M.D., & Smereck, G.A.D. (1992). The consciousness rainbow: An explication of Rogerian field pattern manifestation. *Nursing Science Quarterly, 5,* 72–79.

Andersen, M.D., Smereck, G.A.D., & Braunstein, M.S. (1991). Personalized Nursing LIGHT Model: An effective intervention model to change high-risk behaviors among hard-to-reach urban IV drug users. In *Research in progress* (pp. 4–11). Bethesda, MD: National Institute on Drug Abuse & NOVA Research.

Andersen, M.D., Smereck, G.A.D., & Braunstein, M.S. (1993). LIGHT Model: An effective intervention model to change high-risk AIDS behaviors among hard-to-reach urban drug users. *American Journal of Drug and Alcohol Abuse, 19*(3), 309–325. New York: Marcel Dekker.

Andrews, F.M., & Withey, S.B. (1976). *Social indicators of well-being.* New York: Plenum.

Aristotle. (1984a). Metaphysics. In J. Barnes (Ed.), *The complete works of Aristotle.* Princeton, NJ: Princeton University Press.

Aristotle. (1984b). Nicomachean ethics; Physics; Eudemian ethics. In J. Barnes (Ed.), *The complete works of Aristotle.* Princeton, NJ: Princeton University Press.

Bandler, R., & Grinder, G. (1982). *Reframing: Neurolinguistic programming and the transformation of meaning.* Moab, UT: Real People Press.

Barrett, E.A.M. (1988). Using Rogers' Science of Unitary Human Beings in nursing practice. *Nursing Science Quarterly, 1,* 50–51.

Barrett, E.A.M. (1990). Health patterning with clients in a private practice environment. In E.A.M. Barrett (Ed.), *Visions of Rogers' science-based nursing* (pp. 105–115). New York: National League for Nursing.

Cooper, J.M. (1975). *Reason and human good in Aristotle.* Cambridge, MA: Harvard University Press.

Donahue, M.P. (1985). *Nursing, the finest art: An illustrated history.* St. Louis: Mosby.

Griffin, J.G. (1986). *Well-being, its meaning, measurement, moral importance.* Oxford, England: Oxford University Press.

Hardie, W.F.R. (1965). The final good in Aristotle's ethics. *Philosophy, 40,* 277-295.

Heidegger, M. (1927). *Being and time.* Scranton, PA: HarperCollins.

Kant, I. (1929). *Critique of pure reason.* (N. Kemp-Smith, Trans.). New York: St. Martin's.

Kenny, A. (1965). Aristotle on happiness. *Proceedings of the Aristotelian Society, 66,* 93-102.

Kraut, R. (1989). *Aristotle on the human good.* Princeton, NJ: Princeton University Press.

Lear, J. (1988). *Aristotle, the desire to understand.* Cambridge, England: Cambridge University Press.

Maslow, A.H. (1982). *Toward a psychology of being.* Princeton, NJ: Van Nostrand.

Monan, J.D. (1968). *Moral knowledge and its methodology in Aristotle.* Oxford, England: Oxford University Press.

Nagel, T. (1972). Aristotle on *eudaimonia. Phronesis, 17,* 252-259.

Parmenides. (1965). The way of truth (fragment). In W.K.C. Guthrie (Ed.), *A history of Greek philosophy.* New York: Cambridge University Press.

Rogers, C.R. (1961). *On becoming a person.* Boston: Houghton Mifflin.

Rogers, M.E. (1970). *An introduction to the theoretical basis of nursing.* Philadelphia: F.A. Davis

Rogers, M.E. (1981). Science of unitary man: A paradigm for nursing. In G. Lasker (Ed.), *Applied systems and cybernetics* (pp. 1719-1722). New York: Pergamon Press.

Rogers, M.E. (1983, June). *Charting the future.* Paper presented at the First National Rogerian Conference, New York University.

Rogers, M.E. (1986). Science of Unitary Human Beings. In V. Malinski (Ed.), *Explorations on Martha Rogers' Science of Unitary Human Beings.* Norwalk, CT: Appleton-Century-Crofts.

Rogers, M.E. (1988). Nursing science and art: A perspective. *Nursing Science Quarterly, 1,* 99-102.

Rogers, M.E. (1990). Nursing: Science of Unitary Irreducible Human Beings: Updated 1990. In E.A.M. Barrett (Ed.), *Visions of Rogers' science-based nursing* (pp. 5-11). New York: National League for Nursing.

Shakespeare, W. (1987). *Hamlet.* (G.R. Hibbard, Ed.). Oxford, England: Oxford University Press.

Smereck, G.A.D., Andersen, M.D., & Braunstein, M.S. (1992). LIGHT Model nursing intervention in hospital emergency rooms among IDUs at risk for AIDS. Poster presentation, VIII International Conference on AIDS/III STD World Congress, Amsterdam, The Netherlands, July 19-24; Vol. 2., *Poster Abstracts, VIII International Conference on AIDS/III STD World Congress* (Amsterdam, The Netherlands, June, 1992), p. D402.

*Webster's New World Dictionary of American English* (3rd ed.). (1988). New York: Simon & Schuster.

# 19

# Implementing the Science of Unitary Human Beings at the San Diego Veterans Affairs Medical Center

*Judy Heggie*
*Maryanne Garon*
*Mary Kodiath*
*Ann Kelly*

This chapter consists of contributions of four key members of the Rogerian Task Force at the San Diego Veterans Affairs Medical Center (SDVAMC). Each author has a unique history of involvement with the task force and a different practice perspective. Judy Heggie is the current Chair of the Rogerian Task Force and has been involved in the implementation process for five years. Her current position is Associate Chief, Nursing Service for Education. Maryanne Garon is the immediate past Chair of the Rogerian Task Force and has been involved with the project since 1985. Mary Kodiath presents her interpretation of use of the Science of Unitary Human Beings in her clinical practice as a Nurse Practitioner. She has been at the SDVAMC since 1987 as Director, Chronic Low Back Pain Clinic, and joined the Task Force in 1988. Ann Kelly, a Psychiatric Clinical Nurse Specialist, offers her uses of the model in her work with the homeless mentally ill. One of the initiators of the model at the SDVAMC, she rejoined the Task Force in 1990 after several years' hiatus from the Veterans Administration (VA). These four individual perspectives will give readers a sense of the joys and perils of implementing this model in a large, complex bureaucracy.

## IMPLEMENTING ROGERS' ORGANIZED ABSTRACT SYSTEM—THE SCIENCE OF UNITARY HUMAN BEINGS

### Task Force Chair and Nursing Administrator's View (Judy Heggie)

Early in the 1980s, the Education Department and the Clinical Nurse Specialist Group at the San Diego Veterans Affairs Medical Center decided that a nursing theoretical model would be needed to change the focus of nursing practice from the medical model to a more holistic, nursing-oriented view of the client. Following educational programs on nursing theoretical models and staff surveys to determine nursing staff philosophy of care, Rogers' (1970, 1990) model was selected as the one that best fit with prevailing staff beliefs.

Many steps have been taken since those early days to integrate Rogers' model and nursing care delivery. (See Table 19.1 for the sequence of events.) No one, at that time, realized what a difficult undertaking this would be. The extent of organizational and individual change necessary was not foreseen. Those choosing to assist with this project thought that, through the use of education, behavior could be easily changed. A behavior change was believed to indicate a change in an individual's belief system. At that time, we were naive as to the true meaning of the mutual process of integrality.

No one voiced the necessity of a perspective transformation or paradigmatic shift in the nurses' view of client care as a prerequisite to meaningful behavior change. Mezirow (1981) defined perspective transformation as "an emancipatory process of becoming critically aware of how and why the structure of psychocultural assumptions has come to constrain the way we see ourselves and our relationships, reconstituting this integration of experience and acting upon these new understandings" (p. 6). Perspective transformation requires reflective thinking. Reflective thinking involves an interest in knowledge of ourselves through reflection to understand our ideology—the beliefs that shape our interpretation of reality and are used to justify behavior and action. Reflection on our ideology—sexual, political, religious, racial, occupational, and cultural—helps us understand how these enculturated beliefs limit our vision of ourselves and our relationships (Habermas, 1971). Once we recognize oppressing sociocultural beliefs and we think and see the world differently, we change our interpretive framework. We incorporate

# Table 19.1
## Sequence of Events in Model Implementation

| Stage | Action | Outcome |
|---|---|---|
| *1981*<br>Assessed need. | Need for a nursing theoretical model determined. | Seven nursing theorists discussed. Classes presented. Staff surveyed regarding thoughts on nursing, human beings, health, environment. |
| Models narrowed to two: Rogers and Roy. | Classes offered on Roy's and Rogers' models. Staff surveyed. | Rogers' model selected. |
| *1985*<br>Classes offered on Rogers' model. | Series of classes presented to nursing leadership and staff. Dr. Gean Mathwig addressed the nursing staff. Dr. Martha Rogers spoke to nursing staff. Purple boxes placed on all units with slinky on top to hold articles on the model. Monthly closed-circuit updates on model. Bulletin board displayed theory and model relationship. Video tape developed for use in nursing orientation. Sample nursing modality plans developed. | More nurses became aware of and familiar with the model. |
| *1986*<br>Incorporation of Rogerian concepts. | Therapeutic Touch classes offered. Nursing service philosophy reviewed and changed. Appraisal tool developed. | Therapeutic Touch practiced by select CNSs. New philosophy reflects Rogerian concepts. Appraisal tool tested. Tool shared with community for input. |
| Appraisal tool evaluated. | Determined to be too long and time-consuming for staff. | Tool returned to committee for changes. |
| *1987*<br>Nursing Service decentralized. | Much change in positions and committees. | Model implementation postponed. |

## Table 19.1 (continued)

| Stage | Action | Outcome |
|---|---|---|
| *1988–1989* | New appraisal tool developed by a Clinical Practice committee with input from the Rogers Task Force. | Tool tested and accepted. All staff nurses given education regarding tool. Tool in use on most units. |
| *1989–1990* | Nursing Grand Rounds with a focus on clinical application of concepts. Article published: Heggie, Schoenmehl, Chang, & Grieco (1989). | Limited attendance due to staff shortages and high client acuity. |
| *1990–1991* | Definition of nursing care written. Brown-bag lunch classes to discuss model concepts and application. | Continued to have limited attendance for same reasons as above. |
| *1991–1992* | Articles published: Kodiath (1991); Garon (1991). Computer contests. Education brought to units upon request. | More nurses discussed the model, and increasing numbers were aware of model implementation. |

new understandings into our value system and, with this perspective transformation, real change can occur (Freire, 1990).

For years, we have been presenting classes on Rogers' framework, both content on the postulates and principles of the model, and case studies demonstrating clinical application, and we have acquired a number of "Rogerians." However, their number, in relation to the entire staff, is not sufficient to bring about major staff belief system changes. Many can discuss aspects of the model, such as environment or patterning, but some nurses, when asked to describe a client in a classroom setting, continue to present the person in terms of the medical diagnosis and to focus their care primarily on that aspect. Many nursing staff members have been slow to accept the theoretical model; at times, resistance has been demonstrated by some members of the nursing administration. Examination of this resistance led to the realization that sociocultural belief and value systems, such as use of a task-oriented institutional model or the medical model, was a key factor in inhibiting acceptance and change.

A look at the context of practice in an acute care medical center today provided some insight into the difficulty encountered in model implementation. Today, the practice of nursing in a hospital setting consists of high client acuity, short stays, often insufficient staffing, a search for equipment, malfunctioning equipment, missing medications, phone interruption, upset family members, and a great deal of paperwork (Street, 1992). Nurses often feel they can't cope with one more "stressor." They want someone to "fix" things for them. Many nurses have a diploma or a two-year degree. Many are task-oriented. Some consider adding the use of a nursing model just another burden.

The nursing appraisal of the client at the San Diego Veterans Affairs Medical Center includes Rogerian categories of rhythm, patterning, energy, and mutual care planning. As the Science of Unitary Human Beings evolves, changes are made to update language. For example, with the development of the Rogerian practice methodology (Barrett, 1990), we are in the process of changing the assessment tool to reflect pattern appraisal and deliberative mutual patterning. In an attempt to support the staff and still teach and encourage use of the information gathered, the task force developed a consultation team. This team gives assistance when requests arise for help in understanding and integrating model concepts. We have a group of five nurses who provide staff development for all units requesting information. The purpose of this education is to foster nurses' belief that they have the power to make a difference in their own and their clients' lives. We try to help them understand how using the model's concepts and focusing on the clients' goals will save them time and energy. We emphasize that including the clients and their families in planning care will decrease their stress by placing responsibility for the clients' decisions where it belongs—with the clients. We try to help them view the person–environmental energy fields from the clients' perspective and to understand how important they are to the clients' hospital experience and their recovery after discharge.

Our most recent approach was to run bimonthly contests on the medical center computer through the nursing letter carrier network. The contests dealt with the concepts of pattern and energy fields (individual and environmental). A handout for this contest is presented in Figure 19.1. An additional proposal is shown in Figure 19.2, and selected responses received are excerpted in Figure 19.3. These contests are to held to foster discussion, thinking, and understanding regarding the model.

### Understanding Rogers' Model: Contest for April and May

To help understand how the concepts in Rogers' model can be broadly applied, we're going to examine a portion of the story of Cinderella.

Everyone is probably familiar with the fairy tale "Cinderella." Cinderella lived with her stepmother and was treated as a servant. She was saved from this situation when her fairy godmother appeared and dressed her for the ball the Prince gave to select a wife. Her coach was made from a pumpkin, and the driver from a mouse. Cinderella had to leave the ball before 12 midnight, when her clothes would turn back into rags and her transportation and attendants into pumpkin and mice. The Prince fell in love with her and searched for her, following her disappearance from the ball just before midnight. The Prince's only clue to her identity was the glass slipper she left behind. He searched the city for the appropriate owner, found her, married her, and they lived happily ever after.

Let's analyze part of this story using the Rogerian concepts of *pattern and energy fields, individual and environmental.* Although Cinderella was a servant, she always had the hope of being able to change her environment and her life (servant vs. princess). When her fairy godmother appeared, she served as the means, in the environmental energy field, Cinderella needed to accomplish the change to a new way of life (scrubbing floors, taking orders, feeling oppressed versus feeling loved, having breakfast in bed, and helping the Prince better the lives of their subjects).

This seems very unrealistic, but let's think for a moment about some of the decisions we and our clients make that pattern our individual and environmental energy fields:

1. Do you choose to see a doctor? If so, which one and why that one?

2. Do you take any medication? If so, why, which ones, and how often?

3. What people do you choose to associate with? Does this change? If so, why and when?

These are all choices people make. The choices of food you make become dietary pattern manifestations; the people you associate with become pattern manifestations of support; the area in which you choose to live, work, and play—all are manifestations of your environmental field. The food you eat, the people you associate with, and the environment you are present in are all integral to the mutual process of human and environmental fields. The contest for April and May is to describe a story, client, or situation using the concepts of pattern and energy fields (human and environmental). Send your entry to the Nursing Office in care of Judy Heggie. Good luck!

## Figure 19.1
## Contest Handout

———————————

Through sheer perseverance, our 12-person task force has made significant inroads during the past year. We now receive requests for staff development programs and have increasing response to our contest. Our goal is to reach the critical mass, using every means at our disposal. Our future plans include using the philosophy of perspective transformation to bring about a true integrality of Rogers' abstract system with planning and delivery of patient care.

### Understanding Rogers' Model: Clarification of the Contest for April and May

Responses to the latest contest were limited; perhaps the situation was too abstract and difficult to apply. If so, perhaps the following analogy will help.

Fairy tales, such as "Cinderella," provide theoretical problems similar to those that may be encountered in life. They allow the reader to think through how they would solve the same problem. The story of Cinderella can be applied to anyone living in adverse circumstances who wishes to change those circumstances or to anyone who wishes to change his or her life in a dramatic way. As an analogy, perhaps we can think about an athlete who acquires restrictive cardiac disease. The athlete will need to make dramatic life-style *pattern* changes: changes in dietary patterns, changes in exercise patterns, perhaps changes in relationship and career patterns. Will he or she be able to exercise the capacity to knowingly participate in change? Who or what may increase his or her energy: the support of a nurse, information provided by a physician, visits from a respected social worker, or perhaps an entire health care team or system? What about his or her *environmental* energy field? How will that be involved?

You are important in facilitating client care. How can you help a patient decide what changes he or she needs to make in life-style patterning and environment? How much effort do patients wish to put into changes? What will increase their energy? What depletes their energy? What are they interested in working on (what are *their* goals)? How should their families be involved?

Send in your examples of using Rogers' model in practice. The contest for July and August is to describe a story, client, or situation using the concepts of pattern and human and environmental energy fields.

## Figure 19.2
## Contest Handout Update

---

## Former Task Force Chair and Another Nursing Administrator's View (Maryanne Garon)

*A Critical Perspective on Implementation.*    The San Diego Veterans Affairs Medical Center made the commitment to adopt the Science of Unitary Human Beings as the model of practice in its nursing service over ten years ago. To say that the implementation project is finished would be an exaggeration. A much more accurate description is that we have struggled, we have had resistance from many of the staff, and we have had doubt from some in nursing administration. Throughout the past ten years, nursing administrators and others have asked pointed questions about the benefits of continuing with the adoption of this model. Yet, we are making strides in moving toward full implementation.

Most of us have probably heard the common arguments for using a nursing model: it provides nurses with a common language, it can change how we focus our appraisal of clients, it can direct nursing

The Spinal Cord Injury unit submitted the story of a female veteran, an unwed mother, with a spinal cord injury.

Kate, at one time, was a homeless person who lived around freight cars. At one time, she was in the military; at one time, she fell in love; and at one time, she fell off a freight train.

Presently, Kate lives alone in an apartment hotel with on-and-off help from her mother. The odds against Kate's changing her life are similar to those of Cinderella, but Kate has hopes and dreams that tide her over the big bumps of life. She fills her room with flowers that she admits to sending herself. She talks about knowing the Kennedy brothers and about the days when she used to have blond, well-coiffured hair. Kate reminds us all of how important dreams are when we are likely to get bogged down in the humdrum of hospital life. We need Kate to dream her dreams and tell us stories that provide energy and hope for her and for us.

—*Vilma Divinagracia, RN, CCRN and the SCI staff*

A medical unit submitted the following story.

Mr. M had a history of smoking for 30 years and alcohol abuse for 20 years. He was admitted with a right jugular mass that was positive for small-cell carcinoma. He had pattern manifestations of drinking and smoking. Patients make choices, not necessarily wise ones, and some are detrimental to their health. According to Rogers, man is viewed optimistically and has the capacity to change and to participate creatively in change.

The staff developed a plan to help pattern Mr. M's behavior. They involved his family and the entire health care team. They were patient, encouraging, and supportive. They praised progress and encouraged his effort during relapses. They wrote, "Rogers states that nursing seeks to strengthen the congruence and integrity of the human field and to direct the patterning of the personal and environmental fields to maximize health potential." Mr. M was able to quit smoking two months before his right modified neck surgery. The nurses on the medical floor acted as facilitators of the energy (hope) needed by the patient to make the decision to change his smoking habit.

—*Marlene Freeman, RN, BSN and the 3 West staff*

## Figure 19.3
## Excerpts from Responses to the Rogers' Task
## Force Contest: April and May

---

care, and so on. I would like to approach this from a different viewpoint. Valuing, using, and developing nursing knowledge can be transformative and emancipatory, and can enhance the power of practicing nurses. However, before we proceed with altering how nurses practice, I believe we must carefully consider the social and historical contexts in which nursing occurs. Consistent with my critical theoretical perspective, knowledge is not objective; it is embedded in the social and historical context in which it exists.

Late in the nineteenth century and early in this century, there was much less disparity between the education of the average nurse and the average physician. As hospitals and mental institutions increased, nearly every small hospital started a school of nursing to provide a nursing work force. Eventually, the fate of nurses and nursing schools became intertwined with that of hospitals. Within these institutions, the primarily female practitioners became increasingly subordinated to the male-dominated medical profession. Traditionally, nursing knowledge has been subordinated to medical knowledge (Street, 1992). Furthermore, the value or dominance of medicine has been legitimated by the state through legislation that accords to physicians specific rewards and responsibilities and, historically, has legally subordinated the roles and responsibilities of other health professionals to the physician.

In attempts to establish nursing as a science and a legitimate academic discipline, nurse scholars and scientists also employed the prevailing male-dominated views that reduced scientific knowledge to a narrow, prescribed set of rules dependent on scientific method as the one "proper" way to develop knowledge. This is evidenced by the adoption and proliferation within nursing of the positivism or empirical paradigm in research, theory building, and application of knowledge. These views are based on the belief that knowledge is, or can be, objective and *value-free.*

Within institutions, nurse administrators also accepted the superiority of technical knowledge and the paradigms in which this knowledge is created. Both educators and administrators have "unwittingly perpetuated the oppression of nurses and their clinical nursing knowledge" (Street, 1992, p. 44). In order to create change, we ignored power relations and attempted to clarify and impact individual interpretations. For example, we attempted to teach nurses assertiveness without first examining the power relations that perpetuated verbal abuse of nurses. Or, nurses attempted to increase individual power over practice by becoming nurse practitioners, rather than examining the entire profession's power relationship with medicine.

We believe that the Science of Unitary Human Beings offers unique nursing knowledge that can be power-enhancing and liberating for practicing nurses, in institutions and in individual clinical practice. However, implementation cannot be done *to* nurses, since it then becomes as oppressive as the structures in which they work. We believe that this was a major problem with implementation that the original task force members, in their zeal, did not consider. Some of the backlash from that initial misjudgment continues to stymie us. The original administrators and clinical specialists had the best of intentions. They were excited about the potential of a nursing model—the Rogerian model, to be exact—to improve client care. Previously, some of the methods used to introduce the concepts to the staff were described. The staff nurses, however, had a different perception of the process than did those who initiated the project. The message that the staff heard was, "We have this wonderful new knowledge, and *you,* being ignorant, will be able to receive it from us." The staff nurses dealt with this in the best way they were able, in much the same way powerless people usually react. They didn't buy into it, they thwarted implementation efforts, and they made jokes about it! We were trying to implement the model from the old world-view of "doing to" rather than recognizing the mutual process of change as described by Rogers' Principle of Integrality.

Over the past few years, we have recognized the harm of this past message and have spent much time trying to change our image. We have looked at ways to involve the staff and to alter our approach to one that values and recognizes their clinical knowledge.

I offer an example of how I utilized this model in my practice. I became the Clinical Services Director of the Outpatient Department almost five years ago. This was my first administrative position. I never wanted to be in administration because I never wanted to be like one of "them" (what I later identified as an authoritarian or autocratic leader). However, with my fairly new master's degree and strong beliefs about caring for clients, I believed that I could "improve" the care of a greater number of clients as an administrator than as an individual home care nurse. I had few role models of effective leaders, and I had to examine my own beliefs about leadership to develop my role. First, I had a belief in the importance of vision that involved the creation of an environment that is caring, provides social support, is "proactive," and allows people to take risks and make mistakes. I incorporated my theoretical background, which included knowledge of the continuous mutual process of human and environmental energy fields as well as Barrett's (1986) theory of power. By believing in my ability to knowingly create change in the environmental field of clients (which includes me), this negentropic (although somewhat "entropic-appearing") nursing staff could also change.

I had much help in communicating this vision when I utilized my new friend and colleague, Mary Kodiath, as both a sounding board for me and a facilitator for my staff. Recognition of the importance of an open environment for communication is critical. I be that staff deserve as much information as possible to make decisions, so I consistently communicate the information I receive that has a bearing on their practice. This openness also means that, without judgment, I must be willing to hear their side, their beliefs, and their concerns. This leads to my next belief: in the unique and unitary nature of human beings, I, and all human beings, are unitary energy fields identified by a unique pattern. My mutual process with others must be individualized and unique, and must take into account their "whole" lives, not just their working persona. By understanding this and talking about these concepts with staff, I help them to be more free with what they communicate, more concerned with the unique and unitary nature of human beings, and more caring and supportive of their clients and each other.

Finally, I view the nursing system as a complex whole that is continuing to evolve toward higher-frequency diversifying wholeness. It is a group energy field—certainly a true description of my department. By providing an atmosphere of openness, acceptance, and risk taking, nurses are able to shape their practice in ways that benefit them, the institution, and, most importantly, the clients they serve. (For examples of some of the changes that have been accomplished by Outpatient Department (OPD) nurses, see the next section.)

A surprising manifestation evolved during this period. Neither Mary nor I mentioned the Science of Unitary Human Beings for the first two years that we worked with the OPD staff. Yet, when, in 1989, they nominated me for a nursing service award, they identified the "Rogerian model" as being the major difference in the administration of the department since my arrival. By not lecturing or enforcing but, instead, modeling behavior and enhancing the staff's power to use their own knowledge, the end result has been both a progressive nursing department *and* a commitment to the nursing service's adopted model of Rogers' science.

As administrators, educators, and clinical leaders, we seek to understand the social and historical contexts of nursing practice settings. We must be careful not to further oppress staff nurses by denying their knowledge and value. We must also model the behaviors consistent with a Rogerian-based approach to create environments in which professional nursing can truly flourish.

*Changes Initiated by OPD Staff: 1991–1992.*    Adoption of a Rogerian world-view helped to actualize a number of changes in the Outpatient Department at the SDVAMC. Too frequently, managers, acting from an "old world-view" that includes causality, believe that they can effect change by direct interventions and manipulation. A Rogerian model of "leadership" (which is different from "management") includes a nonhierarchical style, mutuality with staff and clients, and recognition that the leader's integrality with the staff and the unit environment is her or his most powerful tool.

Although it may be argued that these changes might have occurred without the use of the Rogerian model, the expansive worldview encouraged creativity and initiative in a nonhierarchical atmosphere to actualize the staff's mutual vision for improving the work environment and care of clients.

### Using the Science of Unitary Human Beings in a Pain Management Program (Mary Kodiath)

I am the Co-Director of Health Patterning for Persons Who Experience Chronic Low Back Pain. In medical terminology, I am the Co-Director of the Chronic Low Back Pain Rehabilitation Program. In nursing, we assist clients to knowingly participate in the changes occurring in their lives. This is a dynamic process that enhances power and actualizes human potential. It has been defined as health patterning (Barrett, 1990).

*The Client with Chronic Pain.*    The chronic pain client is typically viewed by medical health care providers as a "chronic complainer," someone who is "noncompliant" and often very depressed. When patients with chronic pain ask for assistance from these providers, they typically tell them:

> I feel terrible. This pain has taken control of my entire life. I can't even bend over and tie my shoes without an excruciating pain in my back and down my leg. It has even affected my relationships with my friends. They don't call or come over to my house like they used to. I don't even want to go to parties any more, and I used to be the perfect party person. I don't know what's happening to me. I am a completely different persons since this pain started two years ago. At first, the doctors were really interested. They ordered lots of tests and gave me medication. But after everything came back negative, they now tell me it is all in my head, and I need to live with it. I wish I knew how to live with it. They think I'm crazy, and I'm beginning to think I am, too. My wife and I don't even have sex anymore. I don't even

want her to get close to me. I feel like I'm at the end of my rope
and don't know where else to turn.

Doesn't this describe a client's sense of powerlessness? The
medical health care providers (or any health care provider who uses
the medical model) all too often blame the client because he or she
doesn't know how to "get it together." These health care providers,
in turn, pick up the client's sense of powerlessness and often don't
know how to even begin to help.

In the medical model, for patients who complain of low back
pain, the health care providers have thus far been concerned with
X-rays and about two cms of the spinal column. These clients are often perceived as having a psychological problem since the pain cannot be explained medically.

How is a nursing view different? The client is not seen as having
a psychological or physical problem. Rather, the concern is with the
manifestations of the whole human being.

Persons with chronic pain desperately want an increase in their
quality of life. They are most frequently searching for more meaning
in their lives, and they want to know what changes they should make.
What the clients have been told thus far regarding health patterning
has taken their choices away and has only served to decrease their
knowing participation in change. For example, many chronic pain
clients have been told, "There's no cure, it will only get worse. You'll
have to live with it." When the patients have pain, they've been told
to take a pill and lie down. That means they could spend more than
18 hours a day lying down because the pain never goes away. When
the medication doesn't work, they look for some other "quick fix": a
TENS unit, other medication, a chiropractor, and so on. Are these
wrong? No. But using them as quick fixes will never work because
people tend to give all their power over to the "magic cure." Then,
when there is no cure, they become so discouraged and depressed
that their entire life-style changes.

*Health Patterning.*   Barrett (1990) explained that health patterning involves the two major phases of the Rogerian practice
methodology:

1. Pattern manifestation appraisal, which is "the continuous process of identifying manifestations of the human and environmental fields that relate to current health events" (p. 106);

2. Deliberative mutual patterning, which is "the process whereby the nurse with the client patterns the environmental field to promote harmony related to the health events" (p. 106).

For part of the pattern manifestation appraisal, the psychologist with whom I work uses medical model tools concerned with "parts." Among them are:

1. Sickness Impact Profile
2. Beck Depression Inventory
3. University of California, San Diego Pain Questionnaire
4. PAIRS—Pain and Impairment Relationship Scale
5. Cognitive Impairment (Slater & Kodiath, 1991, pp. 1–8).

I can use all of this information, but I ask for information in a different way. I do an appraisal of the patient's pattern manifestations. For example, I ask people to describe their pain and how they deal with it in their lives. How do they describe their energy awareness? I sometimes graph it with them. Each of them talks about the patterning manifested in their lives related to their pain. The chronic pain syndrome actually has a very strong manifestation of pain behaviors, impaired activities of daily living, and overall impairment based on the "healthy patterning" before the chronic pain commenced.

Most clients in chronic pain feel that they have lost all power to make any changes in their lives. I look at each individual as unique, dynamic, and continuously changing. The new dimension that I offer is that clients can choose the changes they want to make from now on. Pain does not have to have a power grip on them. Clients acquire an increased awareness of what they are choosing to do when they have pain. They feel free to make those choices, and they make them intentionally. Their power has been claimed by them, and they experience new life and new possibilities that continue to evolve.

*Appraisal of Pattern Manifestations.*    I ask the clients to fill out a 24-hour diary for five days. They describe their activity over this period of time, and they state whether they have been alone or with someone else during this activity, and whether the activity has been for pain relief or for some other reason. I also ask them to list their medications, the times of intake, and the dosage amounts. At the end of the day, they record their mood, degree of pain, and feeling of sadness versus happiness. These diaries give me a sense of their patterning throughout the day and night. I have them bring the diaries in and we talk about them. Most clients point out to me that their lives are ruled by the pain: it governs what they do, when they do it, how they do it, and with whom they do it. We begin to talk about what they want their lives to be and we set out a plan for rhythms of rest/activity, playing/working, eating/not eating, sitting/standing/lying down, and other rhythms.

*Harmony.*     As clients begin to develop new rhythms of activity and rest, they talk about their goals. Many want to return to work or to begin playing sports again. Many want to just be able to get on the floor and play with their children. The clients begin to realize that they are choosing what manifestations of health they want in their lives. They begin to pattern their environmental fields accordingly, which in turn promotes harmony. Very often, they feel a greatly enhanced quality of life and less pain. They experience a new sense of life or life power and their lives are dramatically changed in new and refreshing ways (see Table 19.2).

### View of a Clinical Nurse Specialist in a Program for Homeless Veterans (Ann Kelly)

I am a psychiatric clinical nurse specialist assigned to a program called Health Care for Homeless Veterans. The purpose of the program is to provide treatment and services to homeless veterans who have a mental illness and/or a problem with substance abuse. Veterans are first contacted in the community through outreach. Outreach is generally accomplished through placements at emergency

### Table 19.2
### Examples of Clients' Knowing Participants in Change as a Result of the Rehabilitation Program

| Pretreatment | Posttreatment |
| --- | --- |
| 1. Spending more time alone as pain increases. | 1. Independent of pain, planning specific activities each week with friends and family. |
| 2. Having a sense of decreased coherence toward the events in their lives since the pain began. | 2. Events in life "begin to fall back into place" and pain is no longer the center of life. |
| 3. Becoming increasingly isolated in a pain-filled world. | 3. Being introduced to their environment with a fresh perspective: bowling; fishing; playing cards with friends; gardening, and so on. |

assistance facilities—places where individuals or families go for assistance with food, clothing, or shelter. Staff identify veterans, and then I meet with them to explain the program and screen for eligibility. For the most part, individuals self-select participation. There are no limits on the length of time I can work with a client, and success is measured by a person's being in treatment and housed.

My world-view and clinical approaches have changed since working with the Rogerian framework. I have selected several postulates of the model and will share, through case example, what these postulates mean to me and how they are used in my practice.

My personal goal in working with all clients is to help them identify their pattern manifestations (who they are, what they want, how they may get what they want) and assist them in organizing the environment to their liking, whether I like their choices or not. This is not always an easy task, so I rely on theory, faith, and experience.

One example of an experience that has strengthened this view concerns "Roger," who wanted help with housing. He was newly discharged from the hospital after being treated for hepatitis and gastritis, and had been living in a very old van. He acknowledged a pattern of alcohol indulgence. Roger wanted to stay sober but did not want a structured program or environment to help him do this. His stated goals included obtaining an apartment, a job, and the freedom of no further medical problems. We began to work together in a rather traditional manner by establishing a "therapeutic relationship." Each time I saw him, he would say that he wanted to achieve his stated goals and that he had been drinking. He would occasionally try structured programs—for example, a detox alcohol program or a recovery home—and then drop out. During this time, he was seeing me every two to four weeks and was seeing a nurse practitioner for physical concerns. I would provide funds for transportation as long as he continued to see the nurse practitioner and attempt alcohol treatment. Roger continued his use of alcohol and, after a while, the nurse practitioner felt that she could no longer manage his care. At this point, he had diarrhea, which was essentially the shedding of the lining of his digestive track from an excess of alcohol. I continued to be present for him without providing funds. Some time later, he asked to go to a recovery home and stayed there for three weeks prior to having a relapse. Approximately four months later, he connected with me and attempted treatment with a medical model program where he maintained sobriety during three weeks of screening. Four months later, he made it to detoxification through a seven-day intensive medical model program and spent several weeks in a recovery home. He achieved nine weeks of sobriety before he started drinking again. In less than two weeks, he was again in a recovery home, where he is currently working on sustained sobriety. I do not always agree with or like the choices he makes. At one point, I felt that he was killing himself, but I am present for him. I am a change in his environment.

*Environment.* I view myself as being integral with the environment. Therefore, knowledge of my energy field pattern becomes critical. For instance, if I am tired, frightened, or worried, it becomes evident in how I am "present" with the current client. Therefore, I start each session with a moment for personal inventory and relaxation. Essentially, I take a deep breath and see whether I can be present for this client. Rarely, I will not be able to be present. When that is the case, I reschedule appointments.

*Pattern Manifestation Appraisal.* Pattern manifestation appraisal of clients is different with my use of the model. Assessments are now pattern manifestation appraisals. Each pattern is unique and all pattern appraisal is individualized. I do not do a formal mental status exam with each client. It is common for me to ask clients to share with me what they believe I need to know in order to assist them. If clients abuse substances, I will ask about the meaning the substances have for them. I ask them to describe their experience. Why do they want to change, and why today? Conceptually, I believe they are providing me a snapshot or a freeze-frame from a movie of their lives. If the clients are mentally ill, I seek to understand their experience with both their mental illness and the treatment facilities that they have encountered in the health care delivery system. To help clients verbalize goals, I ask what they would want if they had a magic wand that would make all things possible.

*Goals and Plans.* After clients state what they want, I explore what they believe they will need to do to accomplish their goal and how much time they see it taking. I view myself as integral with the environment and often talk about myself as a tool. I teach clients about mental illness, substance abuse, systems, and managing life. At the end of each meeting, we contract for our next meeting and for the activities each of us will do prior to that meeting.

*Deliberative Mutual Patterning.* As I work with clients, I look for continued manifestations of pattern, or what I call rhythms—perhaps a history of homelessness or drug use; how they utilize time or communicate. I explore in more depth their precise view of the world. An example of this concerns a client who sought help for alcohol abuse. He believed that he had Post Traumatic Stress Disorder (PTSD) syndrome from his Vietnam experience. I worked with him in a traditional manner and helped him to get into a recovery home. While he was at the home, he began to communicate in a bizarre manner. He became very fearful and verbalized visual and auditory hallucinations. He was given the medical diagnosis of schizophrenia. I did a more detailed appraisal of his homelessness. His tendency over the previous 12 years had been to remain in one place no longer than six months. His care, his finances, and his life drastically changed with such a transient life-style. We worked together to address the perceptions and beliefs that kept him from getting the things he wanted, which included a steady income and an apartment. I was present with him when he began outpatient treatment and then worked with a special case manager to move him into subsidized housing after he received social security payments. He has lived independently (on and off medication) for over one year.

*Evaluation.*    Evaluation is ongoing and outcomes are easily used and identified. Consistent with Barrett's (1990) knowing participation in change, desired outcomes are client-generated and are appraised at every meeting. My belief that all people have a right to choose their behavior helps me not to feel frustrated with what others might call "noncompliance or failure." I am able to remain open to assist the individual when and if he or she decides to arrange the environment to achieve a change—that is, to change the patterning.

One last example is a client who had never successfully completed a rehabilitation treatment program. He had always been asked to leave for "violation of rules." I saw him weekly and as needed, to work with him in regard to his feelings about wanting to break the rules and to frequently change goals without communicating or understanding his own rationale for doing so. He successfully completed a transitional program and went on to vocational training. He dropped out again because of his unwillingness to follow the rules of the program. However, he communicated to a physician that at one time he had succeeded, so he knew he could succeed again. The physician asked me if I would work with him again if he complied with some rules. I informed the physician that I would work with him regardless of whether he complied with the rules. The client chose to move to the East Coast, where he has established a relationship with a brother. I do not know his situation at this time. It is his life, and I value my opportunity to work with him as he chose to pattern his life.

## SUMMARY

The purpose of this chapter has been to convey the complexity of implementing Rogers' Science of Unitary Human Beings in a large medical center. Although difficult, the implementation has been rewarding to those who have participated and, more importantly, has facilitated science-based practice for the benefit of clients.

## REFERENCES

Allen, D. (1985). Nursing research and social control: Alternative models of science that emphasize understanding and emancipation. *Image: The Journal of Nursing Scholarship, 17*(2), 58–64.

Ashley, J. (1972). *Hospitals, paternalism, and the role of the nurse.* New York: Teachers College Press, Columbia University.

Barrett, E.A.M. (1986). Investigation of the Principle of Helicy: The relationship of human field motion and power. In V.M. Malinski (Ed.), *Explorations on Martha Rogers' Science of Unitary Human Beings* (pp. 173–184). Norwalk, CT: Appleton-Century-Crofts.

Barrett, E.A.M. (1990). Health patterning with clients in a private practice environment. In E.A.M. Barrett (Ed.), *Visions of Rogers' science-based nursing* (pp. 105–115). New York: National League for Nursing.

Freire, P. (1990). *Pedagogy of the oppressed.* New York: Continuum Press.

Garon, M. (1991). Assessment and management of pain in the home care setting: Application of Rogers' Science of Unitary Human Beings. *Holistic Nursing Practice, 6*(1), 47–57.

Habermas, J. (1971). *Knowledge and human interest* (J. Shapiro, Trans.). Boston: Beacon Press. (Original work published in German in 1968)

Heggie, J., Schoenmehl, P., Chang, M., & Grieco, C. (1989). Selection and implementation of Dr. Martha Rogers' nursing conceptual mode in an acute care setting. *Clinical Nurse Specialist, 3*(3), 143–147.

Kodiath, M. (1991). A new view of the chronic pain client. *Holistic Nursing Practice, 6*(1), 41–46.

Mezirow, J. (1981). A critical theory of adult learning and education. *Adult Education, 32*, 3–24.

Rogers, M.E. (1970). *An introduction to the theoretical basis of nursing.* Philadelphia: F.A. Davis.

Rogers, M.E. (1990). Nursing: Science of Unitary, Irreducible Human Beings: Update 1990. In E.A.M. Barrett (Ed.), *Visions of Rogers' science-based nursing* (pp. 5-11). New York: National League for Nursing.

Slater, M., & Kodiath, M. (1991). Comprehensive management of the chronic pain patient; case study. *Holistic Nursing Practice, 6*(1), 1-8.

Street, A.F. (1992). *Inside nursing: A critical ethnography of clinical nursing practice.* Albany, NY: SUNY Press.

Thompson, J. (1987). Critical scholarship: The critique of domination in nursing. *Advances in Nursing Science, 10*(1), 27-38.

# 20

# Implementing Rogers' Science-Based Nursing Practice in a Pediatric Nursing Service Setting

*Cynthia A. Tudor*
*Lisa Keegan-Jones*
*Eileen M. Bens*

## SELECTION OF THE NURSING CONCEPTUAL SYSTEM

With the implementation of *shared governance* at Children's Hospital Medical Center (CHMC) in Cincinnati, Ohio, a task force was created to explore the possibility of adopting a conceptual model into the nursing division. This chapter discusses the selection process, preparation of the nursing division for the implementation, present practical innovations, evaluation strategies, and our visions of nursing at CHMC.

The method of sharing the governance of nursing issues and practices increases the staff nurses' participation in and responsibility for decision making. This organizational system was chosen to distribute the concentration of power more effectively, strengthen staff nurses' involvement in the nursing division's activities, and allow individual units greater participation in decisions concerning their environment (Porter-O'Grady, 1987). It was expected that

We would like to extend our most appreciative gratitude to our consultants, Martha Rogers, MScN, RN, and Elizabeth Ann Manhart Barrett, PhD, RN, FAAN. Their assistance was invaluable in operationalizing our visions.

shared governance would increase the quality of care to the client through staff nurse autonomy in decision making and accountability for practice. To facilitate this process, it was suggested that the nursing division choose a conceptual system on which to base nursing practice. In addition, trends in health care have implied that financial compensation for nurses will eventually be based less on static wage programs and more on the value of actual services delivered. In order to achieve this, the practice must be clearly defined.

The utilization of a nursing conceptual system defines nursing values and the knowledge domain of nursing that guides practice in providing consistent approaches to client care. Nurses are well equipped to define roles and expectations—an increasingly important fact as health care evolves and changes in the future (Porter-O'Grady, 1987). As an autonomous, professional discipline, nursing demands that practice not only be clearly defined, but that it imply a specific purpose, direction, and meaning. A conceptual system guides this direction and lights the way. At the first meeting of the Nursing Practice Council in March 1989, the Conceptual Model Task Force was formed.

The task force members included three clinical nurse specialists, four staff nurses, an education coordinator, and a faculty member from the University of Cincinnati. Our mission was to recommend one or two systems that would be suitable for our institution. The Nursing Practice Council, as outlined by shared governance articles, would ultimately be responsible for the final selection.

When the task force began to meet, the need to construct a method for analysis and evaluation of the conceptual system became immediately apparent. The task force reviewed criteria for analysis and evaluation of nursing systems. It was difficult and bewildering to learn the language of paradigms, metaparadigms, conceptual systems, assumptions, and philosophy, and the differences between models and theories. This process required a rapid synthesis of new vocabulary, ideas, and concepts. All of the members passed this initiation task with a new respect for the idea of a practical utilization of a conceptual system within all levels of the nursing division. As a result, the task force adopted a set of criteria for evaluating a conceptual system, which was subsequently used when discussing the various nursing models (see Table 20.1).

The next six months involved detailed discussion and evaluation of ten nursing frameworks and models:

1. Orem's Self Care Framework (Orem, 1985).
2. Neuman's System Model (Neuman, 1982).
3. Johnson's Behavioral System Model (Johnson, 1980).
4. King's Interacting System Model (King, 1981).
5. Levin's Conservation Model (Levin, 1973).
6. Roy's Adaptation Model (Roy, 1984).
7. Rogers' Science of Unitary Human Beings (1970, 1980).
8. Hall's Nursing Theory (Hall, 1966).
9. Watson's Human Care Model (Watson, 1985).
10. Parse's Theory of Man–Living–Health (Parse, 1981).

As we investigated each of the systems, we began to recognize a paradigm shift that has been slowly occurring over time. The members recalled nursing practice in the past and how it has changed to the present system. The nursing of the past, for example, included the handmaiden to the physician; the mechanistic mode of assessing

## Table 20.1
## Criteria for Selecting a Nursing Conceptual System

1. How well does the system relate to the nursing process?
2. How aligned is the system with the institution and nursing departments?
   a. Philosophy
   b. Mission statement
   c. Goals and objectives
   d. Your own private image of nursing
3. Does a particular system assist nurses in caring for a variety of patient populations? (Applicability to all practice settings within the institution.)
4. What are staff preferences/attitudes toward this particular system?
5. Will there be reasonable ease in teaching this particular system to all levels of nursing staff?
6. Identify the components of each system:
   a. How is *person* defined?
   b. How is *environment* defined?
   c. How is *health* defined?
   d. How is *nursing* defined?
7. Will the system carry us into the future?
8. Is the system comprehensive enough to provide direction for practice, education, research, and administration?

Adapted from *Analysis and Evaluation of Conceptual Models of Nursing* (chap. 2) by J. Fawcett, 1984, Philadelphia: Davis.

clients; the medical model; and fragmenting the child into biological, psychological, and social parts. This hospital has a strong history of utilizing and applying the medical model, which continues to be imitated throughout the entire institution, including the nursing division. We wanted to harmonize the parts into a human being—and a family—irreducibly united, which requires a nursing perspective rather than a medical one. The importance of family-centered care made it necessary to look at the whole family, including the home environment, in order to appraise and individualize care for each child. The family is integral with a child's environment, and a parent is usually the person most capable of making decisions for the health and well-being of the family. As nurses, we need to encourage and respect this approach.

As we analyzed and internalized the information gained from these discussions and began to comprehend the intent of nursing conceptual systems, it became essential to compare the assumptions and content of each system with the philosophical statement of the nursing division, private images of nursing, theoretical notions, and usual ways of practicing nursing at CHMC. We sought congruency between the conceptual system and the values and philosophy of the nursing division.

Choosing a conceptual system would not only change our present actions but would guide the nursing division's future evolution. We wanted to solidify this direction of nursing for our future clients and their families. For example, the growing number of chronically ill children changes the traditional definition of health; recognizing the unity of the person as integral with his or her environment means working toward potentials (rather than complete physical functioning) through patterning of the environment. This idea of unity extends to the entire health professions network. The nurse was envisioned to be integral with a collaborative team of health care providers, working together with families to actualize their potentials.

Our hospital has many diverse departments, so this became quite a challenge. Our nursing units include three intensive care units, a home health care team, outpatient clinics and surgeries, two chronic care/rehabilitation units, and the emergency department and trauma team. Multiple units range from hematology/bone marrow transplant to adolescent, neurosurgical, psychiatric/behavioral, surgical, medical, and operating room units, as well as administrative and education services. We wanted a conceptual system that would unite and integrate all these spheres and facilitate a sense of common commitment and purpose.

It became important to choose a nursing conceptual system that was reflective of our belief in the whole person, which, in our case, includes the parent, family, and home environment. The chosen nursing conceptual system would respect the families' and children's capacities to participate in their health care through involvement and decision making and would encompass all departments of the nursing division.

The systems were evaluated in regard to their content, assumptions, definitions of the metaparadigm, logical congruence, social significance and utility, and future applications and significance. We began to speculate about the staffs' future acceptance of and education in the conceptual system, recognizing that some systems would be easier than others to implement. The emphasis of our discussion, however, focused on exploring each system with the intent to choose the "best fit" for our institution.

On January 4, 1990, the task force finalized its recommendations: Neuman's System Model (1982) and Rogers' Science of Unitary Human Beings (1970, 1980) would be presented to the Nursing Practice Council, whose members are accountable for making decisions that are responsible and informed, in regard to the nursing staff. To this end, the task force thought that it was first necessary to explain and interpret the two systems to the nursing staff, in order to allow information (about the staff nurses' thoughts and preferences) to flow to the Nursing Practice Council members and provide the basis for an informed decision.

The explanation began with a simple inservice program that discussed conceptual systems and introduced the staff nurses to the vocabulary and language of the systems and their service to nursing. The program, entitled, "You, Too, Can Learn to Love Conceptual Models," was videotaped and made available to all nurses. It included information regarding conceptual systems, the metaparadigm, evaluation criteria, and the nursing philosophy statement for the institution. The objective was to introduce the information in such a way that the staff nurses could understand the idea of a conceptual system and begin to see how it would change and improve their practice.

Two more inservice programs followed, each one describing one of the recommended systems. The objective now was to familiarize the staff with the two chosen systems so that each could be discussed among themselves. The members of the Nursing Practice

Council would receive information from the staff to make the final decision. When these objectives were completed, it was apparent that further education was needed. Although the staff had some understanding about the conceptual systems, they had little comprehension of the differences between the two and of their value to nursing. Two more inservice programs, focused on the practical application of each system, were planned and implemented. To promote discussion, articles were distributed throughout the division, and mini inservice programs were given on several units by the task force members.

Through these staff education activities, the staff had the opportunity to learn about the selection process and each system. The staff, however, was not yet ready to listen. To learn a conceptual system with the intent to practically apply the theories and principles requires active participation and commitment. The staff was not prepared to fully understand, nor appreciate, the value of a conceptual system at this time. The inservice programs were primarily utilized to allow the Nursing Practice Council delegates to obtain information about staff preferences for each system in preparation for deciding which would be the best fit with our institution.

On June 29, 1990, the Nursing Practice Council discussed which conceptual system would be congruent with our practice. The council delegates were divided into dyads. Each council member was requested to assess both systems, using the criteria for selection, and then to relate, to the partner in the dyad, his or her understanding of each system and indicate which one was preferred as the choice for the nursing division. Each dyad then presented its discussion to the group at large and elaborated on the personal views expressed as well as unit and staff preferences.

Among the many questions the council attempted to answer were:

How flexible would the system be?

Would it allow for individual creativity, as well as evolving to a pediatric population?

Would it promote measures for growth in the staff and client populations?

Which system would be more accepted by the staff?

How would it change our documentation?

As the council answered these questions, they struggled with uniting personal preferences and staff attitudes.

Both systems are holistic in that they bring together the person and the environment. Each encourages collaboration with family and other health disciplines in guiding the child's care. Both would require a change in documentation. Questions were raised about the ease of understanding the vocabulary of each system, which might have an impact on the acceptance and education of the staff nurses.

Neuman's System Model (1982) was thought to be more concrete and structured, having familiar language and vocabulary. This would make it more acceptable to the staff, especially when initiating the change and providing education. The concept of stressors is familiar to nurses and therefore easily understood and incorporated into our present documentation system.

Rogers' Science of Unitary Human Beings (1970, 1980) is more abstract and less structured, which would allow for and promote creativity on all levels. For the future, this opened unlimited opportunities for improvement and growth. Rogers' view of health and pandimensionality acknowledges all client populations, ages, health potentials, families, and cultures. In addition, the theory of power shares the decision making with the family. The language of the system was perceived to be a major concern in relation to hampering the staff acceptance and education needed to implement the system.

After much discussion, the two systems were both thought to adequately reflect our philosophy and to fit equally well into the nursing division. The consensus of the council was that the system should be chosen through a majority vote. A preliminary vote revealed the group to be evenly split. Further discussion ensued. Upon final ballot, Martha Rogers's Science of Unitary Human Beings (1970, 1980) was adopted!

Many factors were involved in the choice of the Science of Unitary Human Beings. The Science of Unitary Human Beings projects an opportunistic future, allowing the entire nursing division to evolve in multiple directions while maintaining a sense of integrality within itself and with the health care team. In addition, the task force members, several of whom were also members of the Nursing Practice Council, favored this conceptual system, identifying with both its philosophy and its principles. (The task force members had put extra time, effort, and study into this project and were viewed by the council members as having superior expertise; therefore, their knowledge and opinions about a final choice were considered.)

The Nursing Practice Council recognized the initiative and creativity of the project and its implications for the nursing profession, and were willing to begin a new voyage into relatively unknown waters. Few institutions have incorporated a conceptual system, and fewer still have applied the Science of Unitary Human Beings (1970, 1980). None had adopted this system within a pediatric population. We felt like pioneers. As in any new endeavor, we were viewed by others with a mixture of curiosity, amusement, enthusiasm, envy, and, sometimes, contempt. But, like any pioneers, we found the challenge uncertain, energizing, and exhilarating. The delegates realized there would be difficulties ahead but, in their final choice, they viewed the major assumptions and concepts of the Science of Unitary Human Beings to be more aligned philosophically and more congruent with nursing here at CHMC.

## IMPLEMENTATION

Once Martha Rogers' conceptual system had been chosen, the implementation process began. Extensive planning was required with an institution of this size and with a diverse nursing staff. The task force felt that a consultant would be essential to this process, and two consultants were selected. One had expertise in the implementation process, and the other had expertise in the Rogerian system.

In April 1991, the implementation consultant came to CHMC to view different units and to meet with selected staff—the assistant vice presidents of nursing, unit directors, clinical nurse specialists (CNSs), educational services for nursing (ESN), and staff nurses. The visit had three purposes: (1) to assess current nursing systems and operations; (2) to assess current nursing delivery systems and their congruence with Rogers' system; and (3) to begin the change process. During this visit it was emphasized that learning a conceptual model would be a very difficult process that required careful planning.

In May 1991, both consultants arrived for a strategic planning day. In attendance were: the task force, divisional council members, and CNSs. The day began with an overview of Rogers' Science of Unitary Human Beings. We then worked through a visioning process to help us form a more concrete image of what nursing practice would be like after implementation was complete. Among several issues considered during the visioning exercise were: nursing practice and the changes it would bring to children and families; nursing management and management systems; quality assurance; education; research; professional development; and the environment. It was envisioned that nurses would be more powerful and would use more noninvasive modalities. Families would be able to identify nurses' unique practice and would feel comfortable making decisions and contributing to the plan of care. There would be a large focus on nursing research. Out of this meeting came a need to identify specific roles in the planning, implementation, and evaluation of the conceptual system change process. We analyzed the current systems and tried to foresee difficulties that might arise during the process of change. We also began to delineate the responsibilities of the task force, management, and staff. At the end of this day, we indeed had the beginning of our strategic plan.

By July 1991, we had a draft of our strategic plan and a critical path outlined for implementation. Selected structures were identified for developing the education, management, research, and practice systems. The plan included perspective transformation, education, and evaluation. It delineated the roles and responsibilities of the shared governance councils (Practice, Quality Assurance and Improvement, Education, Management, and Research) as well as those of management, the CNSs, the consultants, the task force, and the resource staff. We had selected a range of dates for each section of the plan. During this time, the task force also developed our position statement with respect to the conceptual system. The position statement was based on the following conclusions:

1. We believe in the unitary approach to family-centered care.
2. We believe that children and their families are complex, open systems that are different from the sum of their parts.
3. We believe that the environment is a profound, key factor in regard to the well-being of the child, family, nurse, and nursing practice.
4. We believe that health is a state of being that is defined by the child and family.
5. We believe that nursing is a profession with a distinct body of scientific knowledge.
6. We believe that the central focus of nursing is the child and the family and that the goal of nursing is to assist them in realizing their maximal health potential.

By implementing the conceptual system, we stated, we were hoping to accomplish the following goals:

1. Improved quality of care for the child and family.
2. A family- and child-centered approach to the plan of care.
3. A more systematic approach to nursing care.

4. A consistent method for evaluation of nursing care.

5. A means of more effective communication and increased collaboration among nursing personnel.

6. A method for more clearly defining nursing's unique realm and contribution to care.

7. Promotion of increased professionalism.

8. A guide for nursing research.

9. A means for increased satisfaction and retention of nurses.

By September 1991, our strategic plan was finalized and our fall and winter activities had begun. We had a series of "brown-bag" lunches with a faculty member from the University of Cincinnati College of Nursing and Health, at which we discussed the conceptual system. Our consultant conducted four perspective transformation workshops for the task force, CNSs, assistant vice presidents, council members, and directors.

The perspective transformation process was an important step toward effective implementation. Three objectives were stated at the beginning of each workshop:

1. To verbalize a definition of a conceptual system.

2. To verbalize why CHMC elected to adopt a conceptual system.

3. To develop a beginning understanding of overall goals for CHMC with respect to the conceptual system.

A packet was distributed which included information about the phases of the learning process with respect to a conceptual system, a historical perspective of the current values placed on nursing practice, and how to identify the differences between ideal and real nursing practice (see Table 20.2). Group exercises with each section offered several questions for discussion:

What do nurses know that nobody else knows?

What is different about the ways physicians and nurses describe health?

How do our religious, military, medical, and feminist heritages fit in with nursing as we see it today?

We were also asked to describe an ideal nursing world. By allowing the nurse to examine beliefs and values about the concepts of person, environment, health, and nursing, incorporation of the conceptual system into practice would be facilitated (Rogers, 1991).

## Table 20.2
## Outline of the Perspective Transformation

I. How Nurses Learn a Conceptual Framework: Transformative Learning

II. The Role of the Facilitator in the Learning Process

III. Group Exercises

    A. Creating an awareness of nurses' existing meaning perspectives: How are the concepts of nursing, person, environment, and health defined?

    B. Unveiling the prevailing meaning perspectives of nursing: The private images: How have historical and sociocultural issues shaped the perspectives of nurses today?

       1. Nursing's religious heritage

       2. The medical model

       3. The militaristic/bureaucratic heritage

       4. The feminine heritage

    C. Revealing the discontinuity between the ideal nursing practice and the reality

From "Transformative Learning: Understanding and Facilitating Nurses' Learning and Use of Nursing Conceptual Frameworks" by Martha E. Rogers, August 1991, paper presented at meeting of International Futurists Society, Madrid, Spain.

It was our hope that, once the initial participants completed the workshops, they would function as resources to staff. One task force member and one clinical nurse specialist were assigned to each unit as facilitators in the learning process.

During this time of perspective transformation, the consultant worked with the resource group to further their education of Rogers' Science of Unitary Human Beings. We also had the opportunity to meet with Dr. Rogers and several Rogerian scholars, who gave us invaluable insight into the implementation process.

Throughout 1992, the perspective transformation process continued. As a task force, we had ups, downs, and times of frustration. When it seemed that we were holding the whole world on our shoulders, we found it very helpful to get together as a group to support each other. As expected, different units moved ahead at different rates. Special workshops were held for the assistant vice president and director groups, to help them with specific leadership and management issues related to implementing a conceptual system at the unit level.

As implementation continues and people are more accepting, specific information related to the Science of Unitary Human Beings will be presented. Several different modalities, including workshops, tapes, and group discussions, will be used. As shared governance councils make decisions and changes, the conceptual system will be a major consideration. We are now working on new standards of care and new policies and procedures, and a creative documentation task force has been formed. We conducted a Nursing Grand Rounds presentation, which included didactic information and case studies. It has been important for us to use a low-key approach without difficult vocabulary, in order to bring the concepts to a practical level that staff nurses will find meaningful. We have also found it important to provide some structure within which changes can occur. Since the questions we are most often asked are related to anticipated changes in concrete nursing practices, we are trying to use health patterning plans for CHMC clients in our teaching. Several units are now scheduling times to review health patterning plans and discuss them from a Rogerian practice methodology perspective (Barrett, 1990). In the future, we hope to have scheduled planning meetings on every unit, to foster creativity and to help tailor this process to the unit's needs.

We are beginning to see the fruits of our labor. People are asking for information and are talking about the conceptual system. Every argument is seen as a noteworthy sign of change. We have met resistance where expected and are patiently trying to facilitate staff and management participation in the change process. The coming year will be an exciting one for the nurses, children, and families of CHMC, a year of increasing quality of care and of greater autonomy and respect for nursing practice.

## EVALUATION

As part of our strategic planning process, the task force wanted to carefully evaluate our implementation process, specifically to examine whether particular changes had occurred. The task force took a qualitative and quantitative approach in identifying structural, process, and outcome criteria. Referring to our original position statement, our primary goals for utilizing a model to guide us included: (1) promoting quality nursing care for all patients and families; (2) facilitating a unified and systematic nursing care approach; (3) increasing effective communication and collaboration among nursing personnel; and (4) promoting increased professionalism.

Within the shared governance practice environment, we hoped that the conceptual model would enhance responsibility, autonomy, and accountability for registered nurses. Nurses would more clearly describe their unique realm and their contribution to patient care.

Already, the Division Nurse Practice Council had been asked to consider questions concerning the definition of practice in relation to responsibilities of primary nursing. Nurses on a newly organized rehabilitation unit struggled to define their role within a multidisciplinarian model where, traditionally, speech therapists, psychologists, and physical therapists had very dominant roles. Ultimately, the task force hoped that if nurses could clearly articulate their domain and practice in an environment that is professionally rewarding, job satisfaction and retention might be improved.

We hoped that the model might give clear purpose, direction, and organization to the nursing department. The conceptual system was to be utilized as a way to facilitate and direct goal clarification for nursing practice and to develop nursing philosophies and standards of practice.

Learning and adopting a conceptual model is a very stressful process that challenges all nurses to examine very private and perhaps previously unarticulated beliefs about nursing and the values held regarding the major metaparadigm concepts. Some nurses grieve over a perceived loss of identity since their values and beliefs about themselves as nurses are integral with their perspectives of themselves as people (Rogers, 1989). Rogers' work in transformative learning process also cautions that learning a nursing conceptual framework takes enormous effort and time (Fitch et al., 1991).

The evaluation plan, as organized by the task force, is designed to examine structural, process, and outcome criteria. Structural dimensions that can easily be evaluated include collecting information about the organizational structure in place one year and two years after implementation. Shared governance is currently being evaluated by examining nurse satisfaction, financial analysis, and decision making. Unit structures can be evaluated by examining the councils, delivery system, staff mix, staff complements, numbers of BSN and diploma school graduates, longevity, vacancy rates, turnover, absenteeism, and budgetary constraints. The wide range of variables in a large institution is difficult to control and it will be difficult to interpret many of our evaluation conclusions. The hospital is also implementing a total quality management (TQM) program, downsizing units, and moving to a new clinical building.

Children and family variables may include examining acuity, occupancy, and satisfaction. We are collecting information from our executive council via copies of the nursing articles that describe the governance structure, rules, and regulations; minutes from quarterly meetings; and annual goals from division and unit councils. Information about our staff mix and about how time spent outside of direct care has been distributed (meetings, research, council work), as well as total time utilized, will provide us with essential information. Process dimensions can be evaluated by examining nurses' experiences of learning a conceptual system. We will interview nurses one month after initial education and then every six months for a period of two years. They will be asked specific questions about what the process of learning Rogers' science has been like for them.

Utilizing a critical incident from a family–client practice situation, we will ask nurses to describe that situation in detail. At select intervals, as the nurses describe different situations, a content analysis may reveal the shift to using Rogers' postulates and the timing of the process. We will be looking for the shift to Rogers' propositions, principles, and theories and for shared perspectives of unitary human beings and their environment, health, and nursing.

It may be useful to conduct small evaluation interviews at six-month intervals. The focus would be a group approach with key stakeholder groups of staff nurses, unit directors, educators, clinical nurse specialists, council chairs, and other health care providers at the unit level, including occupational therapy/physical therapy, social workers, and physicians. Nurses may feel rewarded in having the opportunity to implement a professional nursing role and may gain confidence in their ability to describe and communicate their unique contribution.

We will evaluate outcome dimensions by again generating critical incidents and asking staff nurses to analyze, interpret, and formulate a health patterning plan with the child or with the family. The health patterning plan includes the phases of the Rogerian practice methodology: pattern manifestation appraisal and deliberative mutual patterning (Barrett, 1990). The same case study will be utilized with the same group of nurses at 12-, 18-, and 24-month intervals. The variables related to the nurse–client mutual process would change and become more diverse by introducing the Rogerian framework in the activities of the nursing process. In particular, we would expect to see pattern manifestations that are guided by the postulates of the framework. Nursing actions would be guided by deliberative mutual patterning with the child and the family, and noninvasive modalities would be incorporated into everyday practice. We are anticipating that, as staff nurses begin to incorporate the framework into their practice, our current documentation and use of nursing diagnoses will not adequately address the nursing care delivered, and the format for documentation may change. Rogers' Science of Unitary Human Beings sets forth notions about family and child participation and about mutual patterning of the environment. It would be important to measure children's and families' views concerning these changes. A child-and-family survey is utilized on all units. Questions have been added to allow evaluation of the shift in nursing's approach. These data will be collected at yearly intervals.

## SUMMARY

From the beginning of the planning process, we have been extremely sensitive to staff and management views and perceptions concerning this change. The difference in our approach may be unique in that this was a Division Nursing Practice Council decision and was thus driven by the staff. Implementation of past major projects had been through upper management levels. Perhaps, since this is the first major project implemented since shared governance has been initiated, we are meeting some resistance where we may not otherwise have encountered it; or, we might have encountered it at a different time in the process. The resistance to this implementation may be more in the fundamental questions that management and staff ask of the profession and of nursing as a science. Some staff nurses grieve the loss of their perceived role as nurses while they closely examine their practice. Nurses are challenged as professionals to clearly identify their unique realm in an environment that is strongly dominated by the medical model.

The theorizing and the sensitizing have stirred nurses of all educational preparation to identify and question those concepts that help to define the body of knowledge essential to nursing science. We can only speculate as to whether this is unique to our institution or to the profession as a whole. The frustration, from our perspective, of what we thought would be a progressive and exciting journey seems overwhelming in the beginning of implementation. A core group of believers, however, is committed to seeing this through; they realize the enormous amount of invested time and energy required for such a project. Overall, discussion with staff energies us. Their enthusiasm for the project is evident.

We selected Rogers' Science of Unitary Human Beings since we believe the framework to be congruent with our current practice and to be capable of ushering us into the next era of a rapidly changing health care environment. We hope to see our nursing care at CHMC shared by a perspective that shares decision making with the children and their families and enhances knowing participation in their care. Pediatric nurses have identified themselves as strong advocates for children and their families but have struggled not to "direct" or "control" in "knowing what's best for the client." We hope to promote a strong collaborative practice with children and their families, with medicine, and with other health care providers.

As we embark on our next phase of education, we will be introducing the major paradigm concepts of the framework slowly, deliberately, and in a nonthreatening manner. As staff members struggle with the abstraction, we will try to satisfy their intolerance for ambiguity with an opportunity for dialogue, discussion, and application to practice. By depicting familiar clinical situations for staff in the context of the Science of Unitary Human Beings, learning becomes personalized and real. A housewide education program is planned to define the nursing process from the Rogerian perspective with examples of the incorporation of noninvasive modalities. The shift to a nursing model will not be easy: we have been shaped and mentored by our heritage, and we practice in an environment that is strongly directed by the medical model. Eventually, as nurses learn the framework through unit-specific planning and implementation, the task force will be disbanded and activities will be assumed by the division and unit councils. A Rogerian science advisory group may be formed to continue the ongoing work of cultivating interest and research as we learn more and as we strive to provide knowledgeable, compassionate service to all people.

We would emphasize that the planning time is paramount in preparing for the change. This change will not occur rapidly; it will take time to learn and discuss the model. Preferably, this vital time should be spent outside of unit activities or built into daily schedules on the unit. Allowing time for discussion and dialogue and for the staff to express themselves and examine their own values and beliefs is critical. There is a natural tendency to want to learn more about the framework before exploring personal philosophical beliefs about the metaparadigm concepts. Creating some discomfort with the present system is an important step that will allow nurses to be open to the changes that will occur.

Staff and unit involvement, from the beginning, is critical. This involvement cannot be imposed on the staff from management downward. Shared governance provides a structure for staff to be initially involved in practice, education, quality assurance, and research decisions, and gives the clinical nurse a major role in the project. This is unfamiliar and uncharted territory for most of us. It should, however, be an excellent testing ground in operationalizing Rogers' science. Philosophically, nurses agree that the concepts are congruent with their existing practice, but the challenge will be in illuminating those practices that truly represent the Science of Unitary Human Beings and its practical application.

## REFERENCES

Barrett, E.A.M. (1990). Health patterning with clients in a private practice environment. In E.A.M. Barrett (Ed.), *Visions of Rogers' science-based nursing* (pp. 105–115). New York: National League for Nursing.

Fawcett, J. (1984). *Analysis and evaluation of conceptual models of nursing.* Philadelphia: F.A. Davis.

Fitch, M., Rogers, M., Ross, E., Shea, H., Smith, I., & Tucker, D. (1991). Developing a plan to evaluate the use of nursing conceptual frameworks. *Canadian Journal of Nursing Administration, 4,* 22–28.

Hall, L.E. (1966). Another view of nursing care and quality. In K.M. Straub & K.S. Parker (Eds.), *Continuity of patient care: The role of nursing* (pp. 47–60). Washington, DC: Catholic University Press.

Johnson, D.E. (1980). The behavioral system model of nursing. In J.P. Riehl & C. Roy, Sr. (Eds.), *Conceptual models for nursing practice* (2nd ed.) (pp. 207–216). Norwalk, CT: Appleton-Century-Crofts.

King, I.M. (1981). *A theory for nursing: Systems concepts process.* New York: John Wiley & Sons.

Levine, M.E. (1973). *Introduction to clinical nursing.* Philadelphia: F.A. Davis.

Neuman, B. (1982). *The Neuman systems model: Application to nursing education and practice.* Norwalk, CT: Appleton-Century-Crofts.

Orem, D.E. (1985). *Nursing: Concepts of practice* (3rd ed.). New York: McGraw-Hill.

Parse, R.R. (1981). *Man–living–health: A theory of nursing.* New York: John Wiley & Sons.

Porter-O'Grady, T. (1987). Shared governance and new organizational models. *Nursing Economics, 5,* 281–286.

Rogers, M. (1989). Creating a climate for the implementation of a nursing conceptual framework. *Journal of Continuing Education in Nursing, 20,* 112–117.

Rogers, M. (1991, August). *Transformative learning: Understanding and facilitating nurses' learning and use of nursing conceptual frameworks.* Paper presented at the meeting of the International Futurists Society, Madrid, Spain.

Rogers, M.E. (1970). *An introduction to the theoretical basis of nursing.* Philadelphia: F.A. Davis.

Rogers, M.E. (1980). Nursing: A science of unitary man. In J.P. Riehl & C. Roy (Eds.), *Conceptual models for nursing practice* (2nd ed.) (pp. 329–337). Norwalk, CT: Appleton-Century-Crofts.

Roy, S.C. (1984). *Introduction to nursing: An adaptation model* (2nd ed.). Englewood Cliffs, NJ: Prentice-Hall.

Watson, J. (1985). *Nursing: Human science and human care.* Norwalk, CT: Appleton-Century-Crofts.

# Unit IV

## *FOUNDATIONS FOR SCIENCE-BASED PRACTICE*

# 21

# A Rogerian Values Vision: Values of Professional Nurses

*Judith Haber*
*Justine A. Taddeo*

Within a climate of rapid and accelerating change and increasing technology, presidents and deans of colleges and universities, health care administrators, and corporate executives are pausing to examine and assess the bedrock of their organizations and their values (Bruhn & Henderson, 1991; Martin, 1991; Naisbitt & Aburdene, 1990; Porter-O'Grady, 1992). Today, nurses are taking a leadership role in shaping values futuristically rather than accepting those imposed by society. Such a process demonstrates knowing participation in change; the profession is enabled to participate in shaping the nature of its practice for the future. The purpose of this chapter is to present a Rogerian-based vision for the assessment of the values of professional nurses.

## VALUES

Values are enduring beliefs that specify modes of conduct but change over time within a societal/cultural envelope (Burns, 1978). Values provide the basis for the development of attitudes and behaviors and are evident in the patterning of individuals and organizations. Values reflect an extension of critical thinking and are manifested in individual and/or organizational behavior patterns (Barker, 1990). Values are at the heart of the practice process and they are inherent in any practice experience.

If it is believed that values are integral with professional nursing practice, then nurses and the organizations in which they work must commit to engaging in an evolving values pattern appraisal process. The essence of such a process should be the affirmation of nursing's purpose, which, from a Rogerian perspective, would be the promotion of health and well-being of all persons, including the nurse (Rogers, 1992).

Educators, who guide the unfolding of future members of the nursing profession, are perfectly positioned to guide students in exploring, clarifying, and creating value patterns that will be integral with professional nursing practice. Those who function as leaders, managers, and practitioners in the practice setting must nurture human–environment field modalities that support the actualization of organizational values.

## THE EMERGENCE OF THE VALUES OF PROFESSIONAL NURSES' MODEL

Given the belief that educators, as both teachers and learners, are strategically positioned to nurture value formation in students, the nursing faculty at the College of Mount Saint Vincent engaged in an appraisal of their own value patterns (Barrett, 1990a). This included an ongoing appraisal of how these values are or are not manifested in the mutual process among student, faculty, and college. The field pattern manifestation that emerged from the faculty group process was embodied in the Values of Professional Nurses Model illustrated in Figure 21.1. This model, organized in relation to the concepts of person, environment, health, and nursing, demonstrates the continuous unfolding of professional values that the faculty believes are manifested in the mutual process of human and environment fields. The four inseparable slinkies are used to illustrate values and related behavior patterns that are manifestations of the concepts of person, environment, health, and nursing, which are integral with the nursing metaparadigm (Fawcett, 1989). The integrality of the four slinkies embodies a whole that is far more than the sum of the parts, reflecting a Rogerian world-view about values related to professional practice. This model provides for the imaginative and creative use of nursing science. It increases the quantity and quality of our informational capacity, thereby providing multiple options for decision making and action with each other, with students, and with the larger college system.

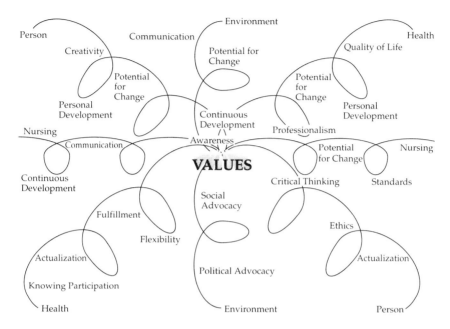

**Figure 21.1**
**Values of Professional Nurses Model**

For example, utilizing the value of knowing participation (see Figure 21.1), the faculty defined knowing participation and engaged in an ongoing dialogue of how this value would be manifested in the human-environmental field pattern of faculty, students, clients, and the health care organization. In our educational setting, students' knowing participation in courses was evident when they defined their own learning objectives, chose their preferred learning style, and participated in a peer review evaluation process. In a parallel manner, staff nurses participated knowingly in their professional development through performance appraisal when they actively participated in defining professional goals and identified strategies for meeting them.

In the practice arena, manifestations of professional values emerge out of the human-environmental mutual process that includes the nurse, the client, and the context, as illustrated in Figure 21.2. This irreducible field can participate knowingly in the

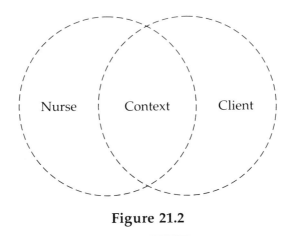

**Figure 21.2**

directions these values take, and, conversely, the direction needs to be integral with the values. This perspective has implications for nurse–client relationships since the value patterns of nurses are integral with shaping practice, continuous professional development, and the ways in which nurses provide care for their clients, whether they are individuals, families, or communities. For example, if health is viewed as a process of actualizing potential for well-being by knowing participation in change, client education becomes valued as a creative process in which the nurse and client mutually engage to facilitate well-being throughout the life process (Barrett, 1990b).

A values pattern process (see Figure 21.3) can be used to conceptualize how an organization can dwell with its values, examine them, and evaluate whether the values it purports to affirm and cherish are actualized in its documents and practice. Assuming that a collaborative process of knowing participation is engaged in by nursing staff and administration, four questions provide a guide for conducting an organizational values pattern appraisal:

1. What are the value patterns of this organization?
2. What would be the manifestations of these value patterns?
3. Which value patterns do we want to actualize?

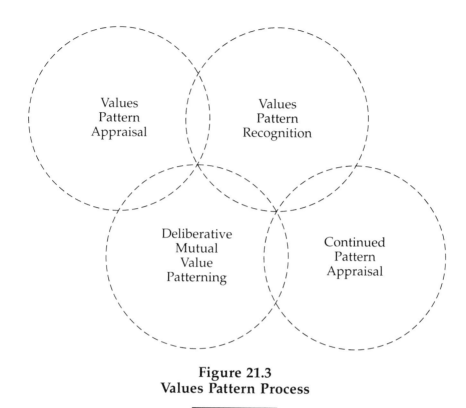

**Figure 21.3**
**Values Pattern Process**

4. What types of programs, policies, and practices do we have/need to develop to facilitate the unfolding of these value patterns?

A values pattern appraisal should reflect whether the affirmed values are manifested, at least on paper, in the mission and/or philosophy of the organization. For example, does the nursing care delivery model uphold the values that are explicated in the philosophy of the nursing department? Whether the model is functional, team, primary, or case management, the policies and procedures of the nursing department should work to support the approach to nursing care delivery. If the values are embedded in these documents, the actualization of them should be observable as manifestations of the human energy field in mutual process with the environmental field, which includes the health care organization.

## ACTUALIZING THE VALUES MODEL
## IN A PRACTICE SETTING

As illustrated in Figure 21.3, students and/or nurses who engage in a values pattern appraisal must first examine their own beliefs and values and expand their network of awareness into one that is integral with each person and manifested by those value patterns that are unique to their human–environment field. Pattern recognition emerges through dialogue about beliefs and values, and, through such dialogue, people engage in deliberative mutual patterning. The patterning becomes more complex and part of a larger whole as they engage in mutual process with the environmental field. The process of continual pattern appraisal and confirmation of alterations is considered evaluatively in the context of continually emerging beliefs, values, and behavior (Cowling, 1990).

As this process comes alive and is operationalized from a Rogerian perspective, let us consider student nurses who are about to graduate and are going on interviews for their first professional position. Prior to beginning the interview process, they should consider and clarify the values that have evolved over the course of their professional education program. Armed with a clarified set of values, the soon-to-be professionals embark on interviews with the goal of engaging in a pattern appraisal and recognition process regarding the integrality of their values and the organizational values. Confirming the "goodness of fit" between the professional nurse and the organization prior to selecting the employment opportunity of choice is a manifestation of the value placed on the Principle of Integrality. For example, a student graduating from ABC University may have developed a value about continuous professional development. When interviewing for a staff nurse position, she would be likely to ask the recruiter questions about staff development programs, tuition reimbursement, education days, offsite conference funding, and inhouse conference offerings. The answers to such questions will reveal the "goodness of fit" relative to this particular value. If, in fact, the organization has a dearth of such activities, the prospective professional would probably be wise to seek employment at another institution, one whose pattern manifestations are consistent with the value about continuous professional development. The human–environmental field is integral in nature and the questions posed by the student may facilitate change in the organization by an awareness of the philosophy of professional development and, perhaps, its relationship to recruitment and retention of professional staff. In like manner, the student will emerge from the interview different from the way she was when the meeting began, because of the mutual process that occurred.

Three organizing concepts have been chosen to examine further the values illustrated in Figure 21.1: (1) Structure and governance, (2) professional development, and (3) practice standards become the focus for questions that potential and actual staff nurse employees of a health care organization might raise within a Rogerian-based Values of Professional Nurses Appraisal Model.

A Rogerian-based values perspective suggests that the structure and governance of an organization should manifest open systems properties. As such, the leadership and management style, the table of organization, and communication channels should have properties of open systems. For example, a shared governance model that emphasizes lateral rather than hierarchical communication, and relationship patterns that are collaborative rather than bureaucratic, creates a climate in which the professional's work and goals are complementary to those of management and to the mission of the organization. This organizational model acknowledges the Principle of Integrality in its emphasis on mutual process among professionals and management within the human–environmental field of the organization (Porter-O'Grady, 1992).

When examining a table of organization, much can be learned about an organization, its values, and the extent to which it manifests open systems properties. The table of organization may reflect a traditional, hierarchical, bureaucratic model that embodies a "top-down" management style. In contrast, as illustrated in Figure 21.4, it could be conceptualized and operationalized as a web of fields in mutual process in which openness is manifested by the dotted lines. Mutual accountability, rather than reporting relationships and lines of authority, is manifested by the dotted two-directional arrows.

Questions that may be raised to facilitate pattern appraisal relative to structure and governance are listed in Table 21.1. An example of pattern appraisal not previously discussed concerns leadership style. In Table 21.1, question 4, four behavioral manifestations of leadership style are presented and should be considered in relation to personal values about the kind of human–environmental field in which a nurse knowingly chooses to practice. Participative leadership behavior most closely embodies the Principle of Integrality; that is, participation by all members of the organization is valued. Mutual accountability is inherent in the mutual process of the management

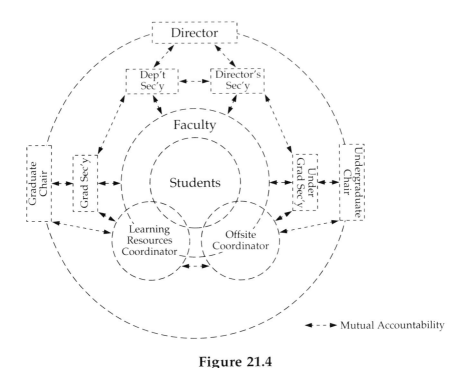

**Figure 21.4**
**Department of Nursing**

and staff. Management and staff are integral, creating unity, whole-ness, and shared purpose (Barker, 1990).

When patterns related to accessing information are appraised, as illustrated in question 9 of Table 21.1, the patterned flow of informa-tion should be characterized by wave patterns, increasing diversity, and no boundaries. Naisbitt & Aburdene (1990) suggested that em-ployees without free access to information cannot take responsibility. With free access, they cannot avoid it. Within a Rogerian conceptual system, information patterns arise from the mutual process of the hu-man field and the environmental field. Human field pattern infor-mation is really information about both; that is, it reveals the administrative-staff-environment in which communication occurs (Cowling, 1990). Information patterns are infinite and can include patient, family, research, financial, and performance information pat-terns. The ability to access information promotes intelligent decision

### Table 21.1
### Questions to Facilitate Pattern Appraisal in
### Relation to Structure and Governance

1. What is the mission and philosophy of the health care organization?
2. What is the philosophy of the Nursing Department?
3. How is the table of organization visually presented? Is it depicted as a hierarchical, bureaucratic model or as a web of integral fields?
4. What leadership/management style is manifested by the organization? Is a directive, achievement-oriented, supportive, or participative leadership/management style evident?
   a. Directive—Does the leader exert a high degree of control, seeking little participation in decision making?
   b. Achievement-oriented—Does the leader set challenging goals for the staff, emphasize excellence in performance, and show confidence that the staff will achieve these high standards?
   c. Supportive—Does the leader demonstrate friendliness, approachability, and concern for others?
   d. Participative—Does the leader consult with staff and take their opinions and suggestions into account when making decisions?
5. Is everyone in the organization a valued member integral with the focus of concern, the human and environment field of the client? How is that manifested in the organization?
6. What are the opportunities for members of the organization to dwell together in discussion and have a voice in shaping policy, developing practice standards, and contributing to the vision of the organization?
7. What is the nature of the Nursing Department governance process? What is the nature of the unit governance process?
8. Is collaboration among disciplines valued? Is it an integral dimension of the evolutionary unfolding of the organization?
9. Are there demonstrated areas of accountability where individuals not only share in decision making but recognize accountability for such participation?
10. How is information made available in the human and environmental field of the organization?

making and knowing participation in change; this is an example of power (Barrett, 1990b).

When actualization of professional potential is an organizational value, evidence of continuous change in employees and in the organizational culture is manifested in the human and environmental field pattern so that it becomes increasingly diverse and characterized by nonrepeating rhythmicities. A value about lifelong learning fosters a greater repertoire of pattern manifestations in the mutual process of human and environmental fields. Indicants of this value would be manifested in policies regarding professional development and criteria for promotion and performance appraisal. The questions in Table 21.2 facilitate a nurse's ability to appraise the extent to which an organizational value about actualization of professional potential and lifelong learning is present. For example, a nurse examining question 2 in Table 21.2 would expect that the value actualization of professional potential would be seen in performance appraisal policies that support the nurse's ability to define his or her professional goals. More specifically, if a clinical or management track is chosen and if professional activities that would enable the nurse to actualize this choice are selected, these choices would be

### Table 21.2
### Questions to Facilitate Pattern Appraisal in Relation to Continuous Professional Development

1. If actualization of professional potential is a value, what are the policies regarding professional development?
2. What is the philosophy and nature of the performance appraisal process?
3. What is the nature of criteria for promotion?
4. What is the nature of the opportunities for:
   a. Advancement in practice positions?
   b. Advancement to management positions?
   c. Participation in decision making?
5. Is community service valued? How is that value recognized in the organization?
6. Is creativity in clinical practice, such as the use of nontraditional healing approaches as a form of deliberative mutual patterning, valued in the organization? How is that value recognized?
7. Is participation in professional organizations valued?
8. If actualizing professional and education potential is a value, what are the policies supporting:
   a. Mentoring opportunities?
   b. Creative scholarship?
   c. Participation in continuing education programs?
   d. Conference presentations?
   e. Tuition reimbursement?
   f. Joint appointments?
   g. Collaborative projects?
   h. Development of professional and personal awareness?
   i. Participation in professional organizations?
   j. Participation in activities that contribute to shaping public and health policy on a local, regional, or national level?
9. What is the nature of the staff development program?
10. Is there a forum for the continued exploration of professional values that could then be enhanced through professional development programs?

continuously appraised. This approach fosters responsibility and accountability by enhancing the power of nurses to be in charge of their practice, embodying knowing participation in change, and supporting professional emergence.

From the perspective of the Rogerian-based Values of Professional Nurses Model, some of the values that are integral with standards of practice include: ethics, advocacy, collaboration, respect for diversity, potential for change, critical thinking, autonomy, accountability, and knowing participation in change. As nurses participate in theory-based practice, practice transforms in terms of the worldview of the practitioner and the values to which he or she is committed. Nurses participate in nurse–client relationships in a manner that brings life to their values. In this case, their theoretical knowledge and values come together and are viewed through the lens of the Science of Unitary Human Beings. Through this lens, both nurses and clients see things differently; they gain an insight that provides meaning in relation to the whole. As the nurse matures, he or she recognizes patterns of practice evolving. Patterns are apprehended differently; they are seen in ways they have not been seen before. Much that is evident is not quantifiable. It is embedded in the whole that comprises the human–environmental field phenomenon of the nurse's practice (Benner, 1984).

In considering a values pattern appraisal relative to practice standards, the nurse needs to look at the nursing care delivery model of the organization. Porter-O'Grady (1992) stated that "the delivery of nursing care model is the foundation for the control of practice" (p. 125). The values mentioned relative to standards of practice may be best supported by a primary care or case management model. Within this kind of model, the professional gains autonomy and greater accountability as he or she assumes the enhanced responsibility associated with models of care delivery. The questions in Table 21.3 highlight some of the issues that may be raised relative to appraising standards of practice. Inherent in all questions is a value about knowing participation in change. For example, a prospective nurse might inquire about the kinds of opportunities open to a staff nurse for participation in the development or change of the measurable practice standards that guide nursing practice in that organization. This nurse might also want to know how the standards of practice are actually implemented. If, in fact, there is a standard about client education, the nurse might want to know about the organizational expectations relative to development and implementation

### Table 21.3
### Questions to Facilitate Pattern Appraisal in
### Relation to Standards of Practice

1. Are there opportunities for participation in the development of measurable practice standards that guide the delivery of nursing care?
2. Are the values manifested in the standards of practice integral with the values of the Nursing Department?
   a. If health and wellness are values, does the organization support health promotion and maintenance programs versus just illness programs?
   b. If mutual process is a value, what kind of nursing care delivery model is employed to facilitate continuous versus episodic care?
3. Are the values reflected in the standards of practice that are integral with the focus and content of staff development programs? Are manifestations of the values reflected in clinical practice?
   a. If the human field is manifested not just by the individual client but by the family and community as well, how do staff development programs promote the perception of the family and community as client?
   b. Is the process of pattern appraisal a shared experience that gains meaning as the nurse and client dwell together?
   c. If mutual process is valued, how do staff development programs promote the collaborative nature of the nurse–client relationship, where the nurse does not impose meaning or arbitrary health ideals on the client's world? How does the nurse dwell with clients in discussion so that clients feel that they have the power to construct their own definition of health and their goals about health?
   d. If the uniqueness and diversity of clients is valued, how do staff development programs promote understanding and acceptance of cultural diversity?
4. Are the orientation programs for new employees competency-based to ensure the acquisition of knowledge and skills consistent with the standards of practice?
5. What kind of staff wellness activities are supported by the organization?
6. Are nurses provided opportunities for peer review relative to the standards of practice?
7. How do the criteria for performance appraisal relate to the standards of care?

of such a program. Do nurses identify the need for and nature of such a program? Or, do pattern recognition and goals for health care emerge from the client's identified perceptions and needs in such a way that the nurse and the client then collaborate in identifying and creating programs that meet the unique needs of each particular client by mutually participating in the knowing creation of change? This approach would provide evidence that this organization values enhancement of client power rather than client passivity, another hallmark of a participative rather than bureaucratic organizational model. As indicated in Table 21.3, question 3d, the nurse would want to make sure that the client's cultural needs are enfolded into pattern appraisal and deliberative mutual processing, thereby indicating valuing of and respect for the diversity embodied in that person's ethnic background and associated health care needs. Equally important is the provision of a forum in which nurses share their own perspectives relative to diversity and their related practice experiences. If, as indicated in question 3a of Table 3, the family, as well as the individual, is the client, then the prospective nurse would want to inquire about how families are included in the pattern appraisal and deliberate mutual processing. Moreover, referral to community resources would be an integral dimension of deliberative mutual patterning rather than something viewed as occurring "after" the hospital illness episode is completed. In essence, the prospective nurse wants to know whether the organization lives its values relative to the purported standards of practice.

Nurse educators who engage in their own continuous values appraisal process are more likely to encourage students as they explore and create their own professional value patterns, which will be integral with professional nursing practice.

The Rogerian values vision presented in this chapter provides a model for the appraisal of professional values in order to determine whether the value patterns of a health care organization are integral with those of the professional nurse. Through this process, nurses discover whether an organization practices its purported values and whether there is knowing staff participation in helping to shape structure and governance, professional development, and standards of practice. Manifestations of deliberative mutual patterning would reflect implementation of organizational values. A process of continuous pattern appraisal would evaluate whether the deliberative mutual patterning unfolds the potential of the organization of which the nurse knowingly chooses to become a professional staff member.

## REFERENCES

Barker, A. (1990). *Transformational nursing leadership: A vision for the future.* Baltimore: Williams & Wilkins.

Barrett, E.A.M. (1990a). The continuing revolution of Rogers' science-based nursing education. In E.A.M. Barrett (Ed.), *Visions of Rogers' science-based nursing* (pp. 303–318). New York: National League for Nursing.

Barrett, E.A.M. (1990b). Rogers' science-based nursing practice. In E.A.M. Barrett (Ed.), *Visions of Rogers' science-based nursing* (pp. 31–44). New York: National League for Nursing.

Benner, P. (1984). *From notice to expert: Excellence and power in clinical nursing practice.* Menlo Park, CA: Addison-Wesley.

Bruhn, J.G., & Henderson, G. (1991). *Values in health care: Choices and conflicts.* Springfield, IL: Thomas.

Burns, J.M. (1978). *Leadership.* New York: Harper & Row.

Cowling, W.R., III. (1990). A template for unitary pattern-based nursing practice. In E.A.M. Barrett (Ed.), *Visions of Rogers' science-based nursing* (pp. 45–66). New York: National League for Nursing.

Fawcett, J. (1989). *Analysis and evaluation of conceptual models of nursing* (3rd ed.). Philadelphia: F.A. Davis.

Martin, W.B. (1991). History, morality, and the modern university. In *Moral values and higher education* (pp. 121–143). New York: Brigham Young University and SUNY Press.

Naisbitt, J., & Aburdene, P. (1990). *Megatrends 2000: Ten new directions for the 1990's.* New York: Avon Books.

Porter-O'Grady, T. (1992). *Implementing shared governance: Creating a professional organization.* St. Louis: Mosby.

Rogers, M. (1992). Nursing science and the space age. *Nursing Science Quarterly, 5*(1), 27–34.

# 22

# Becoming Literate in the Science of Unitary Human Beings

*Mary Madrid*
*Dorothy Woods Smith*

This chapter is designed to provide an overview of paradigms and models, compare an old world-view and a new world-view, and introduce Rogers' nursing model. The relevance of Rogers' abstract model to nursing is illustrated by examples of how nurses have used the model to direct theory development, inspire research, and develop a new way to promote client comfort and health. The usefulness of Rogers' model in planning and providing client care is demonstrated through case studies from nursing practice.

According to Kuhn (1970), "Any new interpretation of nature, whether a discovery or a theory, emerges first in the mind of one or a few individuals. It is they who first learn to see science and the world differently . . ." (p. 144). The term paradigm, as described by Kuhn, represents beliefs and values shared by a community of scientists and unites the majority of the discipline in terms of questions to be asked and phenomena to be explored. A nursing model typically defines people and their environments, nursing and health. Different models, derived within different paradigms, represent different ways of viewing people and the world. Florence Nightingale realized that health and environment are related and that healing takes place within the individual. She described the work of nurses as creating for people an environment that promotes and supports their capacity to engage in healing. It may be that her system of beliefs about people and their environments, and the role of nurses in helping people to heal, was the forerunner of today's nursing models.

In the old world-view, people were seen as three-dimensional mechanistic beings made up of complex arrangements of cells, separate from their surrounding environment. The nature of people was believed to be homeostatic, making adaptations in an attempt to maintain a balanced state of being. The universe was perceived as entropic, implying that everything and everyone would eventually run down and stop. Nursing models conceptualized in the old world-view tended to focus on providing care to treat existing physical diseases and disorders and on restoring people to a previous state of well-being. Concern with biopsychosocial issues indicated an awareness of people as comprising many parts and coexisting with their environments. Concerns about body image incorporated a view of people as three-dimensional, exemplifying the limited scope of the old world-view paradigm.

In 1970, Martha Rogers, a creative and futuristic nurse thinker, published a model of nursing science derived within a new world-view—an organismic world-view in which field theory has replaced cell theory. Human beings are viewed as homeodynamic, integral with the environment, and continually changing through mutual process with the environment. The universe and all kinds of life are perceived as negentropic—in a continual process of becoming. Within this world-view, people are seen as continually changing and able to participate in the nature of that change. Awareness of dimensions other than the physical acknowledges unseen phenomena such as paranormal experiences. Possibilities emerge for the therapeutic use of imagery, meditation, and prayer, and goal setting expands beyond adaptation to encompass growth and transcendence. As nurses perceive the physical as one aspect of a more inclusive human field and realize that healing may or may not include the physical body, the scope of nursing literally takes on new dimensions.

Rogers' Science of Unitary Human Beings has organized these ideas by identifying "building blocks"—postulates that are intrinsic to how human beings and the environment are viewed. The four postulates are: (1) openness, (2) pandimensionality (formerly titled four-dimensional and multidimensional), (3) energy fields, and (4) pattern (see Table 22.1). Thus, in Rogers' (1987) nursing model, all individuals are human fields engaged in ongoing, mutual process with their environmental fields in a universe of open systems. Human beings are viewed as unitary, irreducible wholes, different from

## Table 22.1
## Key Definitions Specific to the Science of Nursing

| | |
|---|---|
| Energy field | The fundamental unit of the living and the nonliving. Field is a unifying concept. Energy signifies the dynamic nature of the field; a field is in continuous motion and is infinite. |
| Pattern | The distinguishing characteristic of an energy field perceived as a single wave. |
| Pandimensionality | A nonlinear domain without spatial or temporal attributes. |
| Unitary human beings (human field) | An irreducible, indivisible, pandimensional energy field identified by pattern and manifesting characteristics that are specific to the whole, which cannot be predicted from knowledge of the parts. |
| Environment (environmental field) | An irreducible, indivisible, pandimensional energy field identified by pattern and integral with the human field. |

the sum of their parts; energy fields are identified by patterns that change continuously and innovatively. Rogers' postulate that human beings *are* energy fields is different from that of human beings *having* energy fields.

Rogers described the nature of change as continuous—a process of becoming, in which some of an infinite number of potentials are actualized. In her model, she identified three "principles of homeodynamics" that postulate the nature of change in human and environmental field patterns. The principles are represented by terms she introduced to nursing: integrality, resonancy, and helicy (see Table 22.2). *Integrality* refers to how change occurs through "continuous, mutual human field and environmental field process" (Rogers, 1990, p. 8). *Resonancy* indicates that, as change occurs,

## Table 22.2
## Principles of Homeodynamics

| | |
|---|---|
| Principle of Resonancy | Continuous change from lower- to higher-frequency wave patterns in human and environmental fields. |
| Principle of Helicy | Continuous innovative, unpredictable, and increasing diversity of human and environmental field patterns. |
| Principle of Integrality | Continuous mutual human field and environmental field process. |

wave patterns become higher in frequency. *Helicy* describes change as innovative and unpredictable, manifested as increasing diversity. Manifestations of field patterning, as shown in Table 22.3, "emerge out of the human–environment field mutual process" (Rogers, 1992, p. 31). Rogers' three principles are not meant to be considered as separate entities; they are to be perceived as integral dimensions of the process of change.

How we view human beings and the environment is the basis for how we think about nursing and health. Examples of how Rogers' abstract model has provided direction for nurses in the areas of theory development, research, and promoting client healing serve to illustrate the usefulness of the model.

Rogers' model has raised questions among nurse theorists and scholars. One Rogerian scholar, Elizabeth A.M. Barrett, derived a theory of power inspired and directed by Rogers' postulate that people are capable of actively participating in the process of change. Barrett (1986), departing from the dominant world-view of power as something that one has and uses to control others, described power as "a way humans engage in mutual process with the environment to actualize some developmental potentials rather than others" (p. 173). She further identified power—the capacity to participate knowingly in change—as a manifestation of pattern characterized by four integral concepts: (1) awareness, (2) choices, (3) freedom to act intentionally, and (4) involvement in creating change. Another Rogerian scholar, John Phillips, is developing a theory of human

### Table 22.3
### Manifestations of Field Patterning in Unitary Human Beings

The evolution of unitary human beings is a dynamic, irreducible, nonlinear process characterized by increasing diversity of energy field patterning. Manifestations of patterning emerge out of the human–environmental field mutual process and are continuously innovative. Pattern is an abstraction that reveals itself through its manifestations.

The nature of unitary field patterning is unpredictable and creative. Change is relative and increasingly diverse. Some manifestations of relative diversity in field patterning are noted below.

| Lesser diversity | | Greater diversity |
|---|---|---|
| Longer rhythms | Shorter rhythms | Seems continuous |
| Slower motion | Faster motion | Seems continuous |
| Time experienced as slower | Time experienced as faster | Timelessness |
| Pragmatic | Imaginative | Visionary |
| Longer sleeping | Longer waking | Beyond waking |

field image in which human beings perceive themselves as different from three-dimensional physical bodies. Phillips (1990) was inspired by Rogers' model, in which human beings are perceived as pandimensional energy fields continually changing through mutual process with a pandimensional universe. He stated: "From a body image perspective, nursing focuses primarily on the dysfunction of parts of the physical body. From a human field image perspective, nursing focuses primarily on the potentials of the person" (p. 15).

Rogers' Science of Unitary Human Beings has helped nurse researchers identify questions to be asked, phenomena to be studied, and patterns to be discerned. Questions asked within this new worldview represent a new way of thinking. Early studies investigated the principles of homeodynamics. For example, Ference (1986) studied resonancy, developing a tool to measure human field motion and testing the idea that, as human beings change, they manifest higher frequency patterns. Barrett (1983) studied helicy, identifying power as a pattern representative of greater diversity. These studies, although focused on a single principle, recognized and were conceptually consistent with Rogers' science in its entirety. More recent studies draw from Rogers' model as a whole. Rogers' (1970) statement that human beings' "unity with nature" and "evolutionary becoming" are intrinsic to the nature of changes associated with traumatic events (p. 80) suggested to Dorothy Smith (1992) that spirituality might be related to the actualization of human field potentials through mutual process with a transcendent dimension or Being. Linking of this idea to the observation that some people reported personal growth, transformation, and transcendence following life-threatening events led to a national study of power and spirituality among polio survivors (Smith, 1992).

Rogers' model gave impetus to the development of Therapeutic Touch (TT), a creative nursing practice modality suggested by theory and supported by research. Developed by Dolores Krieger and Dora Kunz, TT is a human field treatment that has been known to relieve pain (Keller & Bzdek, 1986; Wright, 1987), diminish anxiety (Heidt, 1981; Quinn, 1984), and accelerate healing (Krieger, 1988; Wirth, 1990). In this nursing modality, nurses intentionally and compassionately facilitate changes in the energy field patterning of clients. During Therapeutic Touch, although the nurses's hands need never touch the client's body, people typically experience relaxation and other beneficial changes in their human field pattern. Recent studies have supported the concept of the integrality of the mutual process of human and environmental fields by identifying pattern changes in the nurses who practice TT (Heidt, 1990; Quinn, 1993), as well as in the people whom they treat (Meehan, 1985; Mersmann, 1993). The postulates of Rogers' model (openness, pattern, energy fields, and pandimensionality) form the theoretical matrix that gives rise to the development and testing of creative and innovative treatment modalities.

Our view of people and the environment is the basis for how we provide nursing care. The following case studies, based on Mary Madrid's practice, are presented to illustrate how Rogers' model was used in the nursing care of these individuals. These case studies are intended to serve as exercises through which readers can discover how a nurse's way of looking at the world will be associated with the nurse's care of his or her clients. At the end of each case description, a brief commentary from the perspective of Rogers' model is provided.

## CASE STUDY: DAVID

David was a 62-year-old male who suffered a heart attack while driving a car, crashed into a pole, and sustained multiple injuries. Damage to his spinal cord left him paralyzed below the neck and respirator-dependent. He remained in intensive care for 13 months. The need for halo traction and a respirator continued throughout his hospitalization.

David had been an active businessman and he had a bright, alert mind. It was difficult for him to deal with a situation in which he perceived himself as being powerless, dependent, and immobile. Communication was especially difficult for him, and he found it frustrating when staff members did not readily understand the words he formed with his mouth. His wife and brother were often at his bedside, and he manifested behaviors that reflected happiness and relaxation when they were present: his facial expressions were bright and enthusiastic, his respiratory pattern was smooth and rhythmic. Much of their communication was nonverbal, but it was powerful and effective.

I (MM) worked as a staff nurse on the evening shift, and David was most often assigned to be my patient. Human field pattern appraisal was most important since it gave me the opportunity to recognize behavioral manifestations of human field pattern and initiate nursing actions that would promote David's optimum well-being.

In the old world-view, David would be viewed as a three-dimensional being who would need to cope with his disability and adapt to the limitations of his hospital environment. Using Rogers' model, David was seen as a pandimensional human energy field, different from the sum of his parts and in continual mutual process with his environmental field. His environment, which included his room and the people in it, extended to the atemporal, aspatial universe of imagination, memory, and dreams. As a human energy field, he had an image of himself that was far more extensive, expansive, and whole than that of his body or mind considered alone.

David had had a long day by the time I arrived for work each evening. Pattern appraisal at the beginning of the shift most often demonstrated a sense of fatigue. This was manifested by a tired facial expression, a labored breathing pattern, and a lack of enthusiasm in engaging in conversation. By the time I arrived, the music on the radio, played continuously throughout the day, had lost its pleasurable meaning, and David viewed it as no more than "just another noise that blended in with the other hospital sounds."

To promote rest and a feeling of refreshment, I would give him a bed bath. Conversation was kept to a minimum during this time and he appeared to take the opportunity to think about the events of the day. Upon completion of his bath, he would usually verbalize his feelings about how his day had been and what he had found to be of special interest or concern. His bath was followed by a period of Therapeutic Touch. He would then fall asleep and awake refreshed an hour or two later.

By encouraging David to be slow and articulate with his communication, I developed the ability to read his lips so that conversation between us was effortless. I learned that he had a special interest in Native Americans and that he had spent most of his adult life studying their culture and history. He had become quite an expert.

He often expressed his feelings of boredom and how time seemed to drag as he lay in bed with nothing to do but wait for events such as mail delivery or visiting hours to break the monotony of the day. In an attempt to reduce boredom and promote a feeling of time passing more quickly, I suggested that we have a mutual agreement. On each day that I was to be working, I would look up and share with him the origin of a word or well-known phrase (e.g., "I heard it through the grape vine"). In turn, he would tell me something concerning the culture and history of Native Americans. He enthusiastically agreed. This exchange illustrates the use of deliberative mutual patterning, which, together with pattern manifestation appraisal, comprises the Rogerian practice methodology.

David would be occupied for long periods throughout the day visualizing himself in his library with his books and memorabilia. He would recall the excitement of reading and learning something new about Native Americans, a subject that was so intriguing to him. He recalled how information about these people captured his imagination and how easy it was for him to picture them living out their lives as depicted in writings he had read or at places that he had visited. He delighted in the ability to so clearly bring this information into the relative present for his enjoyment. He did so with such depth and detail, creating mental images of their adventures, customs, and traditions, that he found time racing by. He pondered over the many questions he had about their lives, organizing and synthesizing his knowledge in order to find answers to these questions. He looked forward to sharing his excitement and enthusiasm with me.

As people become more diverse, time is perceived as passing more quickly. This is illustrated by how time dragged when David was bored and raced as he became involved with his creative and imaginative activities. His mental imaging of being in the library or in another culture, his memories of the past, and his anticipation of sharing his excitement with his nurse were evidence of the pandimensional nature of his activities. David was involved in creating changes, identifiable by pattern manifestations that were nonlinear and without temporal or spatial attributes. He was actualizing potentials in the process of becoming, in contrast to just coping to maintain homeostatic adaptation.

David was positioned and turned every two hours. If he was not positioned in a manner that was comfortable for him, he would lie there frustrated and angry because of his discomfort and his inability to change his own position. The task of positioning him to promote comfort, however, was difficult. His not being able to readily verbalize how he wanted to be positioned was as frustrating for the staff as it was for David. He would be turned, and several attempts at positioning his head and the limbs of his body would be made in order to find a position that was "just right" for him. If this was not accomplished after several inquiries of "Is this position OK?" and what the staff perceived to be a "reasonable amount of time and effort," he would lie in a position that was uncomfortable for him.

I noted that whenever he was being positioned, he would be intent on looking at the ceiling. I asked him why he was doing this and found that he had a certain spot on the ceiling that he would use as a focal "comfort spot." If he was positioned so that he could see that "comfort spot," his body would be aligned in a comfortable position. He had spent many hours looking at that ceiling and knew its pattern. He used this pattern as a reference point. Each position had a different "comfort spot." One was a small water spot, another was a jagged crack in the ceiling. I found it useful to have him point out these spots to me so that I could use them to position his head and body comfortably.

Rogers' principles of change are illustrated by David's story: integrality, the continual mutual process of human and environmental fields; helicy—patterning toward greater creativity and diversity; and resonancy—higher-frequency patterning. Nonlinear development is illustrated by the nonrepeating nature of the pattern of changes.

A group analyzing this case study noted that David's nurse showed creativity and diversity in her approaches, and that the continual, mutual process between human and environmental fields could be observed in her pattern as well as in his. The group extended the idea of patterning the environment by suggesting that, to pattern David's physical environment, one might apply stars or illustrations of his choice to the identifying spots on the ceiling, to give him visual pleasure as well as a reference point for caregivers.

## CASE STUDY: CARLOS

Carlos was a 33-year-old Hispanic male who was well-known to the nursing staff in the intensive care unit. Three or four times a year, the police would find him on the street unconscious and would bring him to the hospital. He would arrive in the intensive care unit on a respirator, unresponsive, having seizures, and testing at a toxic alcohol level. His hair would be dirty and matted, his face unshaven, and his moustache unruly. The crusty grime on his clothes and body gave evidence of his unwillingness to bathe or an unavailability of bathing facilities.

On each admission, the sequence and pattern of his behavioral manifestations were similar but not identical to those of prior admissions. He would remain intubated and unconscious for several days. During this time, he would have continual seizure activity that would begin to gradually decrease in frequency and intensity relative to his alcohol level. Other than withdrawing from painful stimuli, he would demonstrate no signs of awareness of his environment.

Approximately two days after the seizure activity ceased, Carlos would "wake up." It usually was not a peaceful awakening. Carlos would be agitated and combative. He would thrash about in his bed and make determined (often successful) attempts to pull out his intravenous lines and/or his endotracheal tube. He would throw anything he could get his hands on and make multiple attempts to climb over the side rails of his bed. As he displayed signs of awakening, the restraints were kept on "stand by," and the staff usually had to apply them soon after he awoke to protect him from injuring himself or others.

Within 24 hours of awakening, he would usually be extubated by choice or by the medical staff. He would be in restraints for several days, cursing and shouting at staff members as they administered care to him. At regularly scheduled intervals, his restraints were released and/or the sites were changed. It was necessary for at least three staff members to be involved in this process. It was a battle to perform even the simplest nursing care since he was continually trying to kick, bite, or punch anyone within reach. He never had any visitors, and no friends or family made telephone calls to the unit to seek information about his clinical status.

The manifestations of his human field pattern would eventually undergo another change. His combative behavior would cease, and he would become quiet and withdrawn. Quite often, he would be found weeping. A great deal of time would be spent with the covers pulled over his head. The nursing staff would try to make conversation with him, encouraging him to take an interest in his environment, but he would ignore their suggestions and burrow deeper under the covers. He seldom made eye contact.

Pattern appraisal demonstrated his feelings of depression and loneliness. He had no energy or interest in participating in activities that would promote movement toward well-being. His behavioral manifestations reflected the pattern of his energy field. His human field image was low in personal esteem and personal worth. He mourned the loss of alcohol. He felt alone and without support systems.

Carlos did not stay long in the unit. When he was "medically stable," he was transferred out of intensive care to another nursing unit. We would not see him again until his next admission.

On this particular admission, when Carlos was about due to "wake up," I thought of a different approach in providing his care. The sequence of pattern manifestations Carlos had displayed was similar to those of prior admissions. Instead of preparing for a battle when he awoke, I initiated deliberate mutual patterning strategies that would pattern the environment in a manner that would promote feelings of security, comfort, and well-being.

Carlos was still intubated; the pattern of his respirations was rhythmic and restful. Slight movements of his arms and legs, an occasional twitch of his eyes or facial muscles, and an intuitive perception communicated his forthcoming arousal. Numerous baths had made his skin clean and shiny, but his hair was still dirty and matted and his face was unshaven.

When he awoke, I wanted Carlos to see himself differently. I had hoped that a fresh, clean physical appearance might be instrumental in changing his perception of his human field image and would assist him in recognizing and actualizing his potentials. I washed his hair, shaved his face, and trimmed his moustache. Whenever I was by his bedside, I spoke to him. I told him what I was doing and how I was looking forward to seeing him awake. A radio playing soft music was placed at his bedside to promote feelings of peace and tranquility.

Since Carlos usually concentrated on finding ways to extubate himself shortly after he awoke, I suggested to the medical staff (who knew him from prior admissions) that attempts be made to extubate him before he awoke and did so himself. This would allow him the opportunity to speak to others and would reduce feelings of fright and agitation. They were receptive to this suggestion and began the process of weaning him from the ventilator. The physical manifestations of his energy field (arterial blood gases, pattern of breathing) indicated that extubation was possible, and it was carried out. To further enhance a feeling of well-being, I used Therapeutic Touch during the last few hours before he awoke; I wanted to promote a relaxed, rhythmic patterning of his energy field. I had an intuitive sense as to when he would awaken, and I paid special attention to clues manifested in his behavioral manifestations so that I was at his side when he became conscious.

The pattern manifestations that emerged from the mutual process of his human and environmental energy field demonstrated the efficacy of the nursing modalities. Carlos seemed surprised when he woke and found me at his bedside, talking to him and holding his hand. He stared at me but made no attempt to withdraw his hand. He smiled when I told him how "handsome he looked cleaned and shaven." He was given a mirror so that he could see the change in his appearance. He looked at himself carefully and then asked me if I could do a better job on his moustache since one side was crooked. I joked about my role as a barber, and he joined in the laughter.

Other staff members came by to observe his behavior. They began to talk to him, telling him how amazed they were to see such a change. Based on historical experience, they told him what they had expected and joked about not having to do "combat duty" on this admission. Carlos seemed pleased with himself and began to engage in conversation with those around him. He remembered some of the staff and apologized to them for his past behavior. Shortly thereafter, he pulled the covers over his head and went off to sleep.

When the change of shift occurred, the night staff did not readily recognize that it was Carlos who was lying in the bed. They excitedly made remarks to him and among themselves on how "great" he looked and how delighted they were to see the changes in his behavior. Carlos basked in this atmosphere of warmth and friendliness. The nature of the mutual process between his human and environmental fields was quite different from what he had experienced on admissions in the relative past. He took delight in joking with the staff and having conversations with them.

The Principle of Integrality is illustrated in Carlos' experience. Although Carlos was in the same hospital as before and some of the same nurses were providing his care, his perception of this hospital experience was different from experiences in the relative past. The pattern of the mutual process between Carlos' human and environmental field on this admission was also dramatically different. Rather than avoiding contact with Carlos, the staff was eager to approach him and express their surprise and delight in seeing him from this new perspective. They were comfortable in his presence and did not feel that it was necessary to be on guard to protect themselves from injury.

Carlos began to express concern about his life-style patterns. He became more reflective and tuned in to information concerning his unique human field pattern. He verbalized these insights. He knew that his drinking was out of control and wished that he could keep a job. He wanted to have in his life people who cared for him, but he had difficulty developing significant relationships.

The use of humor and of affirmations was instrumental in directing change in the rhythm and pattern of Carlos' energy field. Through mutual process, these modalities worked to establish trust and to allow him the opportunity to participate in the process of change. They heightened his ability to see himself from a new frame of reference and encouraged him to exercise behaviors that would enhance feelings of personal respect and worth.

The mutual process of human and environmental energy fields created Carlos' desire to make changes in his life-style pattern. He spoke of the loneliness he experienced after moving to this country and how much he missed his mother, who lived in Puerto Rico. Carlos fondly recalled the loving and caring behaviors his mother had exercised with him. Even as an adult, each night she would gently pull the covers over him, kiss him good-night, and tell him how much he meant to her. This was a special moment for Carlos, and the memory of it was soothing and refreshing.

Carlos spent a considerable amount of time with his head under the covers. The staff continued to use humor as a therapeutic modality. They would "tease" him out from under the covers, but Carlos lowered them with hesitation. I questioned this behavior and asked him to explain why it was so important for him to lie "all covered up." I learned that when Carlos pulled the covers over his head, he would create a pandimensional image of his mother saying good-night.

He could see himself in his mother's house and feel the warmth and love associated with this experience. He felt more vibrant and alive. The description of his feelings demonstrated a change in his human energy field from a lower to a higher frequency. He took comfort in creating this image and would readily resort to pulling the covers over his head when he was distressed or anxious. This behavior would facilitate his ability to engage in this pandimensional experience.

The process of health patterning (assisting clients' knowing participation in change to promote well-being) (Barrett, 1990) continued. Carlos had the capacity to actualize his potential. Health patterning modalities were used to assist him in this process. In order to promote power enhancement so that Carlos would participate knowingly in change, I assisted him in clarifying his goals.

He wanted to see and be with his family in Puerto Rico and hoped to "move back to my country." Economically, this was difficult. He would work for a while, start to save up some money, become discouraged and frustrated, and start drinking heavily again.

Carlos was soon to be moved out of intensive care to another unit. I wanted the health patterning process to continue. There were nurses on the transfer unit who knew Carlos, and I spoke to them about his behavior, his goals, and his interest in pursuing them. In the relative past, he had refused assistance from social workers; this time, he was receptive to having them assist him in entering a program that would help him deal with his pattern of heavy drinking. They would also help him find employment and establish him in a social support group.

Carlos was enthusiastic about these plans. Deliberative mutual patterning continued during the short time he remained in intensive care. Specific goals, defined by Carlos, were identified, and resources were made available that would assist him in accomplishing these goals. He freely and intentionally participated in the process of change directed toward promoting harmony in his human energy field.

He was made aware of the power he had within himself to make choices and was encouraged to draw on his personal strengths to become steadfast in working toward accomplishing his goals. It was suggested that he write out and use affirmations as expressions of intentionality to facilitate feelings of confidence and personal worth.

"Human field image is one manifestation of the mutual process of human beings with their environments" (Phillips, 1990, p. 14). The remarkable change in Carlos' human field image was a "diverse manifestation of [his] human field pattern" (Phillips, 1990, p. 14). It represented the "ever-changing relative present that synthesizes the past, present, and future" (p. 14). Carlos had stopped using the term "good for nothing" when speaking about himself and began to manifest behaviors that conveyed faith in himself and assurance of his ability to be successful in accomplishing his goals.

Carlos was encouraged to keep the image of his mother and his home in Puerto Rico fresh in his mind. It was not always possible for him to "duck under the covers" to elicit images that promoted feelings of refreshment and comfort. Through the use of guided imagery, he was taught to bring pleasant experiences from the relative past into the relative present.

He left the unit determined to "make it all happen." There was a good possibility that he would do just that! Carlos' human field had experienced an accelerated rhythm, and his pattern was more diverse. He had become aware of his situation, he had made choices, and he was participating in the process of creating change. For the first time, he felt that he had the freedom, courage, and strength to act on his intentions toward sobriety and employment and had identified resources whereby he could involve himself in creating those changes. For the first time in a long while, Carlos felt powerful. By recognizing the importance of the client's mutual process with the environment (integrality), the nurse recognized the potential for creating change by introducing specific options for health from which Carlos could choose (helicy), and his choices facilitated higher-frequency, more diverse changes (resonancy).

## REFERENCES

Barrett, A.M. (1983). *An empirical investigation of Martha E. Rogers' Principle of Helicy: The relationship of human field motion and power.* Unpublished doctoral dissertation, New York University, New York.

Barrett, E.A.M. (1986). Investigation of the Principle of Helicy: The relationship between human field motion and power. In V. Malinski (Ed.), *Explorations on Martha Rogers' Science of Unitary Human Beings* (pp. 173–188). Norwalk, CT: Appleton-Century-Crofts.

Barrett, E.A.M. (1990). Health patterning with clients in a private practice environment. In E.A.M. Barrett (Ed.), *Visions of Rogers' science-based nursing* (pp. 105–115). New York: National League for Nursing.

Ference, H. (1986). The relationship of time experience, creativity traits, differentiation, and human field motion. In V. Malinski (Ed.), *Explorations on Martha Rogers' Science of Unitary Human Beings* (pp. 95–105). Norwalk, CT: Appleton-Century-Crofts.

Heidt, P. (1981). Effect of Therapeutic Touch on the anxiety level of hospitalized patients. *Nursing Research, 30,* 32–37.

Heidt, P. (1990). Openness: A qualitative analysis of nurses' and patients' experiences of Therapeutic Touch. *Image: Journal of Nursing Scholarship, 22,* 180–186.

Keller, E., & Bzdek, V.M. (1986). Effects of Therapeutic Touch on tension headache pain. *Nursing Research, 35*(2), 101–106.

Krieger, D. (1988, April). *Therapeutic Touch: Two decades of research, teaching, and clinical practice.* Paper presented at the twentieth anniversary of Council Grove Conferences on Voluntary Controls Program for the Menninger Foundation, Topeka, Kansas.

Kuhn, T.S. (1970). *The structure of scientific revolutions* (2nd ed.). Chicago: University of Chicago Press.

Meehan, T.C. (1985). *The effect of Therapeutic Touch on the experience of acute pain in postoperative patients.* Unpublished doctoral dissertation, New York University, New York.

Mersmann, C. (1993). *Therapeutic Touch and milk letdown in mothers of non-nursing preterm infants.* Unpublished doctoral dissertation, New York University, New York.

Phillips, J.R. (1990). Changing human potentials and future visions of nursing: A human field image perspective. In E.A.M. Barrett (Ed.), *Visions of Rogers' science-based nursing* (pp. 13–25). New York: National League for Nursing.

Quinn, J. (1984). Therapeutic Touch as energy exchange: Testing the theory. *Advances in Nursing Science, 6*(2), 42–49.

Quinn, J. (1993). Psychoimmunologic effects of Therapeutic Touch on practitioners and bereaved recipients: A pilot study. *Advances in Nursing Science, 15*(4), 13–26.

Rogers, M.E. (1970). *An introduction to the theoretical basis of nursing.* Philadelphia: F.A. Davis.

Rogers, M.E. (1987). Rogers' Science of Unitary Human Beings. In R.R. Parse, *Nursing science: Major paradigms, theories and critiques* (pp. 139–146). Philadelphia: Saunders.

Rogers, M.E. (1990). Nursing: Science of Unitary, Irreducible, Human Beings: Update 1990. In E.A.M. Barrett (Ed.), *Visions of Rogers' science-based nursing* (pp. 5–11). New York: National League for Nursing.

Rogers, M.E. (1992). Nursing science and the space age. *Nursing Science Quarterly, 5*(1), 27–34.

Smith, D.W. (1992). *A study of power and spirituality in polio survivors using the nursing model of Martha E. Rogers.* Unpublished doctoral dissertation, New York University, New York. (University Microfilms No. 92-22, 966)

Wirth, D. (1990). The effect of non-contact Therapeutic Touch on the healing rate of full thickness dermal wounds. *Subtle Energies, 1*(1), 1–20.

Wright, M. (1987). The use of Therapeutic Touch in the management of pain. *Nursing Clinics of North America, 22*(3), 705–714.

# 23

# Learning Rogerian Science: An Experiential Process

*Sarah Hall Gueldner*
*Wanda Daniels*
*Maranah Sauter*
*Margie Johnson*
*Brenda Talley*
*Martha Hains Bramlett*

Since the 1970s, students have attempted to grasp, primarily by traditional passive learning methods, the highly abstract and esoteric conceptual system of Rogers' Science of Unitary Human Beings. This chapter describes a unique and successful approach to doctoral-level study of Rogerian science based on creative learning methods. Its success can be attributed to the innovative design of a course in which participants actually experience the concepts of the theory in a variety of nontraditional, illuminating ways. Students learn Rogerian science by living Rogerian science. The chapter first presents an overview of the course under scrutiny and a brief discussion of the importance of creative thinking to theory building. Theory-based literature related to innovative learning methods is considered. Two essays are then presented, the first reflecting the teachers' perspective and the second describing the students' experience.

The authors would like to acknowledge with special appreciation Carl Brown, Emory University, who taught Tai Chi; and Claire Clements, University of Georgia, University Affiliated Program for Persons with Developmental Disabilities, who guided the group in art activities.

## COURSE DESCRIPTION

The Rogerian Conceptual System of Nursing Course described herein is a five-credit doctoral-level course offered by the Medical College of Georgia School of Graduate Studies. Enrollment was recently extended to include Master's students who have demonstrated a particular interest in the system and who are willing to participate fully. Course alumni from previous years are welcomed back, and there are additional guest appearances by Dr. Rogers and other Rogerian scholars. The course is designed to lead students to a fuller understanding of the principles and concepts unique to the Rogerian system.

## TRADITIONAL LEARNING

In the past, most students have learned Rogerian science by traditional passive learning methods—lectures, reading, writing, and films. Passive learning is an effective method for acquiring some types of knowledge, but it does not maximize retention of information (Bevis, 1973) nor can it teach one how to learn, critique, or seek meanings. For internalization to occur, the information must be used in some way (Bevis & Murray, 1990). The abstract nature of the Rogerian system demands a higher level of learning than that acquired by traditional methods.

In addition to its abstractness, the Rogerian system is complex and evolving; therefore, the language is specific and is continuously being refined and polished by Rogerian scholars. Innovations in knowledge frequently change Rogerian thinking as theories are continually being generated and tested (Rogers, 1990). Passive learning techniques are inept vehicles for the type of learning required here: a learning method that gives maximum leeway for the development of divergent and creative thinking skills.

## CREATIVE LEARNING—
## CREATIVE/DIVERGENT THINKING

The ultimate goal of the Rogerian course is the development of cognitive skills requisite to the generation and testing of theories derived from the Rogerian system. Theory development demands creative thinking, which is defined as the ability to produce novel and original ideas and concepts. Once learned, the ability to think creatively persists over time, is associated with a high degree of motivation, and is characterized by the ability to view a problem from a different perspective each time one examines it (Taylor, 1990; Torrance, Reynolds, & Ball, 1978). Divergent thinking (Runco, 1990) is the ability to produce numerous, different ideas when presented with an open-ended problem or task. Runco (1990) suggested that increasing divergent thinking increases creative performance.

## CREATING THE LEARNING ENVIRONMENT

There is compelling evidence that the learning environment has a powerful impact on creative performance (Oliver, 1984; Runco, 1990; Taylor, 1990). Environmental factors that inhibit divergent thinking and creativity are: lack of time; terming open-ended tasks as "tests"; anxiety and fear of failure; premature, unjust, or overly harsh criticism; overemphasis on success; and autocratic discipline and rigidity. Factors that facilitate divergent and creative thinking include: structuring a rich environment that encourages students to think in new ways; modeling of creativity, originality, and spontaneity by the teacher; the teacher's praising and affirming creative thinking when appropriate; and the teacher's giving specific instructions to "be creative."

Divergent and creative thinking may also be enhanced or constricted by the opportunities afforded an individual (Oliver, 1984; Taylor, 1990). Taylor (1990) reported that exposure to unfamiliar environmental conditions elicits, more consistently, more original ideas than commonplace, everyday, familiar tasks and questions. The type of *ideational* strategies required by "unfamiliar stimuli," Taylor added, has a direct bearing on the success of this tactic.

Various types of activities used to increase creative and divergent thinking are reported in the literature. Reading and writing poetry (Hillman, 1980); group imagery (Schwab & D'Zamko, 1988); humor (Ziv, 1988); and discrepant events (Zielinski & Sarachine, 1990), such as discussions about moral dilemmas, in which the outcome is different than was expected, have all been used with varying degrees of success. Almost all of these concepts and principles of creative learning were embedded in the Rogerian nursing course.

## LEARNING ROGERS BY IMMERSION

### Reflections by the Teachers

The Rogerian abstract conceptual system is much too special to be taught using ordinary teaching strategies. A new world-view must be collectively embraced, allowing each member of the class to become more aware of his or her being and of oneness with all other beings and the universe. Unless this task can be achieved, learning about the Science of Unitary Human Beings is without flavor or meaning.

Even the most cursory perusal of the course outline reveals that content is not the distinguishing feature of the innovative learning process described herein. The unique feature rests instead with the environmental climate that is created for the course. Teaching within this model, the most important work of the teacher is to create an environment that leads participants into an exciting new world-view. The environment is patterned to allow each participant to look deeper than ever before into his or her thinking in order to discover the ultimate truths of the universe and see these truths in a personal way.

The learning environment was patterned to enhance internalization of knowledge about the philosophy undergirding the Science of Unitary Human Beings. The course was purposefully *not* held in a classroom; instead, its format varied from traditional academic course work in terms of the setting, scheduling, and assigned learning activities. Specifically, the learning environment was patterned to include:

1. A collection of resources, and time for immersion in relevant literature.

2. An informal atmosphere that allowed participants to come to know each other as team members in the search for new knowledge.

3. Attention to environmental attributes that legitimize and promote new world thinking.

4. Exposure to demonstrations and discussions related to nontraditional therapeutic modalities.

5. Resources to support the immediate expression of scholarly "Ah-hahs" that were sure to be manifested.

6. Freedom and opportunity for expression using a variety of media.

7. A climate of nurturant critique.

8. An abundance of "unitary" toys and food to afford regular relief from the sometimes overwhelming task of assimilating difficult and unfamiliar thinking into a personal world-view.

It was important for the group to spend time together in a Rogerian way—to live within the unitary system. Toward this goal, the environment was filled with high-frequency images and a diverse assortment of options not usually available in traditional academic environments.

### Creating the Reading Environment

The complex and unfamiliar nature of the Rogerian science requires that students quickly become conversant with a wide body of literature that they may not previously have had the opportunity or inclination to read. Since the course must begin and end within an academic quarter (11 weeks), there is not time for students (even doctoral students) to discover, read, and digest enough of the critical literature on their own. Therefore, a collection of the most important readings has been compiled and is made available. The class meets for the first time only briefly, for orientation concerning the nature of the course and to receive course materials, which include selected audio and video tapes and the basic reading packets. Additionally, at least single copies of essential books such as *Flathead* (Abbott, 1952), *Tao of Physics* (Capra, 1983), *Explorations on Martha Rogers' Science of Unitary Human Beings* (Malinski, 1986), and *Visions of Rogers' Science-Based Nursing* (Barrett, 1990) are made available for the group to share at a central location until they can purchase their own.

After the orientation session, the class does not meet again formally for a month. This gives the students time to read the materials, to discover other relevant readings on their own, to become somewhat conversant with the concepts and terminology of Rogerian science, and to be troubled by dozens of questions for which there is no absolute answer!

### Creating a Retreat Atmosphere

The remaining class time is scheduled as either one week-long retreat or two shorter retreats. It is here that the creative process begins. A seminar format is created, which almost ensures that the participants will come to see the world differently. Surrounded by high-frequency images, the group lives together in the Science of Unitary Human Beings. Daily, they grow in their understanding of its principles, and they enable each other to become more and more aware of their oneness with the universe. Expression through music, movement, and art is encouraged.

The most recent class was held on Nag's Head Beach, and each day began with a beginners' Tai Chi session on the beach. The nights often evolved into harmonizing song fests by the ocean, with an occasional spirited round of line dancing. One afternoon, each participant was guided to create his or her own sand casting, using the treasures from the sea that had been washed ashore by the tide. (A qualified non-nurse Tai Chi instructor and an artist were enticed to come along with an offer of free room and board in return for their expertise.)

Structured presentations and dialogue were scheduled for at least two hours each morning, and similar two- to three-hour sessions were held each afternoon. During these seminar sessions, the group examined the principles and concepts unique to the Science of Unitary Beings and critiqued definitions central to the system. Testable hypotheses were formulated, and studies conducted within the system were critiqued. Rogers' work was evaluated in terms of its adequacy as a base for nursing science, and testable theories that flow from Rogerian science were identified. Innovative methodologies were considered, and the state of the science was continually appraised and debated. Practice applications were an integral part of the discussions; they included demonstrations and discussions related to nontraditional modalities, such as Therapeutic Touch and imagery.

Unitary toys (such as kits and giant bubble blowers) were provided for breaks. Together, the group prepared food for most meals (an important feature of the setting, since graduate students almost always have to choose carefully how they will spend their limited financial resources). Mealtimes were marked with foods judged by the group to be unitary, and included an abundance of home-grown tomatoes, corn-on-the-cob, and homemade ice cream topped with fresh peaches. In the evenings, popcorn—that very unitary food that becomes transformed and declares its unitary nature with its deliciously pervasive aroma—took top billing. At least one round of sparklers was a feature of each retreat session.

Together, the group celebrated both the most prominent and the most obscure characteristics of the universe: rainbows, rain, the sun, and the semicircular track of a sea turtle who came ashore overnight to lay its eggs on the sand. On one occasion, the group looked through a telescope at the rings around Saturn and the moons of Jupiter. On another occasion, the group was led by a written piece to marvel at the order of the world from the inside of an onion. The experiences were patterned to include media that call up all of the senses—the sounds of music and the waves, the smell of fireplaces or of the salty air, the taste of favorite foods, and expressive movement. The experience of openness was patterned by relaxing as many traditional environmental barriers as possible. The sessions were held at the beach. (At other retreats, they have been held in mountain cottages and sometimes in homes, but almost never in classrooms.) The sessions were not referred to as classes.

### Facilitating the Mutual Mentor–Mentee Process

When learning about the Science of Unitary Human Beings, there is no substitute for person-to-person contact with the established community of Rogerian scholars. Therefore, course options always include activities that bring the novice and the expert together in dialogue. One class was given the option of attending the Fourth Rogerian Conference, in New York, as an alternative learning activity. On other occasions, seminar time has incorporated participation in the annual Region 7 functions of the Society of Rogerian Scholars. Dr. Rogers herself has been present for several days near the end of each course, after students have had an opportunity to read classic materials and practice articulating the concepts and principles of the science together.

### Written Assignments

Written assignments promote clarity and develop precision of expression therefore, each individual is expected to create a manuscript or some other product that can withstand peer review for either publication or presentation at a regional or national meeting. More than one third of the 50 individuals who have taken the course have had their work published or accepted for publication. Seven have gone on to complete Rogerian dissertation research, and another is progressing toward that goal. Dr. Linda Johnston developed an instrument to measure the concept of human field image within the Science of Unitary Human Beings as her dissertation, and the most recent doctoral graduate, Dr. Margaret Hindman, examined the relationship between humor and field energy. Three alumni of the course have completed, or are presently completing, Master's theses or projects based on the

Science of Unitary Human Beings. Several have presented their work at regional and/or national conferences.

Given that written expression is considered essential to theory development, the course syllabus includes a written assignment. At least one computer (and printer) is available at each retreat so that Ah-hah's can be written down before they are lost. Each year, the computers have been used to compose beginning manuscripts and to print and distribute poems and an address–telephone list of participants. Alternative experiences are always negotiable, however, even for this written assignment. An alternative option that has often been acceptable is a group paper intended for submission to a journal or presentation at a regional or national meeting.

### Creative Expressions

A surprising number of persons have chosen to express their new world-view through creative media. Several students have written poems to convey their new awareness, and one student has seemed to burst into poetry, sometimes composing several poems in one day. Another chose to express her new thinking through stained glass creations. A group from one class has prepared a video tape based on poetry and expressive movement to submit for the next Rogerian conference in New York.

### Manifestations That the Magic Has Happened

There are several observable operational markers that denote when the primary course objectives have been achieved. The expression of the learner comes alive, and his or her dialogue becomes more animated and marked by the sometimes newfound skill of posing rhetorical questions. Participants often begin to wear purple clothes and collect slinkies, and to exchange purple things with each other and Dr. Rogers, to exhibit their new awareness that purple is the highest-frequency color in the rainbow. For fun, they proclaim pseudo-truths within the system, such as, "Chocolate is good for the pandimensionality of my energy field." Depending on their life circumstances, some students progress in their interest and understanding more than others, but the course is designed to ensure that all students grow into a new perspective that enables them, for the rest of their lives, to continue changing in harmony with a new world-view.

## The Student Experience

The Rogerian adventure began at New York University, in the heart of Greenwich Village, where the Fourth Rogerian Conference was held. The cultural as well as the learning environment generated excitement and energy that were difficult to contain. Outdoor cafés, streets filled with quaint shops, the sound of jazz, museums, Broadway, and the Statue of Liberty, along with everything else that makes New York a city like no other, provided the perfect setting for this learning experience.

The conference provided direct and unique exposure to the frontrunners of Rogerian science. Names like Barrett, Fawcett, Krieger, Phillips, Parse, Malinski, Newman, Fitzpatrick, and particularly Rogers, could now be put with faces. The enthusiasm of the spirited collection of scholars was infectious. They spoke with conviction, interpreted the language for us, and presented their discoveries, views, and visions of how nursing within the Science of Unitary Human Beings would help humankind. These presentations facilitated understanding of those aspects of the science that had previously puzzled us.

The atmosphere of the conference encouraged dialogue, even for the Rogerian novice. As students, our questions were encouraged and our thoughts were respected. The choices of topics and presenters were many, and we were able to select those presentations most meaningful to us and at our level of learning. We were impressed to learn that three of the presenters were "alumni" of the course; only a few years ago, they had started like us, yet they spoke the language and dialogued with amazing ease. At the end of the three days, we returned home exhausted yet curious to know more. A clearer understanding of how the human and environmental fields are inseparable and indivisible and how they flow one through the other emerged from this experience, and we conceptualized the Rogerian Principle of Integrality with enhanced experiential awareness.

After the excitement of the conference and the city of New York, a quiet period for independent reflection and further reading was especially rewarding. With newly achieved insight, we were able to direct our energy toward meeting our own individual learning needs. Much learning was pandimensional as we continued to draw on our experiences in New York. We now had time to ponder over our learning and to identify unanswered questions. As our month of independent study came to an end, we found ourselves eager to begin the next leg of our adventure.

Nag's Head, a beautiful beach resort on the outer banks of North Carolina, proved to be the perfect setting for the Rogerian grand finale. Twenty-three inquiring persons gathered at the shore to further explore the Science of Unitary Human Beings. Among the group were doctoral- and master's-level students, doctoral nursing faculty, an environmentalist, an artist, members of the Society of Rogerian Scholars, and Dr. Martha Rogers herself. The group was diverse with regard to talents, experience, and knowledge of Rogerian science, yet all shared a common bond.

The creation of the climate whereby we would come to experience the concepts of the Science of Unitary Human Beings began immediately upon arrival. The faculty and alumni from previous Rogerian courses were very supportive and made us feel comfortable with our uncertainty about Rogerian science. For an entire week, we would experience our integrality with the environment. Our lodging was right on the beach or within walking distance. Our meals, many of which included gifts from the sea, were served on a beachside deck in a most relaxed atmosphere, permitting us not only to enjoy those around us, but also to experience a portion of our world we might have failed to appreciate before.

The activities of the course seemed to evolve rather naturally, yet everything held much meaning. As we moved away from temporality, our constant concern regarding schedules and deadlines became nonexistent. Our focus became pandimensional rather than linear. We too were evolving.

Each day began with a class in Tai Chi, an ancient art of meditation with movement. Each morning, Carl Brown, adjunct faculty at Emory University and Ecological Adviser to Drepung-Loseling College of Tibet—American Campus, taught these beachside classes in such a manner that we were able to hear and see the ocean, the skies, and the sand; to breathe the salty air; to feel the ocean breezes blow. Our heightened awareness of the integrality and mutual process of human and environmental energy fields was invigorating. This gave us balance and power to deal with life stresses as they arose.

After Tai Chi, the group negotiated the activities and time sequence to follow. We spent many hours each day exploring Rogerian science through in-depth discussions as we sought to increase our understanding of its underpinnings. These seminar sessions were spectacular since we had Dr. Martha Rogers right there with us to clarify troublesome areas. Some sessions evolved into a dialogue of questions and answers; others involved listening to the faculty discuss and present theory and thoughts. We felt like sponges. There was so much there to know and experience, and we simply could not get enough.

A number of other Rogerian experiences highlighted the week: a trip to the Wright Brothers' Memorial at Kitty Hawk, making sand castles, finding treasures on the beach, seeing an outdoor drama, *The Lost Colony,* singing and dancing under the stars, flying kites, watching a thunderstorm, and laughing at cartoons that illuminated aspects of Rogerian science. All offered something of value in increasing our awareness as unitary human beings. Martha Rogers even put on a pair of rollerblades.

We were freed from traditional constraints, and many creative ideas surfaced during that week. A classmate, Margie Johnson, came up with an entrepreneurial innovation that she calls "visionary pondering." She explained that patterns will evolve as human beings, from our visual field on earth, continue to explore the vast timelessness of the universe. As *Homo sapiens* becomes *Homo spacialis* and establishes colonies throughout the universe or inhabits those colonies that already exist, Malinski (1986) has proposed that changes in the human body will occur in such a way that the appearance of the visible human field will change. Sustained contact with gravitational patterns in outer space will be associated with circulatory compromise in the lower extremities, making them first weaker, then smaller, as is characteristic of the evolution process. However, mental acuity will strengthen, so that telepathic communication may make vocal generations recognizable to humans on Earth.

Margie noted that, since these changes will evolve continuously at varying speeds of time, the ability to coexist, both here on earth and in our space colonies, will present an extraordinary opportunity for visionary entrepreneurs. For instance, if our space-dwelling relatives do not require the appendages we call legs, how will they move about on earth when they visit? It may be that future entrepreneurs in each spaceport will rent legs and compression suits for those coming and going from one space environment to the other. Likewise, when our friends from outlying planets visit, they may need to have pocket computers that can rapidly translate their thoughts into vocal form so that they can be understood during their visit. As the inhabitants of earth colonize and visit the many planets, they may need special head devices to enhance their ability to receive telepathic messages.

As we continuously evolve and explore the unknown or undiscovered realms of our selves as well as of the universe, we must be visionary planners. Economic independence has always been important to humans. Entrepreneurs of the future will be those of us who dream the "impossible" businesses. The Science of Human Beings affords a philosophical framework within which we can continuously ponder such visionary business opportunities. Such is the thinking of one developing Rogerian—who may just be rich someday!

## CONCLUSION

The combination of creative and traditional learning strategies used in this course has proven far more successful in embodying the essence of Rogerian science than use of traditional methods alone. Experiential activities alternated with periods for reflection provided diverse opportunities for utilization of the skills inherent in creative thinking and necessary for theory building. Synergistic expressions sparked unpredictable and unique bursts of creativity in the learners.

The course was truly an experiential process. We were given warm, rich learning environments; skilled, knowledgeable guides and mentors; and many diverse experiences for the task at hand—using creative thinking to learn about the conceptual system known as the Science of Unitary Human Beings. The original, creative ways in which many graduates of the Rogerian course have organized and shared their understanding of the Science of Unitary Human Beings are the ultimate manifestation of its success. This poem, offered by another of our classmates, is a verifying example.

Meditation

Brenda Talley

Like a silken cloak
the cool sea wind caresses me,
enfolding me into the rhythms of the universe.

I sense every grain of sand
beneath my feet

as my consciousness merges
into the essence of unity.

As air through a butterfly net,
the energies of the universe slip through the
space of my being.

Flowing smoothly, rushing slowly,
vibrant with opalescent energy, serene.
Everywhere, nowhere,
feeling everything and nothing.

Being and nonbeing.
My senses reeling with
the sounds and colors of eternity,
yet not hearing and unseeing.

What has been melts
into what is not yet,
like a wax rose
left too long in the sun.

Slowly I awaken to the
slumber of the present—
the cry of the gull,
the laughter of children.

I see a purple kite fighting
to reach the clouds,
struggling for freedom, but earth-tethered
in the singing winds of now.

I again hear the ocean's rhythm
as waves crash at the shore
and then are not,
but always are.

## REFERENCES

Abbott, E.A. (1952). *Flatbead.* New York: Dover Press.

Barrett, E.A.M. (1990). *Visions of Rogers' science-based nursing.* New York: National League for Nursing.

Bevis, E.O. (1973). *Curriculum building in nursing: A process.* St. Louis: Mosby.

Bevis, E.O., & Murray, J. (1990). The essence of the curriculum revolution: Emancipatory teaching. *Journal of Nursing Education, 29,* 326–331.

Capra, F. (1983). *The Tao of physics* (2nd ed.). New York: Bantam Books.

Hillman, J. (1980, May). *Reading and writing poetry.* Paper presented at the Annual Meeting of the International Reading Association, St. Louis, MO.

Malinski, V.M. (1986). *Exploration of Martha Rogers' Science of Unitary Human Beings.* Norwalk, CT: Appleton-Century-Crofts.

Oliver, A. (1984, June). *Blockages to creativity.* Paper presented at the International Conference: Education for the Gifted ("Ingenium 2000"), Republic of South Africa.

Rogers, M.E. (1990). Nursing: Science of Unitary, Irreducible, Human Beings: Update 1990. In E.A.M. Barrett (Ed.), *Visions of Rogers' science-based nursing* (pp. 5–11). New York: National League for Nursing.

Runco, R.A. (1990). The divergent thinking of young children: Implications of the research. *The Gifted Child Today, 13* (4), 37–39.

Schwab, L.S., & D'Zamko, M.E. (1988). Group imaging for action: Creative thinking and problem-solving. *The Journal of Creative Behavior, 22* (2), 101–111.

Taylor, A. (1990, July). *Integrating critical thinking and creative thinking in the cooperative learning model: Implications for addressing the frame of reference for these two distinct processes.* Paper presented at the National Conference on Cooperative Learning, Baltimore, MD.

Torrance, E.P., Reynolds, C.R., & Ball, O.E. (1978). Images of the future of gifted adolescents: Effects of alienation and specialized cerebral functioning. *Gifted Child Quarterly, 22,* 40–45.

Zielinski, E.J., & Sarachine, D.M. (1990). Creativity and criticism: The components of scientific thought. *The Science Teacher, 57* (8), 18–22.

Ziv, A. (1988). Using humor to develop creative thinking. *Journal of Children in Contemporary Society, 20* (1–2), 99–116.

# 24

# Theory Development Using Quantitative Methods in the Science of Unitary Human Beings

*Jacqueline Fawcett*

Theory development always is based on a frame of reference for the phenomena of interest to a discipline, that is, a conceptual model. This chapter focuses on the influence of one conceptual model of nursing—the Science of Unitary Human Beings—on theory development through quantitative methods. Guidelines for the derivation of theories from the Science of Unitary Human Beings are described, and criteria for evaluating the conceptual-theoretical-empirical structures of theory testing research are identified.

## CONCEPTUAL MODELS AND THEORY DEVELOPMENT

Theory development encompasses the derivation of middle-range theories through intellectual efforts and the testing of those theories by means of empirical research. Viewed from that perspective, theory development proceeds through three, or sometimes four, levels of abstraction (Fawcett, 1993) (Figure 24.1). The most abstract level is the *conceptual model,* a set of abstract and general concepts and propositions that provides a distinctive frame of reference for phenomena within the domain of inquiry of a particular discipline. The Science of Unitary Human Beings draws attention to the unity of human life and emphasizes the mutual human-environmental field

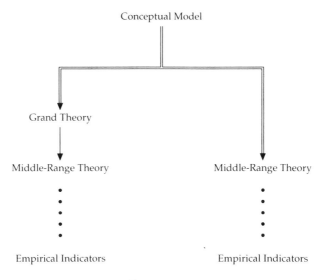

**Figure 24.1**
**Grand and Middle-Range Theory Derivation**

process. The global nature of conceptual model concepts and propositions precludes their direct empirical observation and testing.

The next level of abstraction is the *theory,* a set of relatively specific and concrete concepts and propositions that addresses a relatively circumscribed phenomenon. Theories are classified as *grand* or *middle-range.* Theory development may proceed from the conceptual model to a grand theory and then to a middle-range theory, or the derivation may be directly from the conceptual model to the middle-range theory. Grand theories are more abstract and broader in scope than middle-range theories. They are made up of relatively abstract concepts that lack operational definitions and relatively abstract propositions that are not amenable to direct empirical testing. Indeed, grand theories are developed through thoughtful and insightful appraisal of existing ideas or creative leaps beyond existing knowledge. Middle-range theories, in contrast, are substantively specific; they encompass a limited number of concepts and a limited aspect of the real world. They are made up of relatively concrete concepts that are operationally defined and relatively concrete propositions that can be empirically tested in a direct manner.

On the most concrete level are the *empirical indicators,* the very specific and concrete real-world proxies for middle-range theory concepts. More specifically, they are the actual instruments, experimental conditions, and procedures that are used to observe or measure the concepts of a middle-range theory.

## Guidelines for Theory Development

Conceptual models act as guides for the development of new theories by focusing attention on certain concepts and their relationships, and they place those concepts and their relationships in a distinctive context. More specifically, each conceptual model guides theory development by identifying the phenomena to be investigated, specifying how theories about these phenomena are to be generated and tested, and prescribing the methods to be used to investigate these phenomena. A fully developed conceptual model reflects a particular research tradition that is made up of six guidelines for inquiry that deal with and encompass all phases of a study (Laudan, 1981; Schlotfeldt, 1975):

1. The phenomena that are to be studied.
2. The distinctive nature of the problems to be studied and the purposes to be fulfilled by the research.
3. The subjects who are to provide the data and the settings in which data are to be gathered.
4. The research designs, instruments, and procedures that are to be employed.
5. The methods to be employed in reducing and analyzing the data.
6. The nature of contributions that the research will make to the advancement of knowledge.

Each guideline is derived from the distinctive substantive content and focus of the conceptual model and the model author's view of research. Guidelines for theory development within the context of the Science of Unitary Human Beings are beginning to be developed.

The first guideline of the Science of Unitary Human Beings states that the phenomena to be studied are unitary human beings and their environments (Rogers, 1987). The second guideline states that the problems to be studied are pattern manifestations of the human–environmental field mutual process, especially pattern profiles (Phillips, 1989, 1991).

The third guideline for research based on the Science of Unitary Human Beings states that virtually any setting and any person would be appropriate for study, with the proviso that both person and environment be taken into account. The fourth guideline states that both basic and applied research are needed to continue to develop nursing theory. Basic research, according to Rogers (1987), "is directed toward an increase in knowledge in a given science" whereas applied research "investigates the practical application of knowledge already available" (p. 122). Furthermore, Rogers (1987) supported the use of both qualitative and quantitative methods of empirical research, as well as philosophical inquiry. She did, however, note that "there are incongruities and contradictions between holistic directions in nursing and the forms of inquiry used by nurses. . . . There is a critical need for new tools of measurement appropriate to new paradigms" (p. 122). In fact, three instruments have been directly derived from the Science of Unitary Human Beings. Ference (1979) developed the Human Field Motion Test, Barrett (1983) developed the Power as Knowing Participation in Change Tool, and Paletta (1988) developed the Temporal Experience Scales.

Reeder (1986) maintained that Husserlian phenomenology is an appropriate approach to basic research derived from the Science of Unitary Human Beings. Cowling (1986) noted that existentialism, ecological thinking, and dialectical thinking are appropriate modes of inquiry for studies based on the Science of Unitary Human Beings, as are historical and philosophical inquiries and methods that focus on the uniqueness of each person, such as imagery, direct questioning, personal structural analysis, and the Q-sort. Cowling also noted that, although descriptive and correlational designs are consistent with the Science of Unitary Human Beings, strict experimental designs are of "questionable value," given the fact that "the unitary system is a noncausal model of reality" (p. 73). However, Cowling went on to say that quasi-experimental and experimental designs "may be appropriate to specific theoretical propositions because they provide a mechanism for testing probabilistic change manifested from human–environmental process" (p. 73). In addition, case studies and longitudinal research designs focusing on identification of manifestations of human and environmental field patterns are more appropriate than cross-sectional studies, given Rogers' emphasis on the uniqueness of the unitary human being.

The fifth guideline states that data analysis techniques must take the integrality of person and environment into account, as well as the emphasis on unitary human beings. This view "precludes the use of standard data analysis techniques that employ the components-of-variance model of statistics, for this statistical model is logically inconsistent with the assumption of holism stating that the whole is greater than the sum of parts" (Fawcett & Downs, 1986, p. 87). Cowling (1986) indicated that "multivariate analysis procedures, particularly canonical correlation, can be useful methods for generating a constellation of variables representing human field pattern properties" (p. 73). The problem here, however, is that canonical correlation is a components-of-variance procedure. The sixth guideline states that research conducted within the context of the Science of Unitary Human Beings will enhance understanding of the continuous mutual human-environmental field process and changes in energy field patterns.

## CONCEPTUAL–THEORETICAL–EMPIRICAL STRUCTURES

The guidelines for theory development are operationalized in what I call a conceptual-theoretical-empirical structure (Fawcett & Downs, 1992). As can be seen in Figure 24.2, vertical propositions link the conceptual model concepts (CMCs) to the theory concepts (TCs) and the theory concepts to the empirical indicators

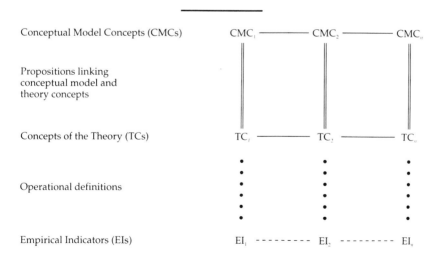

**Figure 24.2**
**General Form of a**
**Conceptual–Theoretical–Empirical Structure**

(EIs). Vertical propositions in the form of representational statements indicate which theory concepts represent which conceptual model concepts. The representational statements typically are phrased as "Conceptual Model Concept$_1$ is represented by Theory Concept$_1$," "Conceptual Model Concept$_2$ is represented by Theory Concept$_2$," and so on. Thus, each theory concept acts as a proxy for the more abstract conceptual model concept. These propositions are depicted by double lines ($=$). Vertical propositions in the form of operational definitions link the theory concepts to the empirical indicators. The operational definitions, depicted by dotted lines (. . . . .), state exactly how the theory concepts are to be observed or measured. The conceptual–theoretical–empirical structure may also include horizontal relational propositions at each level of abstraction. Relational propositions, therefore, state how the conceptual model concepts are related to each other, how the theory concepts are related to one another, and how the scores on the empirical indicators are interrelated. These propositions are depicted by single lines (____). If desired, the sign (positive [+], negative [−], unknown [?]) for the direction of each relationship could be added to the diagram. Arrowheads (◄ ►) could also be added to depict the symmetry of the relationship.

## Theory Testing

A conceptual–theoretical–empirical structure should be constructed prior to the testing of a theory derived from a conceptual model and should be used to evaluate the results of the theory-testing endeavor. First, the theory concepts and propositions are derived from one or more conceptual model concepts and propositions. Second, empirical indicators are selected for the theory concepts, and a research design that will test the propositions is developed. Third, the data obtained from the empirical indicators are analyzed by following the methodological guidelines of the conceptual model. Finally, the empirical research findings are used to make a judgment about the validity of the theory and the credibility of the conceptual model.

Alligood's (1991) study was an excellent example of theory derivation and testing from the Science of Unitary Human Beings. As shown in Figure 24.3, Alligood linked the concepts from the grand theory of accelerating change with the conceptual model principles of helicy and integrality. She then derived a middle-range theory of

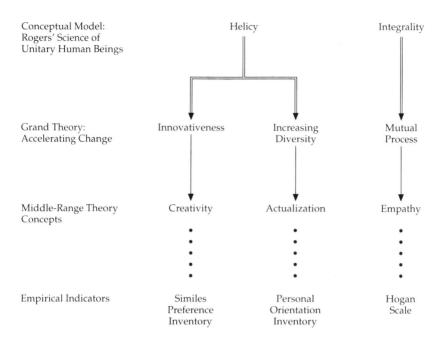

**Figure 24.3**
**Derivation of Grand and Middle-Range Theories from a
Conceptual Model: Alligood's (1991) Theory of
Creativity, Actualization, and Empathy**

creativity, actualization, and empathy from the grand theory of accelerating change. Creativity was selected to represent the grand theory concept of innovativeness, which in turn represented the Principle of Helicy. Actualization was selected to represent the grand theory concept of increasing diversity, which in turn was a second proxy for the Principle of Helicy. Empathy was selected to represent the grand theory concept of mutual process, which in turn represented the Principle of Integrality.

Alligood (1991) proposed the following hypotheses:

1. There is a positive correlation between creativity and empathy.

2. There is a positive correlation between actualization and empathy.

3. Creativity and actualization, combined, account for more of the variance in empathy than either one does separately (p. 89).

Alligood's report included the methods and findings from two cross-sectional surveys, Study 1 and Study 2. The Study 1 sample was made up of 236 men and women between the ages of 18 and 60. In the Study 2 sample there were 47 men and women between the ages of 61 and 92. In both studies, creativity was measured by the Similes Preference Inventory, actualization was measured by the Personal Orientation Inventory, and empathy was measured by the Hogan Scale. Adequate reliability coefficients for the three instruments were obtained for the study samples.

Hypothesis 1 was supported in the younger sample (Study 1), although the magnitude of the correlation was low ($r = .27$). That hypothesis was not supported in the older sample (Study 2); although the correlation between creativity and empathy was slightly larger in magnitude, it was negative in direction ($r = -.32$).

Hypothesis 2 was supported in both samples. The younger sample (Study 1) yielded a correlation of moderate magnitude between actualization and empathy ($r = .39$), whereas the correlation was substantial for the older sample (Study 2) ($r = .68$).

Hypothesis 3 was upheld in the younger sample (Study 1). In contrast, the combination of creativity and actualization did not account for a significantly greater percentage of the variance than either variable alone in the older sample (Study 2).

### Evaluation of Conceptual–Theoretical–Empirical Structures

Alligood's research may be evaluated using the typical elements of a research critique, but that type of evaluation emphasizes only the methodological strengths and weaknesses of a study; the conceptual and theoretical components are neglected. Instead, consider an evaluation schema that focuses attention on the conceptual–theoretical–empirical structure of the study. The evaluation criteria listed in Table 24.1 reflect the guidelines for theory development discussed previously and, therefore, emphasize the derivation of the theory from a conceptual model, the methods used to test the theory, and the interpretation of the research findings with regard to the theory and its parent conceptual model.

Examination of Alligood's report revealed that most of the criteria were met. The conceptual model and grand theory proposed by Rogers were explicitly identified and adequately summarized. The

## Table 24.1
## Criteria for Evaluation of the Linkage of Conceptual
## Models with Theories and Empirical Indicators

- The conceptual model is explicitly identified as the underlying guide for the theory-generating or theory-testing research.
- The conceptual model is discussed in sufficient breadth and depth so that the relationship between the model and the purpose of the research is clear.
- The linkages between the conceptual model concepts and propositions and the theory concepts and propositions are stated explicitly.
- The methodology reflects the conceptual model:
  —The study subjects are drawn from a population that is appropriate for the focus of the conceptual model.
  —The instruments are appropriate measures of phenomena encompassed by the conceptual model.
  —The study design clearly reflects the focus of the conceptual model.
  —The statistical techniques are in keeping with the focus of the conceptual model.
- Discussion of research results includes conclusions regarding the empirical adequacy of the theory and the credibility of the conceptual model.

derivation of the theory of creativity, actualization, and empathy was discussed in detail, and the report included an accurate diagram of the conceptual–theoretical–empirical structure. The use of cross-sectional samples was not completely consistent with the guidelines for research based on the Science of Unitary Human Beings, although the selection of that design could be defended inasmuch as Alligood was not examining changes in patterns, but rather correlates of unitary human development, that is, a pattern profile. The instruments selected are valid measures of the middle-range theory concepts. The use of correlational data analysis techniques, including Pearson product moment correlation coefficients and multiple regression, is in keeping with Cowling's (1986) directives, but does raise a question inasmuch as those techniques are based on the components-of-variance statistical model.

Furthermore, Alligood's discussion of the collective study findings included conclusions regarding the empirical adequacy of the theory. Her explanation for unexpected findings focused on methodological issues, including the need for a larger sample of older subjects and a question about the validity of the instrument she used to measure creativity. She stated: "The theory would suggest a stronger correlation between creativity and empathy than in the findings of these studies. This raises a question of the construct validity for the [Similes Preference Inventory] in this research and suggests the need to consider different measures of innovativeness or creativity in future Rogerian studies" (p. 94). Moreover, although Alligood did not explicitly address the credibility of the Science of Unitary Human Beings, she did acknowledge that some of the results of her research did not support Rogers' contentions and recommended further research, especially with older persons.

Alligood's (1991) recommendation for further research was a typical conclusion when research findings do not support the theory that was tested. However, if we accept the rule of logic stipulating that even one disconfirming case invalidates a theory, we must conclude that Alligood's theory of creativity, actualization, and empathy is not empirically adequate, which in turn raises a question about the credibility of the Science of Unitary Human Beings.

## CONCLUSION

In conclusion, when theories are derived from a conceptual model and tested according to the methodological guidelines of that model, the research results should be used to draw conclusions about the empirical adequacy of the theory *and* the credibility of the conceptual model. If the findings of theory-testing research support the theory, it may be concluded that the theory is empirically adequate, and that it is likely that the conceptual model is credible. If, however, the research findings do not support the theory, both the empirical adequacy of the theory and the credibility of the conceptual model must be questioned. To ignore the negative findings would only perpetuate a view of a conceptual model as an ideology that cannot be questioned. That view is, of course, incompatible with scholarship.

## REFERENCES

Alligood, M.R. (1991). Testing Rogers' theory of accelerating change. The relationships among creativity, actualization, and empathy in persons 18 to 92 years of age. *Western Journal of Nursing Research, 13*, 84–96.

Barrett, E.A.M. (1983). An empirical investigation of Martha E. Rogers' Principle of Helicy: The relationship of human field motion and power. *Dissertation Abstracts International, 45*, 615A.

Cowling W.R., III. (1986). The Science of Unitary Human Beings: Theoretical issues, methodological challenges, and research realities. In V.M.

Malinski (Ed.), *Explorations on Martha Rogers' Science of Unitary Human Beings* (pp. 65–77). Norwalk, CT: Appleton-Century-Crofts.

Fawcett, J. (1993). *Analysis and evaluation of nursing theories.* Philadelphia: F.A. Davis.

Fawcett, J., & Downs, F.S. (1986). *The relationship of theory and research.* Norwalk, CT: Appleton-Century-Crofts.

Fawcett, J., & Downs, F.S. (1992). The relationship of theory and research (2nd ed.). Philadelphia: F.A. Davis.

Ference, H.M. (1979). The relationship of time experience, creativity traits, differentiation, and human field motion: An empirical investigation of Rogers' correlates of synergistic human development. *Dissertation Abstracts International, 40,* 5206B.

Laudan, L. (1981). A problem-solving approach to scientific progress. In I. Hacking (Ed.), *Scientific revolutions* (pp. 144–155). Fair Lawn, NJ: Oxford University Press.

Paletta, J.L. (1988). The relationship of temporal experience to human time. *Dissertation Abstracts International, 49,* 1621B.

Phillips, J.R. (1989). Science of Unitary Human Beings: Changing research perspectives. *Nursing Science Quarterly, 2,* 57–60.

Phillips, J.R. (1991). Human field research. *Nursing Science Quarterly, 4,* 142–143.

Reeder, F. (1986). Basic theoretical research in the conceptual system of unitary human beings. In V.M. Malinski (Ed.). *Explorations on Martha Rogers' Science of Unitary Human Beings* (pp. 45–64). Norwalk, CT: Appleton-Century-Crofts.

Rogers, M.E. (1987). Nursing research in the future. In J. Roode (Ed.), *Changing patterns in nursing education* (pp. 121–123). New York: National League for Nursing.

Schlotfeldt, R.M. (1975). The need for a conceptual framework. In P.J. Verhonick (Ed.), *Nursing research I* (pp. 3–24). Boston: Little, Brown.

# 25

# Multiple Field Methods in a Unitary Human Field Science

*Marilyn M. Rawnsley*

Where, one asks, does this appetite for the Universe, for the wholeness of the world . . . come from? . . . In the very act of living we sense, clearly or cloudily, a world about us which we assume to be complete.

Ortega y Gasset (1960, p. 64)

Trust thyself: Every heart vibrates to that iron string.

Emerson (1949, p. 10)

Imagine that you are a traveler and you have an opportunity to visit a foreign land for the first time. There are several options from which to plan your itinerary. Assuming that time and expense are not issues for you, rank order the following choices according to your preferences. If any option is one that you would never choose, mark it zero. An interpretation of this exercise relative to multiple field methods in the Science of Unitary Human Beings will be illustrated later in this chapter.

## TRAVEL OPTIONS

*Opinion A*                                               Rank (  )

You go to a travel agency and select a tour that is prepackaged and preplanned. The tour identifies common points of interest and provides timetables of daily events, detailed maps, ratings of accommodations, and estimates of expected expenses not covered in the prepaid tour fee. Solo side trips for personal exploration are prohibited; you arrive and leave each stop on the tour according to the plan. When you return from this trip and view your photographs and memorabilia, you probably begin to make specific plans to tour a different place with the same agency.

*Option B*                                              Rank (   )

You check with the tourist board of the place that you will be visiting, or you work with a travel agent who has connections with local groups in the region. You want to stay with a family or group that is native to the specific section of the country where you will spend your time. You plan to select your sightseeing according to the recommendations of those persons who appear to be best informed about what goes on in the area. You may choose to participate with your hosts in their holidays and festivities and other customs. You have an approximate time frame for the duration of your stay there. Most likely, you will plan to experience the insider or native point of view on your next trip to a different place.

*Option C*                                              Rank (   )

You book a round trip airline ticket with an open return date. You arrive in a place that you have read or heard about with no firm plans for what you will do while you are there. Rather than "must see" destinations, you move about the country freely, reminding yourself to "go with the flow" and rely on your perceptions. You stumble across some well-known tourist spots and miss many others. You also have serendipitous discoveries of places that have yet to be appreciated. Sometimes, you revisit spots that intrigue you rather than searching for something different. You depart the country satisfied with the impressions you gained, yet aware that there is much more to see.

*Option D*                                              Rank (   )

You purchase a round-trip airline ticket with a definite departure and return date. You buy travel guides and maps, preplan what you definitely must see, and set out with determination. However, you are careful to allow ample time for side trips to explore or return to areas of interest that emerge during your scheduled stops. For the most part, you accomplish your original goals for the trip. You dutifully log the time and expense and mileage for your trip, taking photographs as planned. However, you also keep a diary of your unplanned excursions, sufficiently describing your rewarding and disappointing experiences and leaving a trail that can be retraced.

*Option E* Rank (  )

You select your destination based on a classic literary or artistic work originating in the region. You plan your itinerary to find out as much as you can about the circumstances within which this work was produced. You retrace the steps of the writer or artist by visiting the birthplace and the personal library or studio, perusing official and unofficial documents, and listening to local folklore. You forgo visiting other areas in the region in order to immerse yourself in the life and times within which this work was created. You allow as much time as you need to understand the context of this classic work, planning subsequent trips before you leave.

*Option F* Rank (  )

You select your destination for these reasons: The landscape is totally unfamiliar to you; the territory has either not been clearly charted or else the previous charting is the subject of considerable controversy. You set out on this adventure, perhaps with two or three like-minded companions. Your shared goal is to explore as much of this territory as possible on this initial trip, marking those areas to which you will return at a later time. Although you take note of markers left by previous explorers, you do not rely on them for your conclusions. Sometimes you and your companions travel together, sometimes separately, depending on what is discovered along the way. When you meet at the end of the journey to review your progress, you will most likely have identified a few sites of most interest, mystery, or promise for further examination. You plan return trips to chart these areas with increased depth and precision, looking toward an ultimate goal of making maps for others.

*Option G*                                                Rank (   )

You really prefer armchair/lounge traveling. You would rather read travelogues and books describing exotic lands or the travel adventures of others than deal with the hassles of actually visiting those places yourself. Although you enjoy occasional vacations, they are, by intent, limited to brief sojourns in habitual places. Any explorations are usually intended to expand your knowledge of familiar territory.

## THE KNOWER AND THE KNOWN

Field methods refer to those forms of inquiry that can be classified within the naturalistic paradigm. The naturalistic world-view is concerned with studying phenomena within context. Since all investigative approaches put explicit or implicit parameters on the scope of the study and all investigators have inherent human limitations on conceptual visibility, no study findings can reveal the "whole." Yet, as Ortega y Gasset (1960) philosophically lamented, life seems comprehensible only within an assumption of wholeness. Naturalistic inquiry addresses the innate human sense of integrality, and the label of holistic is frequently invoked to distinguish these investigative methods from their linear empirical counterparts. Rather than deceive ourselves in deciphering the data they yield, it is prudent to remember that, despite our longings for completeness, the aim of these qualitative approaches is to provide detailed description of "the many specifics that give the context its unique flavor" (Lincoln & Guba, 1985, p. 201).

In all science, it is accepted that the credibility of the data is inextricable from the conditions under which they were gathered. But, unlike empirical designs, which attempt to control conditions to be consistent with the dictates of logical positivism, naturalistic strategies do not set up artificial constrictions in an attempt to isolate the phenomenon being studied from its environs. The critical differentiating characteristic of naturalistic methods, as opposed to those of empiricism, is their acknowledgment of the essential connectedness of the observer and the observed. Within a Rogerian frame, naturalistic inquiry can be explained as the human phenomenon of participating knowingly in the continuous mutual process of increasing diversity of integral human and environmental field patterning to disclose situationally shaded slices of a pandimensional reality. The significance of recognizing the essential connectedness of the knower and the known cannot be overstated; it is a premise of interpretation that is conceptually consistent with the Principle of Integrality in the Science of Unitary Human Beings. Therefore, any given way of knowing or research approach is postulated to be the medium through which the integrality of human and contextual fields is expressed or denied.

The introductory exercise invited the reader to participate with the writer in thinking through the compatibility of alternative methods of inquiry with the aims of the Science of Unitary Human Beings. Examination of each qualitative category discloses subspecifics of design. Judging the compatibility of a conceptual system with identified qualitative strategies requires convincing scholarly arguments that provide intensive and extensive interpretation of each of the variations. Since the focus of discussion is the global relevance of selected field approaches within the Rogerian world-view, there is no attempt here to justify specific strategies through an exhaustive explanation of methodological intricacies. (For an excellent example of the depth of scholarship expected in this effort, see Chapter 26 in this book.) In deference to current and emerging scholars committed to those critical explications, no attempt at dissection of methods is intended here. Instead, the aim of discourse at this level is to provide a common frame of reference for a continuing dialogue of Rogerians—novices and experts—who consider the continuous mutual process of substantive advancement in the Rogerian science to be its fundamental challenge.

A potentially productive approach to this puzzle of method and meaning in science is to address the question: "What are the relationships among the knower, the ways of knowing, and the known?" Essentially, this problem is concerned with epistemological foundations of any systematized world-view; it can be directed toward any organized construction of reality whether or not it is authorized as legitimate by others. However, it is generally accepted that knowledge that claims to be scientifically derived belongs in the public domain of language. This caveat means that ways of knowing that are useful in science are not solipsistic; unlike alternate constructions of reality emerging through a schizophrenic process, scientific statements must meet the criterion of intersubjectivity, or shared meaning, among speakers of the language.

In a Rogerian world, infinity is the horizon for creativity. Nevertheless, when purporting to discuss scientific strategies, attention must be paid to issues of shared meaning. The travel alternatives are intended to illuminate personal field patterning relative to investigative patterning. The options described earlier in this chapter (Options A–G) are constructed as creative analogies for recognized research activities. In a broad allegorical sense, they project an image of research as a scientific adventure, an intellectual journey with multiple routes. Intersubjectivity, then, is germane to interpreting the imaginary travel options.

## METAPHORS AND METHODS

Metaphors are linguistic innovations of synthesis that "invest the process of creation with denotations rather than . . . similarities; they organize perceptions endowed with meaning, supplying reality with an intelligible structure" (Rigotti, 1986, p. 157). Metaphors report the discovery of likenesses, relationships, and correspondences disclosed in the phenomenon of similarity (Bredin, 1992; Embler, 1987). Since "metaphor introduces a dynamic tension into the meaning of a text, it permits change in the interpretation of the text" (Daniel, 1986, p. 192). Conceptual peregrinations in the Science of Unitary Human Beings are facilitated by linguistic innovations that introduce dynamic tension into discourse. The use of travel metaphors for research activities is rooted in a premise consistent with the Rogerian Principle of Integrality. In other words, through ranking travel options that in themselves have no hierarchical status, the reader endorses some hypothetical schematics over others. Through the dynamic tension of metaphor, symmetrical configurations of personal and methodological patterning that indicate resonance of human and contextual fields are disclosed.

At first glance, the use of metaphor as a device to illuminate relationships obscured in similarity may seem a circuitous route to the scientific criterion of intersubjectivity; the transformative power of metaphor initiates a plurality of meanings into the public discourse. Yet the question persists: To what extent do these creative analogies for research deal with the scientific criterion of intersubjectivity or shared meaning?

To answer this question, the travel options were distributed to 14 doctorally prepared faculty in nursing who, while not avowed Rogerians, are researchers conducting studies derived from empirical and/or naturalistic paradigms. These experts were asked to match travel options A–G with a list of nine approaches to research (listed in alphabetical order):

1. Case study method.
2. Consumer of research.
3. Empirical (quantitative) design.
4. Echo method.
5. Ethnographic method.
6. Grounded theory approach.
7. Historical research.
8. Phenomenological method.
9. Triangulation.

Another option, "Nothing I can relate to," was included as a possible tenth response. To minimize matching by a process of elimination, directions included a warning that not all of the nine were necessarily represented, and, although not intended as such, some options might be reflected more than once.

Six travel analogies received between 71 percent and 100 percent agreement with the classification intended by the author. At the suggestion of the experts, all items receiving less than 100 percent were rewritten for clarity. The item that scored only 50 percent agreement was substantively reworked and resubmitted to seven of the original sample of experts. This second review yielded a consensus of 85 percent, indicating agreement of six expert responses on triangulation as the approach evoked by the travel analogy. Truth value beyond face validity cannot be asserted from these data; however, another estimation of authenticity is central not only to this exercise but to all imaginative and theoretical efforts. This source of credibility lies in the underestimated dimension of personal validity.

## PERSONAL VALIDITY

Beginning a discussion with a chimerical journey invites the reader to enter into a discourse with the writer. Drawing from Ricoeur's seminal writings on hermeneutics, Pellauer (1987) explained mimesis as the process through which the world of the text and the world of the reader intersect in a creative spiral of discovery, invention, and more discovery. Catudal's (1990) discussion of personal validity was pertinent to a generic understanding of this creative process. According to Catudal (1990), personal validity refers to interpretation of the written word; it provides a conceptual construction for evaluating the credibility of a point of view committed to the public domain of language. The way of making meaning through textual interpretation is said to be the appropriate medium for seeing connections in a literary, artistic, or theoretical work that does not lay claim to conditions of objectivity.

In essence, personal validity proceeds without reference to pre-ordained or scientific rules of making meaning. Instead, personal validity emerges through translation of the work into the context of the individual's experiential field. From this perspective, clarifying connections between one work and another becomes a shared endeavor that initiates through the writer and progresses through the reader. In a Rogerian framework, personal validity could be explained as the continuous mutual process of the human field, the reader, with the environmental field or text that is available through collective language patterning. Language is the appropriate medium for this process since it is "an example of the Rogerian construct of innovative diversity patterning; it has the dual function of differentiating yet linking the environment and the self" (Rawnsley, 1985, p. 27). What flows from this continuous mutual process is referred to as "perspicuous representation" (Catudal, 1990, p. 18), a lucid interrogatory that incorporates reader and writer by asking simply, "Do you see what I see?"

The discussion to this point has been foundational to interpreting the travel options as creative analogies to research strategies whose relevance to a Rogerian world-view can be visualized. Given the integrality of human and environmental fields—that is, the essential connectedness of the knower, the way of knowing, and what is known—it is postulated that, according to the assumptions and principles of the Rogerian Science of Unitary Human Beings, all systematic inquiry proceeds most harmoniously and productively when the human field patterning, or researcher, resonates with the contextual field pattern, or specific research method. From this premise, it is reasonable to speculate that the correct investigative approach has little to do with disciplinary dogma; arbitrary assignment of value to one method over another is inconsistent with Rogerian integrality. Instead, the criterion issue is the "goodness of fit" of human field patterning and inquiry method patterning as indicated by the researcher's fascination with or gravitation toward a particular investigative process. This resonance of knower and way of knowing mediates the emergence of universal meaning in the form of credible knowledge communicated through the public domain of language.

## METAPHORS AND MEANING

The fantasized travel preferences invite the reader to mingle with the text. This active participatory process is constructed to simulate the engaging of qualitative investigators with the data. Through this continual mutual process, meaning is disclosed rather than imposed. Ranking the travel options permits a metaphorical "Rogerian Rorschach"; the reader projects personal preferences postulated to express resonance of human and environmental fields. Through this exercise in mimesis, the readers, like the field researchers, preempt their right to experience the essential integrality of personal and contextual fields.

*Option A* represents a pattern parallel to observational designs derived from the dominant paradigm of empiricism. With its emphasis on strict adherence to a preplanned program, devaluation of spontaneous revisions while the plan is in progress, preset allocations of time and budget, and evaluation of outcomes linked to future plans, this travel analogy captures the stringency of structure in quantitative designs. There was 92 percent agreement from the experts that this travel option was consistent with a linear empirical approach.

With its emphasis on accessing persons who are native to the region and seeking their "insider" point of view through recommendations, *Option B* was unanimously matched correctly by the experts. Participation in the customs, seeking the emic point of view, and commitment to sharing experiences of living within a different culture were recognized by all of the nursing research reviewers as analogous to the aims of ethnography (Goetz & LeCompte, 1984; Patton, 1990; Sarter, 1988). Whether (1) this recognition is indicative of the clarity of the analogy or (2) ethnography in nursing research is more familiar than other qualitative methods is a question not answered by these data.

*Option C* was intended to reflect a phenomenological approach to studying human experience. In the first review, the travel option was correctly matched with phenomenology by only 10 of the 14 experts (71 percent). When this option was rewritten to emphasize open time frames, lack of definitive planning, flowing with perceptions, serendipitous stumbling through familiar and unappreciated territory, and revisiting scenes, the rate of agreement from the experts reached 85 percent. Since phenomenology is a category for a plurality of philosophical perspectives on inquiry (Patton, 1990; Runes, 1984; Sarter, 1988; Van Kaam, 1969), it is possible that a single analogy does not capture adequately the multidimensional texture of this classification.

The analogy described in *Option D* was initially not apparent to these experts. The combination of definite beginning and concluding dates, preplanning using published guides, and accomplishing preset goals for data collection is reminiscent of the structured approach of studies designed within the quantitative paradigm. However, the freedom to pursue avenues of interest that emerge during the experience is not characteristic of linear empirical models. The descriptive diary that yields a trail that can be followed by interested others resembles methods common to qualitative strategies. Ironically, the nursing experts were split on the initial rating; 50 percent correctly identified triangulation, but no pattern emerged in the remaining responses. After receiving feedback from the reviewers, the travel option was rewritten to its present form and was correctly matched in six of the seven second-round responses (85 percent) as reflecting a convergence of methods (Patton, 1990).

*Option E* received a 78 percent agreement rating on the first review. Although the naming of a classic literary or artistic work was designed to reflect a historical approach, all three dissenting responses chose Case Study as the alternative method. Originally, Case Study was not intended as a match with any of the travel analogies. But historical case studies use techniques such as primary sources and events in context derived from historiography (Merriam, 1988). Therefore, the analogy remained as initially written and the research designation, modified to allow for either interpretation, was changed to Historical/Case Study method. On the second round, all seven experts agreed with this expansion of category.

*Option F* was constructed to mirror a grounded theory approach, which seeks to describe psychological and social structure patterns that are foundational to the area being studied (Strauss & Corbin, 1990). The travel analogy was written to reflect inductive conceptual specification and subsequent attempts at verification that are grounded in the processes through which it is identified (Babbie, 1992; Patton, 1990; Sarter, 1988). Since a grounded theory approach implies sequential abstraction of concepts from actuality, the complex steps of identification and verification lend themselves to collaborative methods of investigation. The metaphors of uncharted or controversial territory, the notion of partnership and/or team explorations, the identification of sites for further examination, and the goal of making maps for others are consonant with grounded theory activities. The reviewers either rated it correctly (10 experts = 71 percent) or chose the option "Nothing I can relate to." Again, the unanswered question occurs: "Is incompleteness of the analogy or familiarity of the reviewers more likely accounting for the rating?"

The final travel analogy, *Option G*, depicts the consumer of research who prefers to ponder the investigative challenges of others. These persons may participate in studies limited to familiar areas of practice, but they are not likely to seek the adventure of primary investigator or partner in complex research situations. They are, however, concerned professionals trying to keep informed either through examining issues in the research literature or participating in limited investigations within their area of expertise. Raters achieved 92 percent agreement.

Due to the apparent parallels between historical and case study techniques, only the echo method remained unmatched. This innovative field strategy, developed in social psychology to elicit values of specific groups, was explicated by Hartmann (1992) in her study of value hierarchies in practicing professional nurses. Since the method was only recently introduced into nursing research literature, the reviewers could not be expected to recognize it within the guise of a travel option; therefore, none was constructed. Briefly, the echo method employs similar raters to "echo" and classify the value statements made by persons in their categorical group, thus disclosing and confirming shared meaning. If values patterning is considered significant to in-depth understanding of unitary human fields, then the relevance of the echo method to Rogerian research warrants further elaboration.

## ROGERIAN RELEVANCE

Table 25.1 indicates the postulated relationships among the methods represented in the travel options. It is evident from the table that each of these methods was generated from a discipline different from nursing. That is, no matter how appealing these strategies may be to researchers disenchanted with the inadequacies of quantitative

**Table 25.1**

**Multiple Field Method Patterning**

| Option/Method | Source | Aim | Rogerian Relevance |
|---|---|---|---|
| A. Empirical | Logical positivism | Quantitative analysis | Statistical patterning |
| B. Ethnographic | Anthropology | Culture in context | Cultural process patterning |
| C. Phenomenological | Existential philosophy and psychology | Experience of being in the world | Embedded personal patterning |
| D. Triangulation | Social science | Multiple method confirmation | Convergence patterning |
| E. Historical/Case Study | Historiography | Events in context | Interpretive event patterning |
| F. Grounded Theory | Symbolic interaction | Basic social–psychological process | Population process patterning |
| G. Consumer of Research | Intellectual curiosity | Applicative knowledge | Professional practice patterning |

*Source:* Compiled by M. Rawnsley (1993)

methods in eliciting correlations of pandimensional probabilities, defecting from the landscape of linear logic to claim residence in the shadows of interpretive ambiguity is not the solution. With few exceptions, a common characteristic of naturalistic inquiry is that it aims at discovery of knowledge rather than verification of knowledge. These approaches, therefore, will not serve to verify the existence of a pandimensional, open-patterned, increasingly diverse universe of integral human and environmental fields. A priori hypotheses will not be confirmed. Instead, rich, thick, detailed descriptions of human experience as they are observed, lived, remembered, and interpreted within a Rogerian world-view will have to suffice.

From this perspective, it cannot be stated with any degree of assurance that research methods classified as naturalistic will ultimately yield findings that truly reflect the epistemological foundations of the Science of Unitary Human Beings. Until such explications emerge, we would be well-advised to continue to encourage and respect those who also struggle with hypothesis testing in empirical designs. Celebrating the significance of those studies, so well represented in the annals of Rogerian research, advances the sophistication of the science and underwrites its collegial integrity.

It is understandable that scholars have become increasingly disillusioned about the linear process of empiricism; however, it would be premature to abandon those efforts and embrace qualitative methods as the panacea to methodological woes in Rogerian research. Exclusionary or dogmatic directives about the only correct way of doing science distract from the common goal. Much difficult conceptual terrain must be charted before Rogerians can feel comfortable translating naturalistic methods into their science. Scholars of the Science of Unitary Human Beings can harness their collective creativity and enthusiasm in the service of advancing the science systematically in ways that have demonstrated success: through substantive questions for study, attention to the rigors of specific methodologies for field inquiry, and courageous dissemination of their work for critique.

Despite our desire to endorse naturalistic methods as the preferred Rogerian way of knowing, let us not be metaphorical lemmings running off the scientific cliff. Science is a process of evolving probabilities. Perhaps the momentum for multiple field methods in this unitary field science will spiral into a new level of abstraction in which thesis and antithesis of methods in empirical and naturalistic paradigms achieve synthesis in a pandimensional reality. True to

Rogerian vision, there is no end to excitement in the Science of Unitary Human Beings. While anticipating the next scientific puzzle to emerge, however, do not be idle. Enjoy the mystery; ponder your rankings of the travel metaphors and design an intellectual sojourn within qualitative research contexts that resonate with your personal patterning. Trust yourself; the Science of Unitary Human Beings eagerly awaits your notes from the field.

## REFERENCES

Babbie, E. (1992). *The practice of social research.* Belmont, CA: Wadsworth.

Bredin, H. (1992). Metaphorical thought. *British Journal of Aesthetics, 32*(2), 97-108.

Catudal, J. (1990). Validity, communication, and interpretation. *Journal of Educational and Philosophical Theory, 22*(2), 8-25.

Daniel, S. (1986). Metaphor in the historiography of philosophy. *CLIO, 15*(2), 191-210.

Embler, W. (1987). Notes toward a theory of metaphor. *Et cetera, 44*(2), 163-170.

Emerson, R. (1949). *Self-reliance.* Mount Vernon, NY: Peter Pauper Press.

Goetz, J., & LeCompte, M. (1984). *Ethnography and qualitative design in educational research.* San Diego, CA: Academic Press.

Hartmann, R. (1992). *Value hierarchies and influence structure of practicing professional nurses.* Unpublished doctoral dissertation, Teachers College, Columbia University, New York.

Lincoln, Y., & Guba, E. (1985). *Naturalistic inquiry.* Newbury Park, CA: Sage.

Merriam, S. (1988). *Case study research in education: A qualitative approach.* San Francisco: Jossey-Bass.

Ortega y Gasset, J. (1960). *What is philosophy?* New York: Norton.

Patton, M. (1990). *Qualitative evaluation and research methods.* Newbury Park, CA: Sage.

Pellauer, D. (1987). Time and narrative and theological reflection. *Philosophy Today, 31*(314), 262-285.

Rawnsley, M. (1985). H-E-A-L-T-H: A Rogerian perspective. *Journal of Holistic Nursing, 3*(1), 25-29.

Rigotti, F. (1986). Metaphors of time. *Et cetera, 3:2*, 157.

Runes, D. (1984). *Dictionary of philosophy.* New York: Rowman & Alleheld.

Sarter, B. (1988). *Paths to knowledge.* New York: National League for Nursing.

Strauss, A., & Corbin, J. (1990). Basics of qualitative research: Grounded theory procedures and techniques. *Qualitative Sociology, 13,* 3-21.

Van Kaam, A. (1969). *Existential foundations of psychology.* Pittsburgh, PA: Duquesne University Press.

# 26

# The Unitary Field Pattern Portrait Method: Development of a Research Method for Rogers' Science of Unitary Human Beings

*Howard Karl Butcher*

The evolution of nursing as a scientific discipline is predicated on the uniqueness of phenomena central to its purpose and the development of innovative research and practice methods consistent with nursing's unique conceptual systems. There is a growing recognition that if nursing is to develop a scientific knowledge base, inquiry within nursing must be guided by nursing conceptual systems (Frederickson, 1992; Leininger, 1985; Malinski, 1986; Newman, 1986; Parse, 1987; Reed, 1989; Roy & Andrews, 1991; M.C. Smith, 1990). The purpose of this author was to derive a method of scientific inquiry consistent with the ontology and epistemology of Rogers' Science of Unitary Human Beings.

Rogers' (1970, 1980, 1986, 1987, 1988, 1990, 1992) Science of Unitary Human Beings focuses on the human–environment mutual process as a dynamic, rhythmical, unfolding process and provides a paradigm for derivation and testing of theories that can enhance the understanding of phenomena central to nursing. The purpose of research within Rogers' nursing science is to "understand the nature of human evolution and its multiple, unpredictable potentialities" (Rogers, 1990, p. 9). An understanding of the nature of human evolution is obtained by uncovering human–environmental patterns of wholeness and interpreting the patterns from the perspective of Rogers' Science of Unitary Human Beings. Examining universal human experiences from a unitary perspective will provide a fresh perspective, raise new questions, and allow for new explanations (Rogers, 1992). Rogers (1992) further stated that "[the Science of Unitary Human Beings] is a new reality and encompasses new ways of thinking, new questions, and new interpretations. . . . It also requires consistency with the system to study it" (p. 33).

## ROGERIAN RESEARCH METHODOLOGY

The continued use of borrowed research methods in Rogerian research is being questioned (Barrett, 1990; Carboni, 1991, 1992a; Cowling, 1986a; Newman, 1990; Phillips, 1988a, 1988b; Rawnsley, 1990). Rogers (1992) stated that research methods must be consistent with the Science of Unitary Human Beings if one is to study irreducible human beings in mutual process with a pandimensional universe. There is recent commentary by Rogerian and other nurse scholars on the need to develop research methods more congruent with Rogers' unitary conceptual system (Carboni, 1991, 1992a; Newman, 1990; Phillips, 1988a, 1988b; Rawnsley, 1990; M.J. Smith, 1988). The Science of Unitary Human Beings "calls for research methods that uncover human/environment patterns of wholeness; thus, new research methods unique to nursing must be designed" (Phillips, 1988a, p. 96). Rawnsley (1990) stated that "inductive designs, including qualitative methods, which seem congruent with the goal of understanding the nature and direction of patterning diversity characteristic of unbounded, integral four-dimensional [pandimensional], resonating human and environmental energy fields has not been addressed" (p. 195). There are no research methods, however, developed specifically within Rogers' unitary science.

## ONTOLOGICAL–EPISTEMOLOGICAL–METHODOLOGICAL CONNECTIONS

The creation of a method is not an isolated activity. The approach to inquiry is shaped by ontological and epistemological beliefs of the system of inquiry. A critical feature of the development of the proposed Rogerian method is the examination of the logical connection between the ontology–epistemology of the conceptual system and the proposed research method. Considerable support exists for establishing congruency of method with ontological and epistemological principles of a particular conceptual system in approaching scientific inquiries (Allen, Benner, & Diekelmann, 1986; Cowling, 1986a; DeGroot, 1988; Guba & Lincoln, 1989; Hesse, 1980; Laudan, 1977; Leininger, 1985; Moccia, 1988; Morgan, 1983; Munhall, 1982; Parse, 1987, 1990; Polkinghorne, 1983; Watson, 1981; Webster & Jacox, 1986).

Morgan (1983) provided a useful framework for examining the connection among ontology, epistemology, and research method. The identification of epistemological tenets and epistemological metaphors using Morgan's (1983) framework serves as a means for developing a research method in harmony with the Science of Unitary Human Beings. Morgan's (1983) framework outlines three components: paradigms, metaphors, and puzzle solving. Paradigm characteristics identify underlying assumptions and a metatheoretical or philosophical view of reality. Identifying assumptions about human beings and the universe in which they live forms the ontological foundation of inquiry. Morgan's (1983) second component, metaphors, is used to identify the epistemological stance with regard to scientific inquiry. Epistemology refers to the nature of how people come to have knowledge in the world. According to Morgan (1983), a scientist's world-view is essentially metaphorical and is expressed in the language and concepts that filter and structure perceptions about a particular phenomenon. Metaphorical thinking is a basic way of symbolizing used to forge knowledge and experience (Cowling, 1986a). Identification of favored metaphors embedded in the conceptual system generates an image of the phenomenon as well as an image for how the phenomenon should be studied. Methodologies are chosen to examine implications of metaphorical insight. Morgan (1983) asserted that "favored" methodology links the researcher to the situation being studied in terms of the rules, procedures, and protocol that operationalize the ontological assumptions and corresponding epistemological metaphors.

## ROGERIAN ONTOLOGY

Ontology defines the nature of reality of a particular world-view. Rogers' ontology has been described by Sarter (1988a, 1988b), Carboni (1991), and Reeder (1993). Rogers' nursing science identifies unitary human beings as nursing's unique perspective and as being irreducible energy fields, different from the sum of parts, and integral with a pandimensional universe. The universe, as described by Rogers, is evolutionary and continuously changing toward increasing diversity and innovativeness within a pandimensional reality. The fundamental unity in the universe is the energy field. Energy fields are irreducible and do not have parts. Energy fields are dynamic, in constant motion, continuously open, and infinite. "Individual boundaries are considered to be imaginary and are identified for pragmatic purposes, recognizing that every energy field is integral with the environment" (Carboni, 1991, p. 134). Human and environmental energy fields are integral and are engaged in a mutual process of continuous change. Thus, process, movement, and wholeness characterize Rogers' ontology (Carboni, 1991).

The major ontological assumptions of Rogers' conceptual system may be summarized as: (1) energy fields; (2) unitary and irreducible nature of the human–environment energy field; (3) human–environment mutual process, which signifies the inseparability of the human and environmental fields; (4) pandimensionality, which connotes the relative nature of space–time, infinite realities, and nonlinear change; and (5) all change is continuous, rhythmical, unpredictable, innovative, and evolving toward increasing diversity.

## ROGERIAN EPISTEMOLOGY

Epistemology is the nature, scope, and object of human knowledge; it describes how human beings come to have knowledge (Power & Knapp, 1990). Guba and Lincoln (1989) asserted that epistemology addresses the question, "What is the relationship between the knower and the known?" (p. 88).

Rogers' epistemology identifies pattern manifestations as the source of knowledge about the continuous mutual human and environmental field process. More specifically, Cowling (1990) identified experiences, perceptions, and expressions as unitary pattern manifestations that provide unique information on each human–environmental field process. These manifestations are personal forms of knowing and are the object of pattern appraisal.

The importance of personal knowledge is emphasized in Rogerian science. Rogers (1970) asserted that humans have feelings and thoughts that reflect wholeness. She explicitly stated that the "subjective world of human feelings must be incorporated into the so-called 'objective science' to provide a more comprehensive epistemology relevant to the study of man's experience" (Rogers, 1970,

p. 87). Rogers' emphasis on the uniqueness of each human field (feelings and thoughts) implies that subjective experience is relevant to understanding the human–environmental field process. Knowledge is derived from knowingly experiencing the human–environmental mutual process.

The scope of knowledge in Rogerian science is best described by the concept of pandimensionality. Knowing is neither objective or subjective; it is pandimensional (Reeder, 1993). Pandimensionality supports the idea that there are multiple realities and multiple modes of awareness. The idea of multiple realities reflects the relative nature of the universe and the uniqueness of each human field pattern. Pandimensionality also opens up the possibility of intuition as an additional source of knowledge that is beyond the objective five-senses view. Knowledges that are metaphoric, literary, poetic, rhetorical, figurative, literal, and symbolic are necessary to express pandimensional realities (Reeder, 1993). Intellectual intuition and imaginative synthesis are processes that can grasp the pandimensional pattern of unity in diversity of humans integral with the universe (Reeder, 1984). Thus, pattern appraisal involves multiple modes of awareness, including intuition and personal knowledge.

Cowling (1986a), based on his interpretation of Morgan (1983), stated that clues for structuring scientific inquiry are usually expressed by metaphors that provide an image of phenomenon. Since the metaphors symbolize a basic way of forging knowledge and experience, they provide further understanding of a theorist's particular epistemological stance. A "kaleidoscope of patterns" and "symphony" are two central epistemologic metaphors, embedded in Rogers' Science of Unitary Human Beings, that further illuminate Rogerian epistemology.

*Kaleidoscope Metaphor.*    The kaleidoscope metaphor illuminates the nature of pattern and, therefore, knowledge. When looking through a kaleidoscope, one sees continuous changing patterns of color and light brought about by the unique relationships among bits of colored glass and reflecting surfaces. As the kaleidoscope is rotated, there is constant change, continuous variation in form, revealing new, creative, and innovative manifestations of the evolving pattern.

Rogers (1970) used the metaphor "kaleidoscope" when describing the continuous changing nature of pattern in the life process of humans (p. 62). Patterning is a key concept in Rogers' nursing science. It is through pattern manifestations that changes in the energy field are experienced. These manifestations provide clues as to what the field pattern is like. Rogers (1970) asserted that "pattern evolves with kaleidoscopic uncertainty coordinate with the nature of the man-environment energy exchange taking place through space-time" (p. 91). Manifestations of patterning emerging "kaleidoscopically" are the source of knowledge. The kaleidoscopic nature of pattern signifies the dynamic, rhythmical, continuously changing, and unpredictable, flowing motion of pattern.

Kaleidoscopic patterns are perceived by pattern appraisal. Pattern appraisal includes the contextual or gestalt features of the phenomena under study. Patterns are continuously changing, and viewing them over time reveals their unfolding and transformational nature. Pattern appraisal involves focusing on rhythm, movement, intensity, configuration, and the meaning of pattern manifestations emerging from the human-environmental field mutual process (Newman, 1986).

*Symphony Metaphor.*     The Science of Unitary Human Beings is replete with musical metaphors. The "symphony" metaphor illuminates the rhythm and nature of pattern as well as the experiential nature of human experience. For example, Rogers (1970) stated, "Life's complexity is a haunting melody" (p. 41). "The life process in man is a symphony of rhythmical vibrations oscillating at various frequencies . . . . The life process may be likened to cadences—sometimes harmonic, sometimes cacophonous, sometimes dissonant; rising, falling; now fast, now slow—ever changing in a universal orchestration of dynamic wave patterns" (p. 101). "Behavioral manifestations of the life process are symphonic expressions of unity and cannot be dichotomized as objective or subjective, as internal or external, as mental or physical" (p. 93).

The Principle of Resonancy also accents the symphony metaphor. Resonance in music is the intensification and prolongation of sound, especially of a musical tone, caused by sympathetic vibration. The Principle of Resonancy describes the rhythmical nature of life. Rogers (1970) asserted that "the rhythms of life are inextricably woven into the rhythms of the universe" and a human being "experiences his environment as a resonating wave of complex symmetry uniting him with the rest of the world" (pp. 100–101). Wave frequencies unify the human and environmental fields. Thus, resonating waves provide the epistemological link between the knower and the known. Human and environmental fields are integral in symphonic unity.

## ROGERIAN MUTUAL PROCESS EPISTEMOLOGY

The kaleidoscope and symphony metaphors describe the nature of integrality of the human and environmental fields. Each metaphor also accentuates the experiential nature of change and human evolution. Knowledge, in the form of experiences, perceptions, and expressions is revealed through continuously changing kaleidoscopic–symphonic manifestations of patterning and are accessed through pattern appraisal. Experiencing kaleidoscopic patterns as symphonic resonating waves illuminates the unpredictable participatory nature of human beings with their environment. The Principle of Integrality implies there is no separation between the observer and the observed, the knower and the known, or the inquirer and the inquired into. Furthermore, an inevitable element in the inquiry process is a mix of the inquirer with a variety of other persons associated with the inquiry. Table 26.1 summarizes the tenets of Rogers' ontology and epistemology. The unitary ontology is derived from Rogers' major postulates and principles. Participatory metaphors link the ontology to the mutual process epistemology.

## TOWARD A FAVORED ROGERIAN
## RESEARCH METHODOLOGY

Rogers' unitary ontology, mutual process epistemology, and participatory metaphors serve as a guide in the development of the Unitary Field Pattern Portrait research method (see Table 26.1). To ensure harmony in the ontology–epistemology–methodology relationship, the creation of a Rogerian method of scientific inquiry must recognize

### Table 26.1
### Rogers' Ontology, Epistemological Metaphors, and Tenets

| Ontology "Unitary" | Epistemological Metaphors "Participatory" | Epistemological Tenets "Mutual Process" |
|---|---|---|
| Energy fields | | Pattern manifestations |
| Irreducible wholes | Kaleidoscope | Knower and known integral |
| Integrality | Symphony | Pattern appraisal |
| Continuous change | | Multiple modes of awareness |
| Pandimensionality | | Experience, perception, expression |

the integrality between the investigator and the phenomenon investigated; it must also utilize multiple ways of knowing in appraising kaleidoscopic–symphonic pattern manifestations emerging in the form of experiences, perceptions, and expressions from the human–environmental field mutual process. Rogerian inquiry must focus on human energy fields as irreducible wholes in mutual process with the environment. Therefore, context becomes an essential focus of Rogerian inquiry. The methodology would need to capture the participatory nature of the creation of multiple realities and incorporate the rhythmical, unpredictable, noncausal nature of continuous change.

### Sources for Developing a Rogerian Research Method

Two major sources consistent with Rogers' ontology and epistemology provided a foundation for developing the Unitary Field Pattern Portrait research method: Guba and Lincoln's (1989) Constructivist methodology and Cowling's (1990, 1993) Unitary Pattern-Based Practice Methodology. To provide a comprehensive understanding of the foundation of the Unitary Field Pattern Portrait research method, each is described here.

*Guba and Lincoln's Constructivism.*    When discussing the epistemology of the "new paradigm thinking in science," Capra and Steindl-Rast (1991) asserted that "the people who are in the forefront of this research tend to say that a school known as 'constructivism' is the appropriate epistemology" (p. 123). Guba and Lincoln (1989) explicated a "constructivist" ontology, epistemology, and methodology consistent with Capra's new paradigm thinking in science.

The constructivist paradigm is essentially phenomenological (Lincoln, 1992); in fact, Lincoln uses the terms *constructivist* and *phenomenological* interchangeably. Phenomenology is the rigorous science of experience (Ihde, 1977). According to Lincoln (1992), the constructivist paradigm is called the "constructivist" view in psychology, and other disciplines in the social sciences call it the "naturalistic" paradigm. The constructivist/phenomenological paradigm asserts a "relativist ontology" in which there exist multiple socially constructed realities by individuals as they attempt to make sense of their experience (Guba & Lincoln, 1989). Truth, therefore, is defined as the best informed and most sophisticated construction reached by consensus among those individuals most competent to form such a construction (Guba & Lincoln, 1989). Thus, realities exist in the form of mental constructions that are socially and experientially based, local, and specific in nature. The epistemology of the constructivist paradigm, according to Guba and Lincoln (1989), is "monisitic, subjectivist" (p. 84). The inquirer and the inquired-into are fused into a single, dynamic, monisitic entity whose integrality shapes and creates the process and results of the inquiry. Realities exist with the respondents; thus, subjective engagement is the only way to access constructions held by individuals. Thus, the findings that result from inquiry are created by the mutual process between the researcher and the researched.

There is a striking congruence between the constructivist paradigm and Rogers' Science of Unitary Human Beings. Guba and Lincoln's (1989) constructivist paradigm, like Rogers' ontology and epistemology, is concerned with patterns, interpretation, multiple realities, unpredictability, mutual process, continuous change, subjectivity, complexity, irreducible wholes, mutual shaping, naturalism, tacit knowledge, value-laden facts, and qualitative methods (Guba, 1990; Guba & Lincoln, 1989; Lincoln & Guba, 1985). Table 26.2 illustrates congruence between Guba and Lincoln's (1989) "constructivist" paradigm and Rogers' Science of Unitary Human Beings.

### Table 26.2
### Comparison between Guba and Lincoln's Constructivist Paradigm and Rogers' Nursing Science

| Constructivist | Rogerian Science |
|---|---|
| Humans in natural context | Human–Environmental energy field |
| Multiple realities | Pandimensionality |
| Mutual simultaneous shaping | Mutual process |
| Mutual causality | Noncausality |
| Relativism | Pandimensionality |
| Subjectivity | Subjectivity–Objectivity |
| Interconnectiveness | Unitary |
| Continuous change | Continuous change |
| Complexity | Diversity |
| Inseparability | Integrality |
| Dynamic change | Resonancy |
| Indeterminacy | Unpredictability |
| Openness | Openness |
| Indivisible wholeness | Irreducible wholes |
| Interpretation | Pattern appraisal |
| Intuition and tacit knowledge | Multiple modes of awareness |

*Constructivist Methodology.*    Guba and Lincoln (1989) proposed a research method that flows from a relativistic ontology and subjectivist epistemology. The congruence between Constructivism and Rogerian science provides a basis for a fit between Guba and Lincoln's (1989) constructivist/phenomenological methodology and development of the Unitary Field Pattern Portrait research method. Lincoln (1992) stated: "[A] constructivist methodology uses qualitative methods that attempt to grasp phenomena in some holistic way or to understand a phenomenon within its own context or to emphasize the immersion in and comprehension of human meaning ascribed to some set of circumstances or phenomena, or all three" (p. 376). Guba and Lincoln (1989) specified four "entry conditions" that provide a basis for constructivist inquiry: (1) natural setting, (2) human instrument, (3) qualitative methods, and (4) the use of tacit knowledge (p. 177).

Constructivist inquiry is pursued in a natural setting since multiple realities are dependent on the time and context of the constructors who hold them. In constructivist inquiry, the researcher does not assume in advance that he or she knows enough about the focus of inquiry a priori to know what questions to ask. It is not possible to pursue one's subjective construction with a set of predetermined questions based solely on the researcher's construction of the phenomenon. Rather than a preframed instrument or questionnaire, the highly adaptable human instrument is used in constructivist inquiry. Only the human instrument is capable of grasping and evaluating the meaning of data. Given that the human instrument is used in constructivist inquiry, qualitative methods are the most appropriate means to collect data. "Humans collect information best, and most easily, through the direct employment of their senses: talking to people, observing their activities, reading their documents, assessing the unobtrusive signs they leave behind, responding to their nonverbal cues and the like" (Guba & Lincoln, 1989, pp. 175–176). Constructivist inquiry incorporates tacit (intuitive, felt) knowledge in addition to propositional knowledge (knowledge expressible in language form) because: (1) multiple realities can only be appreciated this way; (2) much of the mutual process between the investigator and the respondent occurs at the intuitive or felt level; and (3) tacit knowledge mirrors more fairly and accurately the value patterns of the investigator (Lincoln & Guba, 1985).

A central aspect of Guba and Lincoln's (1989) constructivist methodology is the mutual shaping of construction through the "hermeneutic–dialectic circle" (p. 173). "Constructivists are hermeneutic, at least in the sense that individual constructions are elicited and refined through iterative interactions between and among investigator and respondents . . . they are also dialectic in the sense that different constructions are compared and contrasted in an effort to come to a consensus that is both informed and more sophisticated than any of the constructions held previously" (Lincoln, 1992, p. 380). There are four elements in the hermeneutic-dialectic circle: (1) purposive sampling, (2) the continuous interplay of data collection and data analysis, (3) grounded construction, and (4) emergent design.

Respondents are selected for the study using purposive sampling. Purposive sampling serves a purpose other than representativeness and randomness. The goal of sampling in constructivist inquiry is to achieve the broadest maximum variation of the sample in order to provide the broadest scope of information. The interplay of data collection and data analysis is achieved through the sharing of constructions with respondents as data collection proceeds. For example, during the interview, the second respondent may read the construction of the first respondent for comment and critique. Data, analyzed at one point, may become part of the agenda for the subsequent interviews. As data collection proceeds, analysis of the data proceeds at the same pace. "As successive respondents are asked to comment on the constructions already developed, a joint construction begins to emerge about which consensus can begin to form" (Guba & Lincoln, 1989, p. 179). The joint construction is "grounded" in all the previous constructions because it is derived through the hermeneutic–dialectic process. The hermeneutic aspect consists of depicting the meaning of individual constructions as accurately as possible; the dialectic aspect consists of comparing and contrasting each respondent with one another and with the inquirer's constructions. The final element of the hermeneutic-dialectic circle is emergent design. As the data collection proceeds, the constructivist continuously seeks to refine and extend the design. As the inquirer becomes better acquainted with what is salient, the sample becomes more directed, data analysis more structured, and the construction more definitive. Through mutual shaping of the construction by all respondents, the constructions are synthesized into a "joint construction" or unified whole providing a rich, dense, vivid, and thick description. The hermeneutic-dialectic circle aims to bring a variety of constructions into as much consensus as possible to produce the most informed and so-phisticated joint construction (Guba, 1990).

*Phenomenological Methods.*  Significant support exists among Rogerian scholars of the congruence of phenomenological methods and the Rogerian paradigm. Cowling (1986b) suggested that "phe-nomenology may provide a means to address the qualitative, experi-ential features associated with unitary human change" (p. 74). Reeder (1984, 1986) provided a convincing argument demonstrating the congruence between Husserlian phenomenology and Rogers' Sci-ence of Unitary Human Beings and stated:

> Given the congruency between Husserlian phenomenology and the Rogerian conceptual systems, a sound, convincing rationale is established for the use of this philosophy of science as an alternative for basic theoretical studies in Rogerian nurs-ing science. . . . Nursing research in general requires a broader range of human experience than sensory experience (whether intuitive or perceptive) in the development and test-ing of conceptual systems for gaining better access to multi-faceted phenomena . . . . Husserlian phenomenology as a rigorous science provides just such an experience. (Reeder, 1986, p. 62)

According to Reeder (1986), phenomenological methods better re-flect the Rogerian paradigm. They are not limited to sensory experi-ence, but include multiple modes of awareness inherent in a pandimensional universe. Phillips (1989b), another Rogerian scholar, asserted that phenomenological research leads to knowledge about the whole by uncovering the meaning of the human–environmental mutual field process. In phenomenological research, there is "no need to deal with such polarities as subjective–objective, since the living experience emerges from the interconnectiveness of the two, where reality is experienced as a whole" (Phillips, 1989b, p. 5). Throughout the phenomenological research process, the researcher is an active participant in the integral nature of people and their en-vironments. "This participation enables the researcher to search for patterns within descriptions, and the emerging patterns are probed to create pattern profiles of the lived experience" (Phillips, 1989b, p. 5). Furthermore, since phenomenological research uses imagina-tion and intuition as a conceptualizing process, it brings into aware-ness the pandimensional universe where one no longer depends on only the physical attributes as indicators of experiencing the world (Phillips, 1989b). The researcher is able to explore what is genuinely discoverable and what is potentially there but not often seen, and is able to uncover the whole of experience of the infinite human field (Ihde, 1977; Phillips, 1989b).

Lincoln and Guba (1985, pp. 39–44) identified 14 criteria for doing research within the constructivist/phenomenological paradigm (see Table 26.3). Carboni (1992b) proposed criteria for Rogerian inquiry that correspond with Lincoln and Guba's 14 criteria. Carboni's criteria were slightly modified to provide a guide for the development of the Unitary Field Pattern Portrait research method.

Each of the criteria of Rogerian inquiry listed is utilized in the creation of the Unitary Field Pattern Portrait research method. In addition, Cowling's (1990) pattern-based practice methodology, which highlights the construction of pattern profiles and expressions, experiences, and perceptions as features of unitary field pattern, provides the second major source for developing the processes of the Unitary Field Pattern Portrait research method.

*Cowling's Unitary Pattern-Based Practice Methodology.* Cowling's (1990) description of unitary pattern-based practice clarified the

## Table 26.3
### Criteria of Constructivist and Rogerian Inquiry

| Criteria of Constructivist Inquiry | Criteria of Rogerian Inquiry |
| --- | --- |
| Creation | Creation |
| Natural setting | Natural setting |
| Focus-determined boundaries | Focus on human energy fields and well-being |
| Human instrument | Human instrument |
| Utilization of tacit knowledge | Utilization of all forms of knowledge |
| Qualitative methods preferred | Qualitative methods preferred |
| Emergent design | Emergent design |
| Purposive sampling | Intensity sampling |
| Inductive data analysis | Creative pattern synthesis |
| Grounded theory | *A priori* nursing conceptual system |
| Idiographic interpretation | Evolutionary interpretation |
| Negotiated outcomes | Shared description and co-creation, and shared understanding |
| Case study reporting mode | Unitary Field Pattern Report |
| Trustworthiness and authenticity | Trustworthiness and authenticity |

identification of indices of human–environmental field patterning. Cowling (1990) identified human energy field pattern emerging from human and environmental field mutual process as the central focus of nursing practice. He states that the human field is appraised through manifestations of pattern in the form of experiences, perceptions, and expressions. Experiences, perceptions, and expressions are not elements in a particulate sense; rather, they describe unitary human beings who are continuously experiencing, perceiving, and expressing in unity (Cowling, 1993).

Experience involves sensing the world in a natural and unprocessed way (Cowling, in 1993). Human beings are able to experience energy field patterns in a variety of ways. Building on Cowling's unitary description of experiences, perceptions, and expressions, Carboni (1992a) stated that experiences may be empirical, five-sense, solipsistic experiences or pandimensional, transpersonal experiences. Empirical five-sense experiences are restricted to the physical body; solipsistic experiences are what Bohm (1980) described as "thought-bound." Experiences that emerge from transcendent or pandimensional awareness are transpersonal in nature and occur when the physically bound and thought-bound self transcends beyond body and mind limitations (Carboni, 1992a). Perception is simultaneous or contiguous with experiencing and involves apprehending experience. Perception is observing, reflecting, knowing, constructing, and making sense of what is occurring, and involves having an awareness of pattern manifestations (Cowling, 1993).

Energy field patterns are expressed in a variety of forms that range from the direct to the very subtle (Carboni, 1992a). Expressions are manifestations of experiencing and perceiving (Cowling, 1993). Expressions may be in the more direct form of language, which tends to be embedded in linear time. This time-bound, causal structure of language tends to divide things into separate entities that are conceived as fixed and static (Bohm, 1980; Carboni, 1992a). Pattern information, however, may be more subtle and expressed in a form of language that transcends three-dimensional limitations. Metaphors, song, dance, poetry, visualizations, and pictorial formats are more subtle unitary manifestations of human–environmental field patterning. Less known nonverbal and nonphysical pandimensional expressions of thoughts and feelings, like telepathy and clairvoyance, are additional forms of unitary field pattern expressions (Carboni, 1992a). Pattern is grasped only through its expressions, which provide clues and are indicators of the underlying unitary pattern (Cowling, 1990).

Guba and Lincoln (1989) and Cowling (1990, 1993) also asserted that knowledge is derived from pattern information using multiple modes of awareness. Intuition and paranormal experiences facilitate pattern recognition. The primary source for validating pattern appraisal information is the client (Cowling, 1990). Self-knowledge represents another form of pattern information and is valued in the process of validating the inferred pattern appraisal (Cowling, 1990). Phillips (1991) also affirmed that Rogerian researchers must attend to "personal knowledge" and posited that "personal knowledge is related to the meaning of the experience in relation to the environmental field" (p. 142).

Cowling (1990) described the process of constructing a unitary pattern profile as a means of capturing the essence and nature of a person's mutual process in the environment. For research purposes, Phillips (1989a) suggested that "pattern profiles," described by Cowling (1983), can provide a better qualitative understanding of changing pattern manifestations. According to Cowling (1990), pattern profiles are descriptions of the features, qualities, and properties of manifestations of patterning emerging from the human–environmental mutual field process and they reflect the person's experience, perceptions, and expressions. The pattern profile incorporates features, qualities, and properties emerging from the pattern information and reflects the participant's experience, perception, and expressions. The profile may be in a listing, diagrammatic, or narrative form. Field pattern profiles provide a means for uncovering the nature of change evolving from the human–environmental field mutual process related to human health and well-being. Phillips (1989a) stated that pattern profiles "will get at the rhythmic nature of change and the creative emergence of pattern manifestations of the whole" (p. 59). A synthesis of participants' pattern profiles to create a "unitary field pattern portrait" will serve as the essence of the Unitary Field Pattern Portrait research method.

Cowling's (1990) Rogerian practice methodology is essentially a phenomenologically based practice method. Boyd (1988) identifies experiences, perception, expression, and modes of awareness as central phenomenological concepts. Thus, Cowling's (1990, 1993) emphasis on experiences, perceptions, and expressions as the focus of pattern appraisal fits well with Guba and Lincoln's phenomenological-constructivist methodology.

## THE UNITARY FIELD PATTERN PORTRAIT
## RESEARCH METHOD

The Unitary Field Pattern Portrait research method is specific to nursing and was developed for research guided by Rogers' Science of Unitary Human Beings. The method is similar to other interpretive phenomenological methods, such as Moustakas' (1990) heuristic research, and is distinct from all other methods in its theoretical underpinnings and its specific processes. The Unitary Field Pattern Portrait research method (described in a later section of this chapter) is a unique synthesis of Guba and Lincoln's (1989) constructivist methodology and Cowling's (1990, 1993) Unitary Pattern Practice methodology and provides a means to investigate significant human-environmental phenomena specific to nursing's concern. The research method flows directly from Rogers' unitary ontology and mutual process epistemology and incorporates the 14 characteristics (printed in **bold type** in the following discussion; see also Table 26.3) of Rogerian inquiry.

### Assumptions

The key assumptions underpinning the Unitary Field Pattern Portrait research method are:

1. Descriptions of nursing phenomena from a unitary perspective enhance nursing knowledge and contribute to theory development within the Science of Unitary Human Beings.

2. Human beings can describe their own experiences, perceptions, and expressions in ways that uncover an understanding of a particular phenomenon.

3. Experiences, perceptions, and expressions are unitary pattern manifestations emerging from the human-environmental energy field mutual process.

4. The researcher, through creative synthesis, logical conceptualizing, and semantic consistency throughout the processes of the method, creates a portrait of a particular phenomenon that reflects its dynamic kaleidoscopic and symphonic human-environment patterning.

5. The researcher interprets the portrait provided by the concepts and principles of Rogers' Science of Unitary Human Beings as a means to create a "unitary field pattern portrait" of the phenomenon.

## Purpose of the Method

The purpose of this research method is to **create** a unitary field pattern portrait illuminating the dynamic kaleidoscopic and symphonic pattern manifestations emerging from the human–environmental mutual process as a means to enhance understanding of phenomena related to human well-being, and to integrate this knowledge with Rogers' Science of Unitary Human Beings. Research using this method contributes to increasing understanding of the dynamic nature of kaleidoscopic and symphonic change related to well-being and human betterment.

## Focus of Inquiry

The focus of inquiry within the Science of Unitary Human Beings and the Unitary Field Pattern Portrait research method is **irreducible human energy fields** in mutual process with their environmental energy fields. A unitary view of wholeness takes into account the unfolding, rhythmical, flowing motion in the human–environmental dynamic web of mutual process.

Manifestations of patterning evolving from the kaleidoscopic and symphonic human–environmental field process are indicators of the unitary nature of change. In the Unitary Field Pattern Portrait research method, the researcher selects significant common human–environmental phenomena in the life process associated with the well-being of unitary human beings as the specific focus of inquiry.

## Processes of the Method

Processes of the proposed Unitary Field Pattern Portrait research method (see Table 26.4) include: initial engagement, a priori nursing conceptual system, immersion, pattern appraisal, field pattern profile construction, hermeneutic–dialectic circle, unitary field pattern portrait construction, and theoretical unitary field pattern portrait construction. Moustakas' (1990) heuristic research served as an inspiration in developing the initial engagement and pattern synthesis

## Table 26.4
## Processes in the Unitary Field Pattern
## Portrait Research Method

1. Initial Engagement: Formulation of a Research Question
   A. Significant common human–environmental phenomenon related to well-being

2. A Priori Nursing Conceptual System
   A. Rogers' Science of Unitary Human Beings
   B. Objectives of the investigation

3. Immersion
   A. Intensity sampling
   B. Selection of natural setting

4. Pattern Appraisal
   A. In-depth interviews: focus on experiences, perceptions, and expressions
   B. Field notes

5. Field Pattern Profile Construction
   A. Creative pattern synthesis

6. Hermeneutic–Dialectic Circle
   A. Repeat process 5 until saturation of patterns
   B. Shared description and creation of shared understanding with participants

7. Field Pattern Portrait Construction
   A. Creative pattern synthesis

8. Theoretical Field Pattern Portrait Construction
   A. Evolutionary interpretation

phases, while the hermeneutic–dialectic process was derived from Guba and Lincoln's phenomenological–constructivist methodology.

### Initial Engagement

In initial engagement, through intense interest and passionate searching, the investigator discovers a research question of central interest to the well-being of unitary human beings. The general research question of a proposed study is stated as: What is the unitary field pattern portrait of [name the phenomenon]?

Experiences, perceptions, and expressions are manifestations of pattern that incarnate the phenomenon's unitary human–environmental field mutual process and, therefore, are considered the primary entities of study. The field pattern portrait is mutually shaped by all participants in the investigation and aims to create a rich and thick description of experiences, perceptions, and expressions of a specific human–environmental phenomenon related to the well-being of unitary human beings.

## A Priori Nursing Conceptual System

All research flows from some theoretical perspective (Cull-Wilby & Pepin, 1987; DeGroot, 1988; Guba & Lincoln, 1989; Moccia, 1988; Phillips, 1988a; Sandelowski, 1993; Thompson, 1985; Tinkle & Beaton, 1983). Sandelowski (1993) pointed out that qualitative methods, including phenomenology, are guided prior commitments to "overarching world-views" (p. 215). The Science of Unitary Human Beings serves as the researcher's **a priori nursing conceptual system** and articulates the study's theoretical perspective. Rogers' conceptual system is explicitly identified at onset of the study.

## Immersion

The investigator immerses as fully as possible in the phenomenon of concern. In this phase, the researcher becomes steeped in the research topic. During immersion, the researcher is absorbed in literature, poetry, music, journal writings, dialogues with self and others, art work, or any host of processes that draws the researcher closer to the topic of inquiry to reveal its meanings (Moustakas, 1990). The notion of immersion is supported by Rogers' mutual process epistemology. The researcher and the researched-into are inseparable. Findings of the inquiry are created out of the **mutual process between researcher and the researched**. This intense immersion in mutual process allows one to encounter, examine, and fully participate in a rhythmic flow with the phenomenon in order to depict the experience in its many aspects, core themes, and essences (Moustakas, 1990).

*Participant Selection.* The Unitary Field Pattern Portrait research method uses **intensity sampling**. Patton (1990) stated that "an intensity sample consists of information-rich cases that manifest the phenomenon of interest intensely (but not extremely)" (p. 171). Extreme or deviant cases may be so unusual as to distort the manifestations of the phenomenon of interest. Following the logic of intensity sampling, the researcher will seek excellent or rich examples of the phenomenon. Since entities of study are experiences, perceptions, and expressions of significant common human–environmental phenomena related to human well-being, any person who identifies himself or herself as experiencing the phenomenon is a potential participant.

*Natural Setting.*     Pattern appraisal takes place in the **natural setting** of the phenomenon's occurrence. The setting pattern appraisal process may be a specific environmental setting, which provides a particular focus of the study.

## Pattern Appraisal

Pattern appraisal is the process of collecting data and identifying manifestations of pattern emerging from the human–environmental mutual field process (Barrett, 1988). The **human instrument** is used in pattern appraisal. The researcher acts as a human instrument by obtaining descriptions of the phenomenon through an in-depth interview conducted in a person-to-person encounter of researcher and participant. Pattern appraisal involves focusing on rhythm, movement, intensity, and configuration of pattern manifestations (Newman, 1986). Human and environmental field patterns are appraised through manifestations of the pattern in the form of experiences, perceptions, and expressions (Cowling, 1990). The appraisal process occurs within the natural setting of the phenomenon under investigation. The researcher enters into a dialogue with the participant, focusing on the expression of the participant's experiences and perceptions of the phenomenon of concern.

An important ingredient in the interview process involves efforts directed toward creating an atmosphere of trust and relaxation. In mutual process with the participant, the investigator actively listens, conveys unconditional acceptance, and remains fully open to the human–environmental field process. The researcher uses an informal conversational interview style that fosters spontaneous generation of questions and conversations. Such an informal conversational interview is consistent with the rhythm and flow of mutual process and aims toward encouraging expression, elucidation, and disclosure of the phenomenon. An open-ended approach allows participants the time and space to explore the topic in a manner that promotes discovery, depth, richness, and meaning. The researcher takes the role of facilitator, clarifier, and evoker of depictions of the phenomenon. Seeking depth and clarity concerning the phenomenon facilitates a rhythm of exploration that uncovers pandimensional patterns of mutual process with the environment.

Pattern appraisal is designed to gather rich, dense, and vivid descriptions and interpretations of the experiences, expressions, perceptions, feelings, thoughts, and meanings of the phenomenon of concern. Although depth and clarity are sought, the researcher does not probe if persons indicate that they do not wish to speak about some particular aspect of the phenomenon. Throughout the pattern appraisal process, the researcher **utilizes all forms of knowledge**, including tacit knowing, intuition, and pandimensional modes of awareness while engaged in mutual process with participants.

The focus of pattern appraisal is on unitary pattern manifestations in the form of experiences, perceptions, and expressions. Although general questions may be formulated in advance, genuine dialogue cannot be planned. The unfolding of the field pattern portrait reflects an **emergent design** since the inquirer will not know in advance what pattern manifestations are likely to emerge, and thus will not know which questions to ask subsequent participants.

Some examples of general questions concerning the experience of the phenomenon being researched are: "Please talk to me about what it is like to experience. . . ." "Describe for me any feelings you may have had when feeling. . . ." "What is the feeling of being [specific phenomenon] like?" "Now please try to be more specific about the thoughts and feelings you have when. . . ." "Please relate what you have just said to feeling. . . ." Each of these questions is meant to nurture mutual exploration and discussion of the phenomenon being studied. Examples of open-ended questions concerning the participant's perceptions may be: "Please talk to me about how you know when you are [specific phenomenon]?" "How do things change when you feel [specific phenomenon]?" "Can you tell me what helps you most when you are [specific phenomenon]?" "Do things around you look different when you are [specific phenomenon]?"

When appraising participants' expressions, the researcher may ask: "What happens when you experience this?" The researcher will search in mutual process for a metaphor that represents what the phenomenon is like, and/or find a way the participant could represent the phenomenon in a picture or diagram, or even draw a picture with the participant. The researcher asks the participant to identify a single word or phrase that captures the essence of the research topic. In addition, the researcher can ask the participant to explore the following words in relation to the phenomenon: energy, flow, will, unity, family, continuous, harmony, movement, wholeness, change, flux, openness, process, rhythm, sharing, participating, power, imagination, and awareness. Other key words or metaphors may emerge during pattern appraisal. Participants may be asked, subsequently, to explore and describe their meaning in relation to the research phenomenon.

To supplement interview data, the investigator may ask participants to explain any personal documents, diaries, journals, logs, notes, poetry, and art work they may have that offers additional understanding of the phenomenon. These artifacts may be collected, if the participant wishes, and would be used during the second phase of pattern synthesis.

The researcher remains focused on appraising as much as possible about the experience in the person's own words while remaining sensitive and focused on the participant's experience. Pattern appraisal continues until the person reports that there is nothing further to say about the phenomenon. Each interview is taped and transcribed verbatim. In addition to pattern appraisal information, the researcher keeps field notes and maintains a Reflexive Journal to be used later for pattern synthesis.

*Field Notes.*    In addition to the descriptive subjective data collected through interviews of each participant, the researcher records field notes, organizing them into three categories: Observational Notes, Theoretical Notes, and Methodological Notes. This organization provides a means of effectively reflecting on and processing the data as they occur (ongoing synthesis) and as they ultimately come together in the final synthesis (unitary field pattern portrait and theoretical construction). Consistent with characteristics of Rogerian inquiry, the mutuality of the researcher and the participants is reflected in the content of the field notes.

Observational Notes include objective descriptions of what the researcher observed. Basic information—such as the site of the interview, what the environmental setting was like, what activities took place, and any observations of important nonverbal expressions or other manifestations of energy field patterning that occurred during pattern appraisal—is recorded in a separate notebook immediately after each interview.

Theoretical Notes are divided into two subcategories, **Deductive** Theoretical Notes and **Inductive** Theoretical Notes. After each interview, the researcher ponders what has been perceived and experienced during pattern appraisal and inductively assigns interpretations of meaning to these perceptions and experiences. During the process of writing these notes after each interview, the researcher also interprets, envisions, and explores the emerging data deductively from the perspective of Rogers' Science of Unitary Human Beings.

Methodological Notes reflect instructions to the researcher and serve as reminders or critiques of the researcher's own methodological tactics. They also reflect all methodological decisions made in accordance with the changing emergent design. The Observational, Theoretical, and Methodological Field Notes are recorded in separate notebooks and organized in order of each interview.

*Reflexive Journal.*   The researcher maintains a reflexive journal during the course of the inquiry. Reflexivity is critical thinking that examines values, beliefs, and interests embedded in the researcher and seeks to understand and integrate them into the study (Lamb & Huttlinger, 1989). The researcher uses the Reflexive Journal to acknowledge personal experiences and values, values of participants, and other values inherent in the context of Rogers' unitary paradigm. Personal visionary insights, intuitions, inferences, mystical insights, feelings, ideas, and reflections are recorded in the Reflexive Journal. Coordinate with the Rogerian characteristics of inquiry, inclusion of a Reflexive Journal recognizes that inquiry is value-bound and allows values to participate in the interpretation of data.

### Field Pattern Profile Construction

There are two phases in pattern synthesis that will lead to a description of the phenomenon. Focus in the first phase of pattern synthesis is the construction of a field pattern profile at the end of data collection for each participant. The field pattern profile is a rich description of the experiences, perceptions, and expressions in the participant's language. Themes and patterns will emerge from the data. These patterns are synthesized into a unified description of the phenomenon's human–environment field process through the process of **creative pattern synthesis**.

*First Phase of Creative Pattern Synthesis.*   Creative pattern synthesis describes the **qualitative** processing of data within the Unitary Field Pattern Portrait research method. However, the Unitary Field Pattern Portrait research method uses a phenomenological data processing similar to the method described by van Manen (1990) rather than the process of content analysis described by Lincoln and Guba (1985). Data are processed within a unitary science using synthesis rather than analysis (Rogers, 1992, personal communication). A selective or highlighting approach (van Manen, 1990) is used to iden-tify thematic statements. In the selective or highlighting reading approach, the researcher will ask, "What statements or phrases seem particularly essential or revealing about the phenomenon?" (van Manen, 1990, p. 93). A field pattern profile is constructed by synthe-sizing the thematic statements and phrases into a descriptive narra-tive that expresses the experiences, perceptions, and expressions for each individual participant. It is important to note that the field pat-tern profile is in the participant's language. Once the field pattern profile is constructed, the researcher arranges for a short meeting with the participant to share the field pattern profile for comment, revision, and validation.

### Hermeneutic–Dialectic Circle

A unique feature of this methodology is mutual creation of the emerging field pattern profile. After the first field pattern profile is validated by the first participant, the researcher can begin pattern appraisal with the second participant. The process described above is repeated with the second participant except that, at the end of the second interview, the second participant is asked to comment on the first field pattern profile. The comments of the second participant on the pattern profile are incorporated into the construction of the sec-ond participant's field pattern profile.

After validation of the second participant's field pattern profile, the researcher synthesizes the two field pattern profiles into one uni-fied, mutually derived field pattern profile using the hermeneutic-dialectic process. The process is dialectic because there is a compari-son and contrast of possible divergent views with an aim of achiev-ing a higher-level synthesis of all participant field pattern profiles. The process is hermeneutic (interpretive) in that each participant considers and interprets the construction of others in relation to his or her own experience. After the interview of the third participant, that participant is asked to comment on the synthesized construction of the first and second participants.

The process of constructing (1) a pattern profile for each par-ticipant and (2) a synthesized, mutually created construction is con-tinued until pattern saturation occurs. Saturation is reached when no further new information emerges from participants and when pat-tern synthesis reveals no new pattern information to be added to the mutually constructed pattern profile. Pattern saturation is reached when there is redundancy in pattern information. Redundancy refers to duplication of content with similar experiences, perceptions, and expressions of the meanings, ideas, and descriptions of the phenomenon. When pattern saturation is reached, pattern appraisal is complete.

**Shared description and creation of shared understanding** occurs through the hermeneutic-dialectic process and aims to provide the most informed and sophisticated mutually created descriptive construction of the experiences, perceptions, and expressions of the phenomenon. Shared description and creation of shared understanding result from the sharing of the mutually constructed pattern profile with each participant throughout the pattern appraisal process.

### Unitary Field Pattern Portrait Construction

The second phase of pattern synthesis involves the construction of a unitary field pattern portrait through a second phase of **creative pattern synthesis**. Field pattern portrait construction begins after pattern saturation is reached. During field pattern portrait construction, the researcher gathers all participant field pattern profiles, the mutually shaped pattern profile, all Observational Field Notes, and other artifacts collected during the course of investigation. The researcher immerses into and dwells with all the pattern information to illuminate the deeper nature of the human–environmental field process. Themes and metaphors, which are manifestations of field pattern related to the phenomenon, are identified and coded into common categories. The researcher stays with the immersion process with intervals of rest until universal patterns, qualities, features, and themes of the phenomenon emerge. Using creative pattern synthesis, the researcher dynamically compares manifestations of field patterning across all field pattern profiles and the mutually shaped pattern profile. Vivid patterns, common to all field pattern profiles, emerge and are nested together. All patterns are combined and synthesized into one unified descriptive portrait that is grounded in experiences, perceptions, and expressions in the field pattern profiles of all participants.

The researcher again immerses into the portrait and reflects on the portrait in light of all the descriptive information collected. The researcher uses imaginative, tacit, intuitive, and contemplative sources of knowledge and insight to discover the essence of the phenomenon and synthesize the themes and essential patterns. The unitary field pattern portrait is grounded with the experiences of the participants since it accentuates the flow, spirit, and life inherent in the experiences, perceptions, and expressions emerging from pattern appraisal (Moustakas, 1990). The unitary field pattern portrait exemplifies the essence of the dynamic kaleidoscopic and symphonic nature of the phenomenon by providing a rich, dense, vivid, accurate, alive, thick, and clear description of universal essences and features of the phenomenon. The unitary field pattern portrait is in the form of an aesthetic rendition of universal patterns, qualities, features, and themes that embrace the phenomenon.

### Theoretical Unitary Field Pattern Portrait Construction

To accomplish theoretical unitary field pattern portrait construction, the researcher gathers the unitary field pattern portrait, Theoretical Field Notes, and Reflexive Journal. The researcher, using **creative inductive and deductive pattern synthesis**, immerses into and dwells with the patterns in light of Rogers' Science of Unitary Human Beings. Creative inductive and deductive pattern synthesis links the patterns inductively identified in the field pattern portrait to the deductive interpretations guided by the researcher's a priori nursing conceptual system. Interpretation, guided by Rogers' Science of Unitary Human Beings, is termed **evolutionary interpretation**. Evolutionary interpretation involves interpreting the field pattern portrait in light of Rogers' principles of resonancy, integrality, and helicy, and the concepts of pandimensionality, pattern, openness, and energy fields to create a theoretical unitary field pattern portrait of the phenomenon.

Theoretical field pattern portrait construction explicates the conceptual description of the phenomenon, thereby connecting the field pattern portrait to the structure of Rogers' nursing science. Theoretical construction advances the evolution of nursing science by lifting the field pattern portrait from description to the level of theory and is expressed in the language of Rogerian nursing science. The theoretical unitary field pattern portrait of the phenomenon is in the form of a definition linking major concepts and principles in Rogers' nursing science. Lastly, theoretical construction moves the field pattern portrait toward positing ideas for further research and nursing practice possibilities.

## UNITARY FIELD PATTERN REPORT

The processes and conclusions of the proposed study are presented in a format emphasizing the unitary and creative aspects of the inquiry. Carboni (1992b) provided a description of the presentation of research findings in what she called a "Unitary Process Report." Like Carboni's Unitary Process Report, the **Unitary Field Pattern Report** is a dynamic and comprehensive account of the research and is presented as a complex tapestry-in-process, one that is open to new and emergent insights. The Unitary Field Pattern Report provides a vibrant image of the depth of the data in all its kaleidoscopic and symphonic complexities and will furnish the basis for assessment of the conclusions by the reader. Particular attention is given to describing the process of pattern synthesis by revealing the synthesis of pattern information from unitary manifestations to pattern profile construction; from pattern profiles to construction of the unitary field pattern; and from the unitary field pattern portrait to the theoretical unitary field pattern portrait. The Unitary Field Pattern Report includes:

1. A description of the natural setting within which the study took place.

2. A description of Rogerian nursing science, emphasizing how it guided all processes of the investigation.

3. A thorough description of the methodological procedures and processes of the study as they unfolded.

4. Verbatim examples illustrating themes emerging from pattern profile construction.

5. Presentation of the Unitary Field Pattern Profiles of two or three participants who clearly exemplify the group as a whole.

6. Presentation of the mutually shaped pattern profile.

7. A presentation of the kaleidoscopic and symphonic unitary field pattern portrait in the form of an aesthetic rendition of universal patterns, qualities, features, and themes that embrace the phenomenon of the phenomenon.

8. Presentation of the theoretical construction of the phenomenon as viewed from Rogers' Science of Unitary Human Beings.

9. A discussion of the study's contribution to the evolution of Rogers' nursing science, nursing practice, and nursing research.

In concert with the aim of all Rogerian research to understand the nature of human evolution and its multiple, unpredictable potentialities, all perceptions and experiences illuminated in the Unitary Field Pattern Report are presented and discussed from a Rogerian evolutionary perspective. This means that all descriptions and interpretations center on manifestations of field patterning of human–environmental energy fields and the changing kaleidoscopic and symphonic patterns that unfolded during the investigation.

## SCIENTIFIC RIGOR

The Unitary Field Pattern Portrait method is a formal method of research as described by Kaplan (1964), with specific assumptions and processes. Since there is a high degree of congruence between the constructivist–phenomenological paradigm and Rogers' unitary-transformative paradigm, Lincoln and Guba's (1985) criteria for **trustworthiness and authenticity** are used to examine the scientific rigor within the Unitary Field Pattern Portrait research method. The logical–positivist criteria for scientific rigor (generalizability, verification, validity, statistical significance) and other terms for testing hypotheses are incongruent and inappropriate measures of scientific rigor in phenomenological–constructivist research methods. Lincoln (1992) stated that there are two major criteria to ensure rigor in research findings within the constructivist–phenomenological paradigm: trustworthiness and authenticity. The Unitary Field Pattern Portrait research method uses the trustworthiness criteria of credibility, confirmability, dependability, and transferability, as described by Guba and Lincoln (1989). The authenticity criteria for scientific rigor were developed specific to inquiry within Rogers' Science of Unitary Human Beings (Butcher, 1993).

## SUMMARY

The Unitary Field Pattern Portrait research method is a system of inquiry developed in harmony with the ontological and epistemological tenets of Rogers' Science of Unitary Human Beings and is a unique synthesis of Guba and Lincoln's (1989) constructivist-phenomenological inquiry and Cowling's (1990, in press) unitary pattern-based practice model. The method provides Rogerian researchers a rigorous process for developing theoretical structures of phenomena within Rogers' unique nursing science perspective that are grounded in the experiences, perceptions, and expressions of persons experiencing the investigated phenomenon. The theoretical structures developed via the Unitary Field Pattern Portrait research method will enhance the understanding of the nature of phenomena related to well-being within a unitary perspective. Other Rogerian systems of inquiry need to be developed. The challenge for Rogerian researchers is to continue to develop and use unique Rogerian research methodologies that uncover human–environmental patterns of wholeness.

## REFERENCES

Allen, D., Benner, P., & Diekelmann, N.L. (1986). Three paradigms for nursing research: Methodological implications. In P. Chinn (Ed.), *Nursing research methodology: Issues and implementation* (pp. 23-38). Rockville, MD: Aspen.

Barrett, E.A.M. (1988). Using Rogers' Science of Unitary Human Beings in nursing practice. *Nursing Science Quarterly, 1,* 50-51.

Barrett, E.A.M. (1990). Rogerian patterns of scientific inquiry. In E.A.M. Barrett (Ed.), *Visions of Rogers' science-based nursing* (pp. 169-187). New York: National League for Nursing.

Bohm, D. (1980). *Wholeness and the implicate order.* Boston: Routledge and Kegan Paul.

Boyd, C.O. (1988). Phenomenology: A foundation for nursing curriculum (pp. 65-87), Curriculum revolution in nursing: Mandate for change. New York: National League for Nursing.

Butcher, H.K. (1993). *A unitary field pattern portrait of dispiritedness in later life.* Doctoral dissertation proposal, University of South Carolina, College of Nursing, Columbia, SC.

Capra, F., & Steindl-Rast, D. (1991). *Belonging to the universe.* San Francisco: HarperCollins.

Carboni, J.T. (1991). A Rogerian theoretical tapestry. *Nursing Science Quarterly, 4,* 130-136.

Carboni, J. (1992a). Instrument development and the measurement of unitary constructs. *Nursing Science Quarterly, 5,* 134-142.

Carboni, J. (1992b). *Coming home: An investigation of the enfolding-unfolding flux of human field-environmental field patterns within the nursing home setting and the enfoldment of a health-as-wholeness-and-harmony by the nurse and client.* Doctoral dissertation proposal, The University of Rhode Island College of Nursing, Providence, RI.

Cowling, W.R. (1983). *The relationship of mystical experience, differentiation, and creativity in college students.* Unpublished doctoral dissertation, New York University, New York.

Cowling, W.R. (1986a). Methods: A reflective model. In P.L. Chinn (Ed.), *Nursing research methodology: Issues and implementation* (pp. 67-78). Rockville, MD: Aspen.

Cowling, W.R. (1986b). The Science of Unitary Human Beings: Theoretical issues, methodological challenges, and research realities. In V. Malinski (Ed.), *Explorations on Martha Rogers' Science of Unitary Human Beings* (pp. 65-77). Norwalk, CT: Appleton-Century-Crofts.

Cowling, W.R. (1990). A template for unitary pattern-based nursing practice. In E.A.M. Barrett (Ed.), *Visions of Rogers' science-based nursing* (pp. 45-65). New York: National League for Nursing.

Cowling, W.R. (1993). Unitary practice: Revisionary assumptions. In M. Parker (Ed.), *Patterns of nursing theories in practice* (pp. 199-212). New York: National League for Nursing.

Cull-Wilby, B.L., & Pepin, J.L. (1987). Towards a coexistence of paradigms in nursing knowledge development. *Journal of Advanced Nursing, 12,* 515-521.

DeGroot, H.A. (1988). Scientific inquiry in nursing: A model for a new age. *Advances in Nursing Science, 10*(3), 1-21.

Frederickson, K. (1992). Research methodology and nursing science. *Nursing Science Quarterly, 5,* 150-151.

Guba, E. (1990). The alternate paradigm dialogue. In E. Guba (Ed.), *The paradigm dialogue* (pp. 17-27). Newbury Park, CA: Sage.

Guba, E.G., & Lincoln, Y.S. (1989). *Fourth generation evaluation.* Newbury Park, CA: Sage.

Hesse, M. (1980). *Revolutions and reconstructions in philosophy of science.* Bloomington: Indiana University Press.

Ihde, D. (1977). *Experimental phenomenology.* New York: Putnam's.

Kaplan, A. (1964). *The conduct of inquiry: Methodology for behavioral science.* New York: Harper & Row.

Lamb, G.S., & Huttlinger, K. (1989). Reflexivity in nursing research. *Western Journal of Nursing Research, 11,* 765-772.

Laudan, L. (1977). *Progress and its problems: Towards a theory of scientific growth*. Berkeley: University of California Press.

Leininger, M.M. (1985). *Qualitative research methods in nursing*. New York: Grune & Stratton.

Lincoln, Y.S. (1992). Sympathetic connections between qualitative methods and health research. *Qualitative Health Research, 2*, 375-391.

Lincoln, Y., & Guba, E. (1985). *Naturalistic inquiry*. Newbury Park, CA: Sage.

Malinski, V. (1986). *Explorations on Martha Rogers' Science of Unitary Human Beings*. Norwalk, CT: Appleton-Century-Crofts.

Moccia, P. (1988). A critique of compromise: Beyond the methods debate. *Advances in Nursing Science, 10*(4), 1-9.

Morgan, G. (1983). *Beyond method: Strategies for social research*. Newbury Park, CA: Sage.

Moustakas, C. (1990). *Heuristic research: Design, methodology, and applications*. Newbury Park, CA: Sage.

Munhall, P.L. (1982). Nursing philosophy and nursing research: In apposition or opposition? *Nursing Research, 31*, 178-181.

Newman, M.A. (1986). *Health as expanding consciousness*. St. Louis: Mosby.

Newman, M.A. (1990). Book review: E.A.M. Barrett (1990), Visions of Rogers' science-based nursing. *Nursing Science Quarterly, 4*, 41-42.

Parse, R.R. (1987). *Nursing science: Major paradigms, theories, and critiques*. Toronto: Saunders.

Parse, R.R. (1990). Parse's research method with an illustration of the lived experience of hope. *Nursing Science Quarterly, 3*, 9-17.

Patton, M.Q. (1990). *Qualitative evaluation and research methods* (2nd ed.). Newbury Park, CA: Sage.

Phillips, J. (1988a). The looking glass of nursing research. *Nursing Science Quarterly, 1*, 96.

Phillips, J. (1988b). The reality of nursing research. *Nursing Science Quarterly, 12*, 48-49.

Phillips, J. (1989a). Science of Unitary Human Beings: Changing research perspectives. *Nursing Science Quarterly, 2*, 57-60.

Phillips, J. (1989b). Qualitative research: A process of discovery. *Nursing Science Quarterly, 2*, 5-6.

Phillips, J. (1991). Human field research. *Nursing Science Quarterly, 4,* 142-143.

Polkinghorne, D. (1983). *Methodology for the human sciences: Systems of inquiry.* Albany: State University of New York.

Power, B.A., & Knapp, T.A. (1990). *A dictionary of nursing theory and research.* Newbury Park, CA: Sage.

Rawnsley, M.M. (1990). Structuring the gap from conceptual systems to research design within a Rogerian world-view. In E.A.M. Barrett (Ed.), *Visions of Rogers' science-based nursing* (pp. 189-207). New York: National League for Nursing.

Reed, P.G. (1989). Nursing theorizing as an ethical endeavor. *Advances in Nursing Science, 11,* 23-31.

Reeder, F. (1984). Nursing research, holism and philosophies of science: Points of congruence between E. Husserl and M.E. Rogers. Ann Arbor, MI: University Microfilms International.

Reeder, F. (1986). Basic theoretical research in the conceptual system of unitary human beings. In V. Malinski (Ed.), *Explorations on Martha Rogers' Science of Unitary Human Beings* (pp. 45-64). Norwalk, CT: Appleton-Century-Crofts.

Reeder, F. (1993). The Science of Unitary Human Beings and interpretive human science. *Nursing Science Quarterly, 6,* 13-24.

Rogers, M.E. (1970). *An introduction to the theoretical basis of nursing.* Philadelphia: F.A. Davis.

Rogers, M.E. (1980) Nursing: A science of unitary man. In J. Riehl & C. Roy (Eds.), *Conceptual models for nursing practice* (2nd ed.) (pp. 329-337). Norwalk, CT: Appleton-Century-Crofts.

Rogers, M.E. (1986). Science of Unitary Human Beings. In V.M. Malinski (Ed.), *Explorations on Martha Rogers' Science of Unitary Human Beings* (pp. 3-8). Norwalk, CT: Appleton-Century-Crofts.

Rogers, M.E. (1987). Rogers' Science of Unitary Human Beings. In R.R. Parse (Ed.), *Nursing science: Major paradigms, theories, and critiques* (pp. 139-146). Philadelphia: Saunders.

Rogers, M.E. (1988). Nursing science and art: A prospective. *Nursing Science Quarterly, 1,* 99-102.

Rogers, M.E. (1990). Nursing: Science of Unitary, Irreducible, Human Beings: Updated 1990. In E.A.M. Barrett (Ed.), *Visions of Rogers' science-based nursing* (pp. 5-11). New York: National League for Nursing.

Rogers, M.E. (1992). Nursing science and the space age. *Nursing Science Quarterly, 5,* 27-34.

Roy, C., & Andrews, A. (1991). *The Roy adaptation model: The definitive statement.* Norwalk, CT: Appleton-Lange.

Sandelowski, M. (1993). Theory unmasked: The uses and guises of theory in qualitative research. *Research in Nursing & Health, 16,* 213-218.

Sarter, B. (1988a). *The stream of becoming: A study of Martha Rogers' theory.* New York: National League for Nursing.

Sarter, B. (1988b). Philosophical sources of nursing theory. *Nursing Science Quarterly, 1,* 52-59.

Smith, M.C. (1990). Struggling through a difficult time for unemployed persons. *Nursing Science Quarterly, 3,* 18-28.

Smith, M.J. (1988). Perspectives of wholeness: The lens makes a difference. *Nursing Science Quarterly, 2,* 94-95.

Thompson, J.L. (1985). Practical discourse in nursing: Going beyond empiricism. *Advances in Nursing Science, 7*(4), 59-71.

Tinkle, M.B., & Beaton, J.L. (1983). Toward a new view of science: Implications for nursing research. *Advances in Nursing Science, 5*(2), 27-36.

van Manen, M. (1990). *Researching lived experience: Human science for action-sensitive pedagogy.* Albany: SUNY Press.

Watson, J. (1981). Nursing's scientific quest. *Nursing Outlook, 7,* 413-416.

Webster, G., & Jacox, A. (1986). The liberation of nursing theory. In J. McCloskey & H. Grace (Eds.), *Current issues in nursing* (pp. 26-35). Boston: Blackwell.

# Dwelling in the Diffuse: A Critical Response to Butcher's Unitary Field Pattern Portrait Research Method

*Marilyn M. Rawnsley*

> For a holistic tradition, the important thing is to find large-scale connections. (Feyerabend, 1978, p. 100)

A respondent's charge is to query scholars, not to praise them. The intent of a critical response is to advance a particular argument—to provide a generic frame of reference for further discussion. In this instance, however, I would be remiss to proceed directly to questions without preliminary comment on the general excellence of Butcher's (1993) effort.

## FRAMING ROGERIAN RESEARCH

Butcher has articulated a well-developed and persuasive rationale for endorsement of a specific qualitative strategy he calls Unitary Field Pattern Portrait research method. The method is drawn from a synthesis of ideas from several acknowledged Rogerian scholars (Carboni, 1992; Cowling, 1990; Phillips, 1991; Rawnsley, 1990; Reeder, 1993) incorporated into a perspective of naturalistic inquiry (Lincoln & Guba, 1985). In brief, the Field Pattern Portrait research method is proposed as a participatory mutual process through which unitary human energy fields (investigator and investigated) engage in multiple modes of awareness to disclose contextual patterning or individual human field profiles consistent with the pandimensional premise of the Rogerian world-view. Through a series of such encounters with different human fields, what is postulated to emerge through the medium of the researcher's energy field is a unitary field portrait pattern of echoes resonating through variations of human experience synthesized as a central theme.

This dialectical approach incorporates an intrinsic intersubjectivity, or shared agreement of meaning, as participants are encouraged to consider and consolidate previous participants' experiential accounts into their respective contextual scheme. From this rich data set, a conceptual hall of human field mirrors is constructed to allow multiple reflections to merge into a composite human field hologram or unitary field pattern portrait. These phenomena are identified and named in accordance with Rogerian nursing science constructs. Thus, it can be concluded that Butcher is describing a classical process of theory building in which designation of phenomena is the essential first phase.

Since Butcher provides sufficient detail for Rogerian researchers to devise a rigorous audit trail to meet the criterion of confirmability in their studies, no further analysis of the elements of method is addressed at this time. After all, the most convincing evidence of the scientific merit of the method will be the number and caliber of studies generated to support or dispute Butcher's claims of compatibility of method with the Science of Unitary Human Beings. Of special interest will be examination of the ways in which the research approach, guided from a Rogerian perspective, shapes the interpretations of data. Will these investigators be operating in the context of discovery as the qualitative strategies suggest? Or does the "a priori" conceptual system indicate preference for the context of justification?

If only Rogerians were as monetarily blessed as they are conceptually rich; adequate funding could permit several scholars to study similar data patterns from a variety of perspectives. It is generally accepted that any given data set can be explained by alternative hypotheses generated from different world-views. What is sought is the "best" or most complete explanation of the selected phenomenon. Feyerabend (1975) encouraged use of ad hoc hypotheses to decipher the same data sets; in this way, inferences consistent with revolutionary ideas can be assessed alongside more traditional views. On balance, competing explanations will be judged by the extent to which inferences from the data, or theoretical hypotheses, address the "virtues" of conservatism, generality, simplicity, modesty, and re-futability (Quine & Ullian, 1970, pp. 42–53). In a Rogerian sense, refutability can be expanded according to Feyerabend's (1975) no-tion of the "self-inconsistent observation reports . . . [useful] . . . where a theory entails assertions about possible initial conditions" (p. 278). Since the Science of Unitary Human Beings is all about ini-tial conditions of open, mutually patterning pandimensional energy fields, it might be fruitful to explore further this methodological in-novation. The most plausible explanation is the one that transcends time, not only accounting for observations that occurred in the past—that is, before the particular world-view was articulated—but also providing reference for observations that have yet to unfold.

Evaluating the credibility of emergent studies using the Field Portrait Pattern research method will be the challenge for future crit-ical respondents. Therefore, the focus of this discussion diverts to a heuristic mode, addressing questions suggested during contempla-tion of Butcher's scholarly explanation. Two issues are salient: the validity of paradigm status for the Science of Unitary Human Beings and the degree of confidence in its epistemological metaphors.

## PARADIGM STATUS

Kuhn's (1970) clarification of paradigm continues to be the gold standard in what is commonly referred to as "normal science." In essence, a Kuhnian paradigm refers to an unprecedented break with past and current world-views of a discipline, frequently accounting for events that had so far eluded explanation. The scientific impact of such a spectacular conceptual shift is to render existing investiga-tive methods inadequate; new strategies need to be invented to examine phenomena as described within this different perspective. In contrast, a regular paradigm offers new explanations through variation in perspective that does not substantively alter the basic world-view of phenomena central to the discipline. Although this conceptualization may suggest new research strategies, it is not es-sentially incompatible with existing methods (Reynolds, 1971).

Given this cursory synopsis of what constitutes great ideas or paradigms, Butcher's premise that the Science of Unitary Human Be-ings is a paradigm for derivation and testing of theories concerned with phenomena central to nursing is most curious. Is he saying that Rogers' conceptual system is a variation on a perspective or world-view called "nursing," which has phenomena central to its domain?

If so, then Butcher is within the purview of those Rogerian scholars who design hypothesis-testing studies using sophisticated statistical techniques; he argues for the qualitative side of the methodological coin. In other words, while a phenomenological or constructivist strategy as outlined by Lincoln and Guba (1985) may not appear to be inconsistent with the Rogerian world-view, it was initially developed to study phenomena within a discipline other than nursing science. Therefore, it is a research strategy that has been modified rather than invented.

Butcher also gives credence to the Science of Unitary Human Beings as a "new reality." If this is so—if the constructs of this conceptual system are actually claiming a different world-view, a dramatic break with previous and current orientations to phenomena said to be central to the domain—then all scientific bets are off. A modified qualitative approach seems innately appealing in a holistic framework, but it cannot solve the problems that are created by the new theoretical puzzle; the boundaries of this Rogerian puzzle as a Kuhnian paradigm of reality are not yet defined. What is hopeful is that carefully crafted naturalistic inquiries will move closer to a methodological breakthrough, and that qualitative research activity will energize creative catapults into new ways of knowing inspired by serendipitous findings.

Butcher maintains that the criterion of authenticity, or the truth value of the method, was developed to be specific to inquiry with the Rogerian Science of Unitary Human Beings. In characterizing the conceptual system clearly and unequivocally as postulating a different reality, namely, as a science of the essence of human fields as known through pattern manifestation, Butcher summons all Rogerian scholars to rethink their paradigmatic positions.

## PARTICIPATORY METAPHORS

The participatory metaphors of kaleidoscopic and symphonic patterning pose another intriguing intellectual problem. Metaphor is a powerful symbolic device in theory development. According to Ricoeur's (1981) seminal work linking phenomenology and contemporary linguistics, metaphor is a semantic novelty emerging through a dialectic of the world of events and the world of ideas. Words have multiple meanings at the lexical level; specific meaning is accomplished through contextual sifting. Ricoeur (1981) referred to this creative construction of meaning disclosed through metaphor as creating a condition of the possible. But to what purpose? Is the elaboration of language simply a different way of saying the same thing? Ricoeur (1981) asked and answered this challenge in a question: "Why should we draw new meanings from our language if we have nothing new to say, no new world to project?" (p. 181).

If Rogers' conceptual system is projecting the new world it claims to see, then metaphor is the appropriate medium of its discourse. However, kaleidoscopic and symphonic patternings do not seem sufficient to achieve the creative construction of meaning that generates a condition of the possible. Linguistically, these descriptive terms for human field patterning seem to be similes—comparison terms that provide an alternate image without projecting a new reality.

Remembering that metaphors create a condition of the possible opens the conceptual lens of discovery. Such metaphors disclose meaning; they emerge through the dialectical tension existing between the world of events and the world of ideas. Through the phenomenological constructivist method he describes, Butcher proposed to do just that: to synthesize meaning through examination of the way participants describe the phenomenon of study as they experience it. Such a process, reflecting Kuhn's (1970) third approach to articulation of a paradigm as an exploration that "deals with the qualitative more than the quantitative aspects of nature's reality" (p. 29), seems highly relevant to the authenticity of method that Butcher intends. Moreover, metaphors that project this new Rogerian reality should naturally flow from interpretation of the findings. Then, epistemological questions of the origin and structure and validity of knowledge, that is, how we know what we know, can be more adequately addressed from within the conceptual framework.

Endings are illusory in a pandimensional world. Concluding this response then, is simply a pause in an ongoing discourse.

## REFERENCES

Butcher, H.K. (1993). *A unitary field pattern portrait of dispiritedness in later life: Development and testing of a research method guided by Rogers' nursing science.* Doctoral dissertation proposal, University of South Carolina, College of Nursing, Columbia, SC.

Carboni, J.T. (1992). Instrument development and the measurement of unitary constructs. *Nursing Science Quarterly, 5,* 134–142.

Cowling, W.R. (1990). A template for unitary pattern-based nursing practice. In E.A.M. Barrett (Ed.), *Visions of Rogers' science-based nursing* (pp. 45-65). New York: National League for Nursing.

Feyerabend, P. (1975). *Against method.* London: Verso.

Feyerabend, P. (1978). *Science in a free society.* London: Verso.

Kuhn, T. (1970). *The structure of scientific revolutions.* Chicago: University of Chicago Press.

Lincoln, Y., & Guba, E. (1985). *Naturalistic inquiry.* Newbury Park, CA: Sage.

Phillips, J. (1991). Human field research. *Nursing Science Quarterly, 4,* 142-143.

Quine, W.V., & Ullian, J.S. (1970). *The web of belief.* New York: Random House.

Rawnsley, M.M. (1990). Structuring the gap from conceptual systems to research design within a Rogerian world view. In E.A.M. Barrett (Ed.), *Visions of Rogers' science-based nursing* (pp. 189-207). New York: National League for Nursing.

Reeder, F. (1993). The science of unitary human beings and interpretive human science. *Nursing Science Quarterly, 6,* 13-24.

Reynolds, P. (1971). *A primer in theory construction.* New York: Macmillan.

Ricoeur, P. (1981). *Hermeneutics and the human sciences.* New York: Cambridge University Press.

# The Sea . . . the Universe . . . and We.

*Sarah Hall Gueldner*

The sea . . . and we . . . are one with the universe,
And the illusion of separateness is created only
By minute differences in the configuration of our molecules.

Nowhere more than where ocean meets land
Is man's oneness with the universe more apparent.
Our history and our future are one with the present
At the ocean's edge.
We pour over the sand,
Marvelling at the shells . . .
Artifacts of an earlier time . . .
That wash ashore twice each day,
As they have done for millions of years . . .
As if mocking the artificial clock time
That holds such power over contemporary mankind.

We emerged from the ocean,
And are clearly drawn back to it.

Intricate footprints left by the high-tech soles of running shoes
Wind along the waters' edge
Alongside footprints left by the bare feet of men, birds, and dogs.
The remains of primitive jellyfish, left behind at high tide,
Rest beside rows of geometrical track marks
Left by four-wheel-drive vehicles
That in the springtime

Carry groups of spirited young
(future caretakers of the universe)
Up and down the beach.

Upshore white clouds from the smokestacks of civilization
Boil by-products into the sky,
To rest again dissolved in the ocean water,
And in the lungs of man,
And in his drinking water.

Downshore the space shuttle stands poised for takeoff,
Each time thrusting us further into our future,
Which is also our past.
The ocean, the shells, the smokestacks,
The sea gulls, the shuttles,
The universe . . . and we . . . are one.
A truth to be remembered as we create our present,
Which also embodies our past
And unfolds to become our future.

# Someday

*Brenda Talley*

Someday,
when we are nothing
and so become all that there is,
when we are the mists of the Milky Way—
as smoke in the wind—
we will dance in the stars.
Someday,
when memories of yesterdays
are no more than whispers
drifting on the stream
vague reminders of the times
we have touched.
Someday,
this dance will be ours
and we will waltz in the echoes
of time and space,
moving gracefully through
the starlit shadows of a thousand tomorrows.

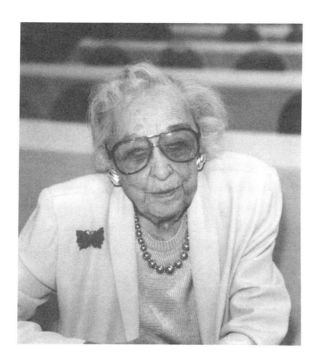

# A Memorial

Martha E. Rogers passed on two months before the release of this publication (May 12, 1914–March 13, 1994). She was our dear friend and mentor, deeply loved by us and countless others who knew her. Her humanness and dedication to promote human potential has inspired and enriched the lives of people from all walks of life. It is impossible to express her greatness with words or to describe her life's work in this brief afterword. Martha's writings and deeds speak for themselves.

Her pandimensional presence was always with us to encourage and support us during the writing of this book. It remains with us and with you, dear readers, as we carry on her work of advancing the Science of Unitary Human Beings.

The chapter, Nursing Science Evolves, her last published writing, is an important contribution to nursing. Martha Rogers truly used her infinite potential to the fullest and she encourages us to do the same.

# Index

35.95